Lawrence Martin, MD, FACP, FCCP, heads the Pulmonary Division at Mount Sinai Medical Center in Cleveland, Ohio, and is also an assistant professor of medicine at Case Western Reserve University School of Medicine. In 1983 he received Mount Sinai's prestigious Goodman Award for excellence in teaching.

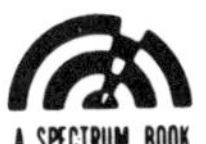

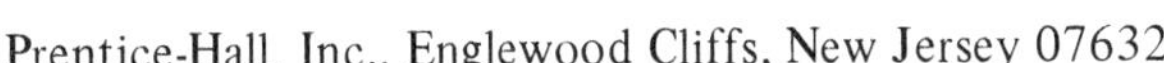
Prentice-Hall, Inc., Englewood Cliffs, New Jersey 07632

Lawrence Martin, M.D.

BREATHE EASY

A GUIDE TO LUNG AND RESPIRATORY DISEASES FOR PATIENTS AND THEIR FAMILIES

Library of Congress Cataloging in Publication Data

Martin, Lawrence, 1943-
Breathe easy.

"A Spectrum Book."
Bibliography: p.
Includes index.
1. Lungs–Diseases–Miscellanea. 2. Respiratory organs –Diseases–Miscellanea. I. Title.
RC756.M274 1984 616.2 84-2119

ISBN 0-13-081746-5
ISBN 0-13-081738-4 (pbk.)

This book is available at a special discount when ordered in bulk quantities. Contact Prentice-Hall, Inc., General Publishing Division, Special Sales, Englewood Cliffs, N.J. 07632

A SPECTRUM BOOK

Printed in the United States of America

10 9 8 7 6 5 4 3 2 1

ISBN 0-13-081746-5

ISBN 0-13-081738-4 {PBK.}

Prentice-Hall International, Inc., *London*
Prentice-Hall of Australia Pty. Limited, *Sydney*
Prentice-Hall of Canada, Inc., *Toronto*
Prentice-Hall of India Private Limited, *New Delhi*
Prentice-Hall of Japan, Inc., *Tokyo*
Prentice-Hall of Southeast Asia Pte. Ltd., *Singapore*
Whitehall Books Limited, Wellington, *New Zealand*
Editora Prentice-Hall do Brasil Ltda., *Rio de Janeiro*

To my father and mother, who quit smoking before it was too late;
to my wife Ruth, who quit the year we married; and
to my children, who know enough never to start.

Contents

Foreword

A wise physician once said that patients with chronic disease should be their own doctors and that they should use their physicians as consultants. I think that this is true. The multiple and unpredictable changes that occur in the course of an illness frequently require the patient to make decisions. Furthermore, in a disease like asthma, the variation in the nature and intensity of symptoms is so great that each patient should know more about his or her own disease than the physician.

It is a very healthy sign of our times that physicians are losing some of their aura of infallibility and inscrutability. They are encouraging patients to ask questions, to understand why things are done, and to help treat themselves. Informed consent is much more than a signature on a form.

Dr. Martin has provided a valuable and needed service to patients and to their physicians. His book contains an enormous amount of information about lung disease. It is accurate, it is up-to-date, and it is relevant. Complicated concepts are explained clearly without oversimplification or loss of accuracy. A gifted teacher, Dr. Martin has the ability to promote curiosity and to stimulate learning. As a result, it is possible not only to look up specific points but to read the book and actually learn.

Breathe Easy teaches about the lung: what it is, how it works, and the myriad diseases that affect it. This book enhances understanding in addition to providing advice. It also contains a great deal of factual information which is skillfully organized and presented. It will be of great value to patients with pulmonary disease and to anyone interested in learning more about the lung.

M. Henry Williams, Jr., M.D.
Professor of Medicine
Albert Einstein College of Medicine

Preface

WHO IS THIS BOOK FOR?

If you have lung disease, or know someone who does, and ever wonder about it, this book is for you. This includes anyone who:

- Has a diagnosed lung condition, whether or not under treatment, and wishes to learn more about it.
- Has symptoms that suggest lung disease: shortness of breath, wheezing, or chronic cough.
- Smokes cigarettes or cigars, and is curious about how smoking may be affecting his or her health.
- I. a concerned relative or friend of patients suffering lung disease or lung symptoms.

Using a question-and-answer format, this book covers all common lung diseases, as well as some uncommon ones. The questions include those most frequently asked in several years of consultative practice in pulmonary medicine.

Lung disease is a major American health problem, resulting in widespread disability and many premature deaths. Most people are at least superficially familiar with common lung diseases: asthma, bronchitis, emphysema, pneumonia, lung cancer. But how much is really known about these conditions? Can they be prevented? How are they best treated? Even more basic, how can someone obtain proper medical care? When is a specialist necessary? How can *you* find good care for *your* condition? These are a few of the many questions asked and answered in this book.

LUNG DISEASE IN PERSPECTIVE—WHAT IS THE PROBLEM?

The following table lists the major causes of death in the United States. If we lump chronic obstructive pulmonary diseases together with pneumonia and influenza, it appears lung disease is the fourth leading cause. In fact, the mortality from lung disease is much higher than these widely published statistics indicate, since about 25 percent of all cancer deaths are from *lung* cancer.

Major Causes of Death in the United States*

	Number of Deaths
All causes	1,982,240
Heart Diseases	755,510
Cancer—all types	435,760
Cerebrovascular disease (including Stroke)	159,100
Accidents (including auto accidents)	94,320
Chronic obstructive pulmonary diseases and allied conditions	59,820
Pneumonia and Influenza	49,040
Diabetes	33,130
Chronic liver disease and cirrhosis	27,180

*Source: U.S. Department of Health and Human Services. Mortality figures are for 1982.

In addition, our lungs are particularly vulnerable to disease that begins elsewhere in the body. For example, patients who suffer from shock, head injury, hemorrhage, multiple bone fractures, drug overdose, and many other nonpulmonary conditions may actually die from *lung failure* late in their hospital course. Thus, many of the deaths attributed to other causes—particularly accidents and trauma—occur because of lung failure. This often cannot be reversed even though the body's other organs function adequately and the patient is hospitalized in a modern intensive care unit. An estimated 50,000 to 75,000 such deaths occur each year. Thus one could say, with some justification, that lung disease accounts for over 250,000 deaths a years, making it the third leading cause.

Even this juggling with published mortality figures ignores the other major problem from lung disease: its morbidity. "Morbidity" refers to all negative aspects of illness while the patient is alive: discomfort, pain, lost work days, lost wages, and the like. If we include common respiratory infections along with asthma, chronic bronchitis and emphysema, then respiratory disease accounts for more morbidity than any other health problem in this country. The economic costs of respiratory disease are enormous, measured in the billions of dollars annually.

For you, the patient, such statistics have little direct importance. While mortality and morbidity data may influence how the federal government responds to a health problem, for the patient it still comes down to personal questions. What can be done to make me feel better now? What can I do to allow me to live a longer, healthier life?

The philosophy of this book is simple: The more fully you understand your health problem, the better off you are. And the better will be your relationship with any doctor. One caveat—this is emphatically not a do-it-yourself book. It is designed as an aid and guide for patients already receiving competent medical care, or who plan for such care if and when the need arises.

HOW TO USE THIS BOOK

This is a resource book for patients with lung disease. In it you should find answers to most questions about your condition or the condition of a loved one. It is unlikely you will want to read this book straight through. It is written so you can begin at any particular chapter or question and skip around, as necessary, to find just the information you need.

There are two ways to go right to the information you want. First, you may scan the Table of Contents to find the chapter and specific question that interests you. Alternatively, you can use the Index at the end of the book to locate information on any particular disease, condition, symptom or test. In reading through any portion of this book you will find ample cross references to additional questions, other chapters, or to the appendices.

Of course, if you want to read the book from beginning to end, that's OK too. You will find the book designed so that each section flows logically from the preceding one.

ACKNOWLEDGMENT

The following people helped make this a better book, and to them I owe a profound "thank you": Drs. Donald Epstein, David Rosenberg, Reuben Swimmer, and M. Henry Williams, Jr., for reviewing the manuscript and making many useful suggestions; Debra Shirley, for her illustrations as well as many helpful editorial comments; and Maribeth Rainey, who assisted me mightily with the typing and preparation of the manuscript.

Lawrence Martin, M.D.
Cleveland

CHAPTER ONE

How Our Lungs and Respiratory System Work

WHAT IS THE FUNCTION OF THE RESPIRATORY SYSTEM?

The function of this system is rather simple: to bring in oxygen and get rid of carbon dioxide. Since oxygen and carbon dioxide are gases, the process is called gas exchange.

Oxygen is necessary for normal metabolism; lack of it leads to death in a few minutes. Carbon dioxide is a waste product of metabolism; if breathing stops, carbon dioxide will quickly accumulate to a toxic level in the blood. Thus, our lungs, the paired organs that exchange these gases with the atmosphere, are considered vital since their total failure is quickly fatal.

We normally have two lungs, one in the right side of our chest cage and one in the left (see Figure 1-1). Between them is the heart, a midline organ that tilts slightly to the left in the chest cage. (You can feel your heart beating by placing your finger tips under your left breast.)

Although gas exchange takes place in the lungs, the respiratory system also includes two other vital components: the central nervous system area that controls our breathing and the chest bellows.

The part of the central nervous system that controls breathing is located in the mid-brain, also known as the brain stem. It is an area more primitive than the area of the brain responsible for thinking and motor movements, known as the cortex. The mid-brain control of breathing is automatic and functions whether

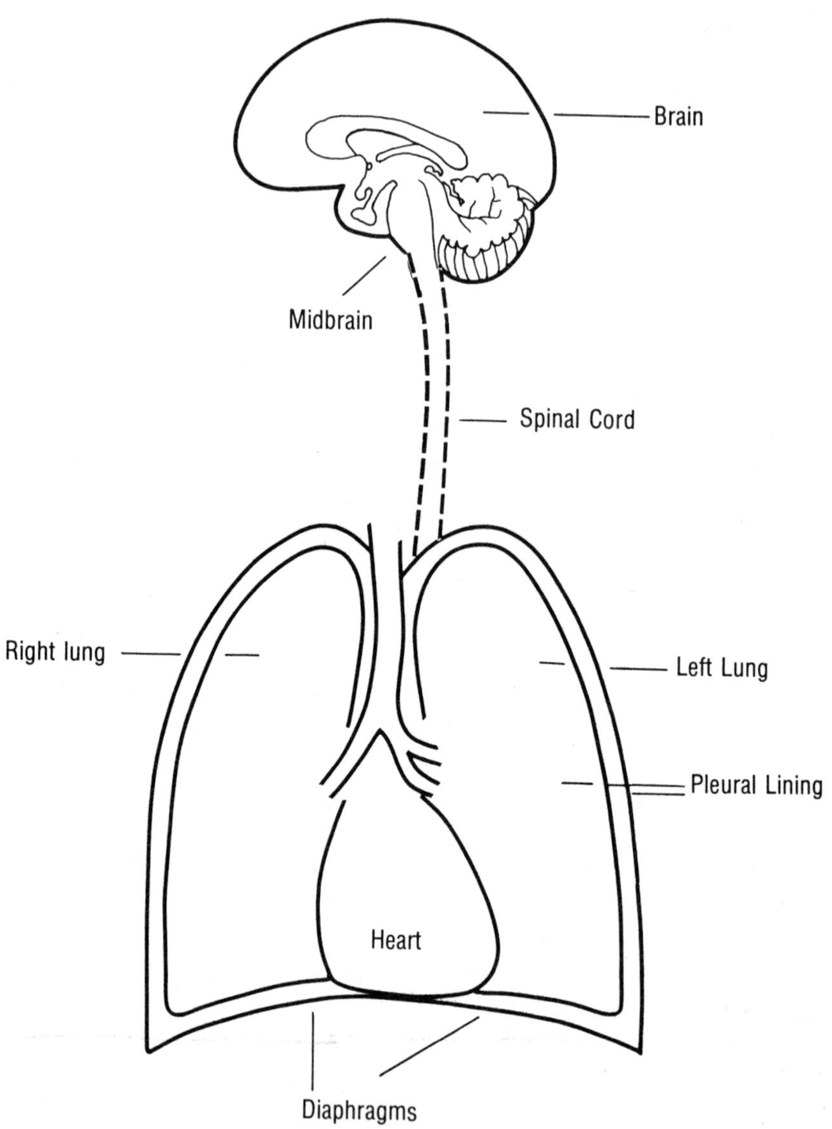

FIGURE 1-1 Schematic view of the respiratory system. In this drawing the front of the body is facing the reader.

we think about it or not. However, it may be altered by drugs or disease. A relatively common cause of respiratory depression is an overdose with narcotics or sedatives.

The chest bellows component of the respiratory system includes the *thoracic cage* that contains the lungs; the diaphragms, the major muscles of breathing; and the pleural membranes, thin tissues that line both the outside of the lungs and the inside of the thoracic cage. The thoracic cage (or chest cage) consists of the ribs that protect the lungs from injury; the muscles and connective tissues that tie the ribs together; and all the nerves that lead into these muscles.

Approximately ten to sixteen times a minute, while at rest, our mid-brain sends nerve impulses to the diaphragms and thoracic cage muscles to contract. This contraction expands the rib cage, leading to the expansion of the lungs inside. With lung expansion we inhale a breath of fresh air containing 21 percent oxygen and almost no carbon dioxide (see Figure 1-2). After full expansion the order to inhale ceases and our thoracic cage passively comes back to its resting position, at the same time allowing the lungs to shrink back to their resting size. During this stage of exhalation (or expiration) we exhale (expire) a breath of stale air, containing about 16 percent oxygen and 6 percent carbon dioxide.

In healthy people this breathing cycle is silent, automatic, and effortless. In the process, oxygen is delivered from the atmosphere into our blood and carbon dioxide is excreted from our blood into the atmosphere.

Although respiratory disease is often thought of as synonymous with lung disease, malfunction of any component of the system can cause a respiratory (breathing) problem. For example, if the brain center controlling breathing is depressed, as may occur with drug overdose, total failure of the system can occur with normal lungs! Similarly polio, a common disease before the discovery of the vaccine, can cause respiratory system failure by damaging the nerves leading to the thoracic cage muscles. In polio victims with respiratory failure the brain and lungs are intact, but the chest cannot expand to move air in and out.

All parts of the respiratory system must work for normal breathing. Yet, despite the importance of all respiratory system components, there is good reason why the lungs are usually thought of when one hears about respiratory disease. Lung disease accounts for the vast majority of respiratory illness. Emphysema, bronchitis, asthma, pneumonia, lung cancer—all originate in the lungs. Our lungs are the only internal organ directly in contact with the atmosphere, making them vulnerable to all pollutants, including cigarette smoke, as well as airborne viruses and bacteria. Because most respiratory illness is in fact *lung disease*, some understanding of lung function and anatomy as it applies to gas exchange should enhance your appreciation of respiratory problems.

HOW DOES GAS EXCHANGE OCCUR?

Overview

Oxygen and carbon dioxide, symbolized O_2 and CO_2 respectively, are colorless, odorless gases. The atmosphere, or air around us, contains approximately 21 percent oxygen and 78 percent nitrogen. There is almost no CO_2 in air (less than 0.3 percent); the carbon dioxide we exhale is negligible in the entire atmosphere. The nitrogen is inert and does not take part in gas exchange. The remainder of air is made up of some rare gases, such as argon, that are also inert and play no role in gas exchange.

To accomplish gas exchange the air we inhale is delivered to tiny sacs (alveoli) deep inside our lungs (Figure 1-3). Oxygen from the air diffuses across a thin membrane into tiny blood capillaries surrounding the alveoli. At the same time CO_2 diffuses from the blood into the alveoli and out of the lungs with each exhalation. The combination of one alveolus (containing air) and its surrounding capillaries (containing blood) is called an alveolar-capillary unit. Both lungs contain an esti-

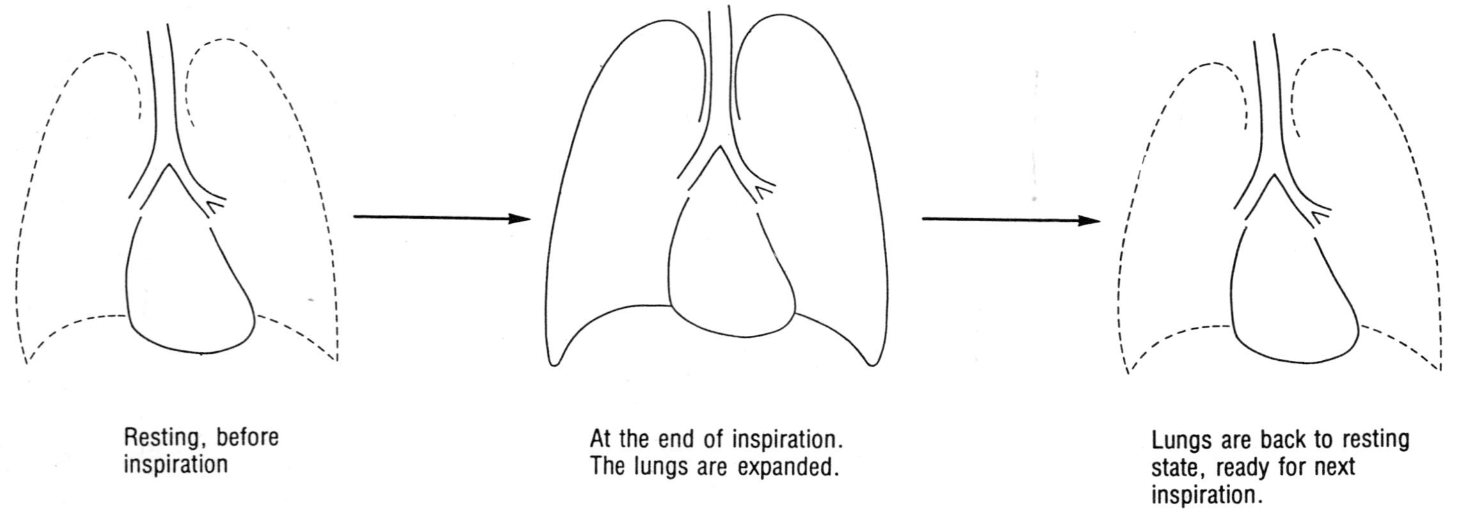

FIGURE 1-2 Inspiration and expiration: a normal breathing cycle. This cycle is normally repeated about 10-16 timers per minute.

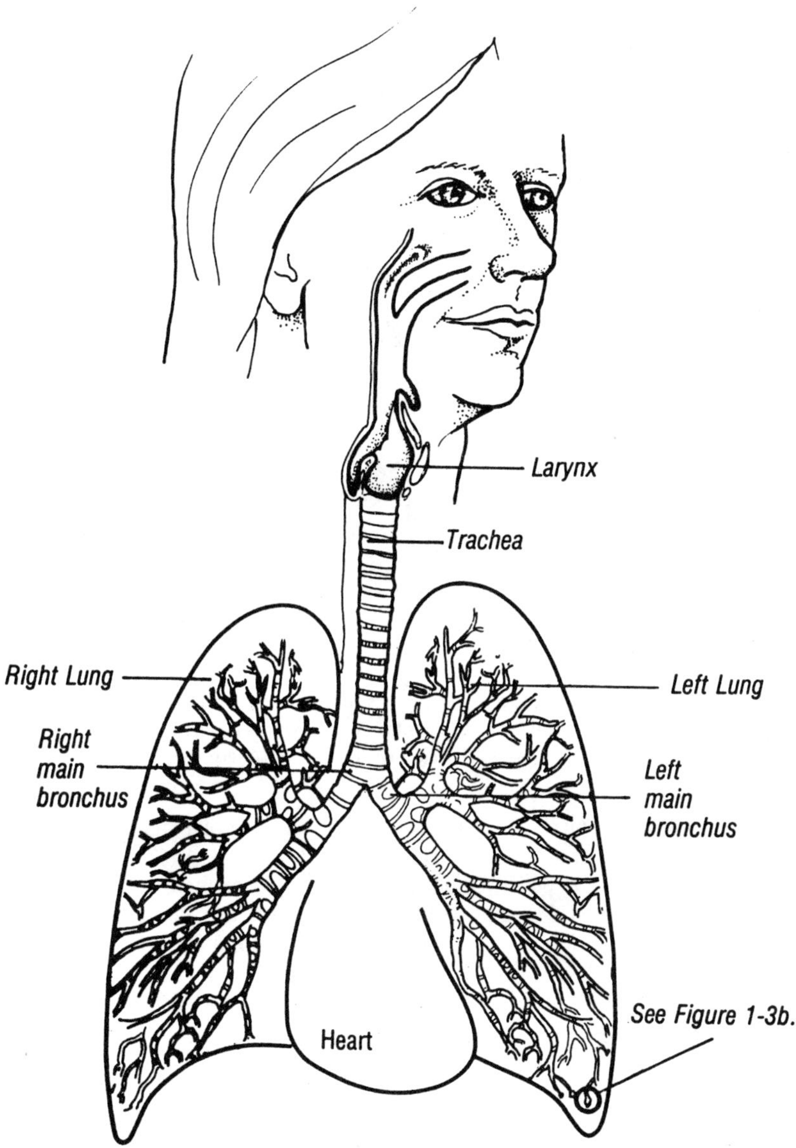

FIGURE 1-3a Diagram of upper airway and tracheobronchial tree. Air enters through the mouth and nose, then travels down the larynx (voice box) and trachea (windpipe). Air then enters the lungs, which consist (in part) of multiple branching airways called bronchi. These end in clusters of air sacs—the alveoli. Each alvcelus is surrounded by blood capillaries, which take up the oxygen and give off carbon dioxide. A 3-dimensional view and cross-section of alveoli are shown in Figures 1-3b and 1-3c.

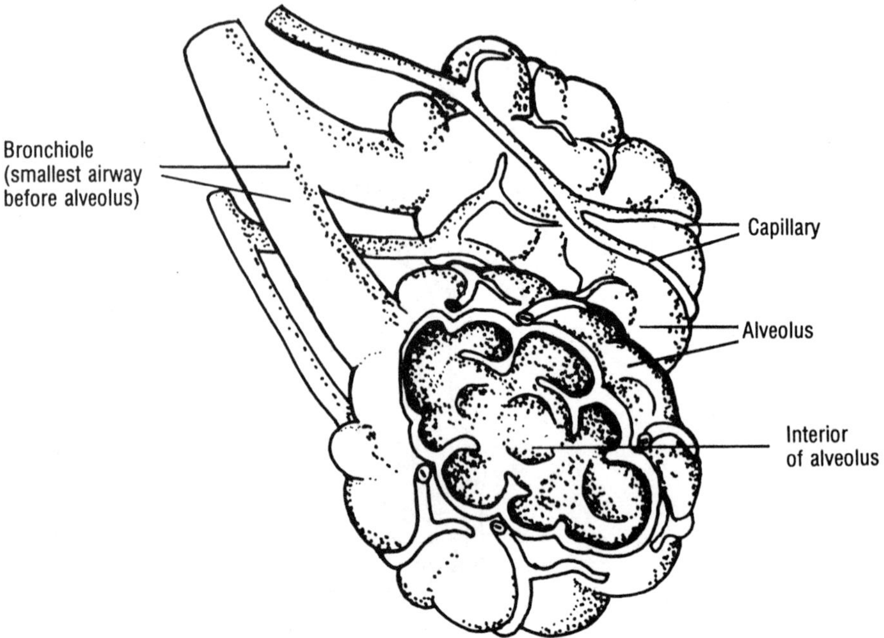

FIGURE 1-3b Each a veolar sac or "alveolus" is surrounded by one or more pulmonary capillaries. This alveolar-capillary unit is where oxygen (O_2) and carbon dioxide (CO_2) are exchanged with the atmosphere. See Figure 1-3c.

mated 300,000,000 units! The surface area of the alveolar membranes, if placed end to end, would cover a tennis court!

This overview can be expanded by dividing gas exchange into the processes of alveolar ventilation (bringing air into the lungs for transfer of oxygen and carbon dioxide) and pulmonary circulation (bringing blood to the lungs to take up

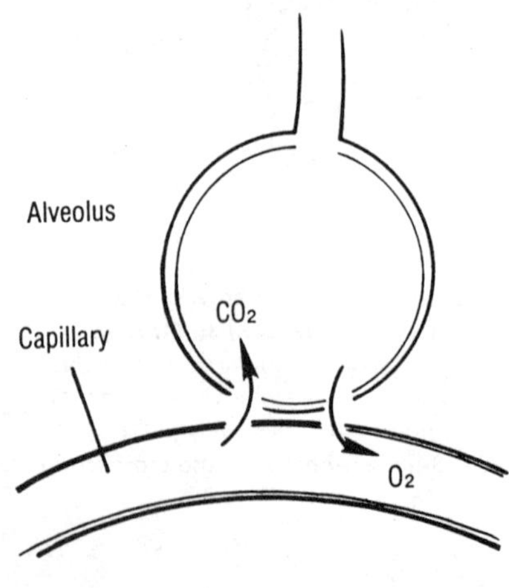

FIGURE 1-3c
Cross-section of single alveolar-capillary unit. As blood flows past the alveolus, CO_2 is given off and O_2 is taken up.

the oxygen and give off the carbon dioxide). For completeness circulation of the blood beyond the lungs (systemic circulation) will also be discussed.

Alveolar Ventilation. We inhale the air around us with each breath. The air enters our mouth and nose (Figure 1-3). In the nose and upper airway many of the dust particles are filtered out, purifying the air. Air from the mouth and nose come together in the throat and begin the journey down into the lungs. First air enters the larynx (voice box) and then the trachea (just below the Adam's apple). The trachea is the largest of the air tubes that deliver the air deep into the lungs. The trachea divides into two large air tubes, the right and left major bronchi. The trachea and bronchial tubes that branch from it are lined with cartilage. This provides a firm structure so the airways stay open when we inhale and exhale.

The airways above the carina are collectively called the upper airways or upper respiratory system. Air entering the upper airway is warmed to body temperature and humidified (water vapor is added to it).

The right and left major bronchi represent the first of over 20 divisions of airways to come (Figure 1-3). With each division the airway becomes narrower, but the number of airways increases geometrically. By the 20th division there are a huge number of individual, tiny airways and air has been distributed to each of them. Also at the 20th division, where the diameter of each airway is less than 1 mm, *air sacs* (called alveoli) appear; this is where gas exchange actually takes place. Eventually, each airway ends in a grape-like cluster of these alveoli.

At the alveolar-capillary membrane gas exchange takes place. Oxygen is delivered to, and carbon dioxide removed from, the capillary blood (Figure 1-3). This gas exchange converts the oxygen-poor blood entering the pulmonary capillary into oxygenated blood. At the same time the room air we inhale (21 percent O_2, no CO_2) has been converted into stale air (16 percent O_2, 6 percent CO_2) that we exhale.

Each minute, under resting breathing conditions, we breathe in approximately 6 liters of fresh air. About 1/3 of this air stays in the mouth, throat, and large airways where no gas exchange takes place; this region of our lungs and upper airway is referred to as 'dead space' because the air in these spaces doesn't give up O_2 or take up CO_2. The remaining 4 liters of fresh air breathed each minute are distributed to the hundreds of millions of alveoli and this air constitutes the alveolar ventilation.

Pulmonary Circulation. Each minute our heart pumps approximately 5 liters of blood to the alveoli, distributing blood among the hundreds of millions of capillaries that surround the equally large number of alveoli. Because the lungs are three dimensional, one alveolar sac may be surrounded by several pulmonary capillaries. The alveolus and its accompanying capillaries constitute the gas exchange unit. If there was no blood flow around the alveolus or there was blood flow without an accompanying alveolus, there would be no gas exchange. Alveolar ventilation is but one part of respiration; the other necessary part, deliverying blood to the capillaries surrounding the alveoli, is called pulmonary circulation.

The total circulation of the blood in our body is a circular affair (Figure 1-4). Blood flowing to and from the lungs constitutes only one part of this circle. Arbitrarily, we can start this circle with one of the four chambers of the heart, the

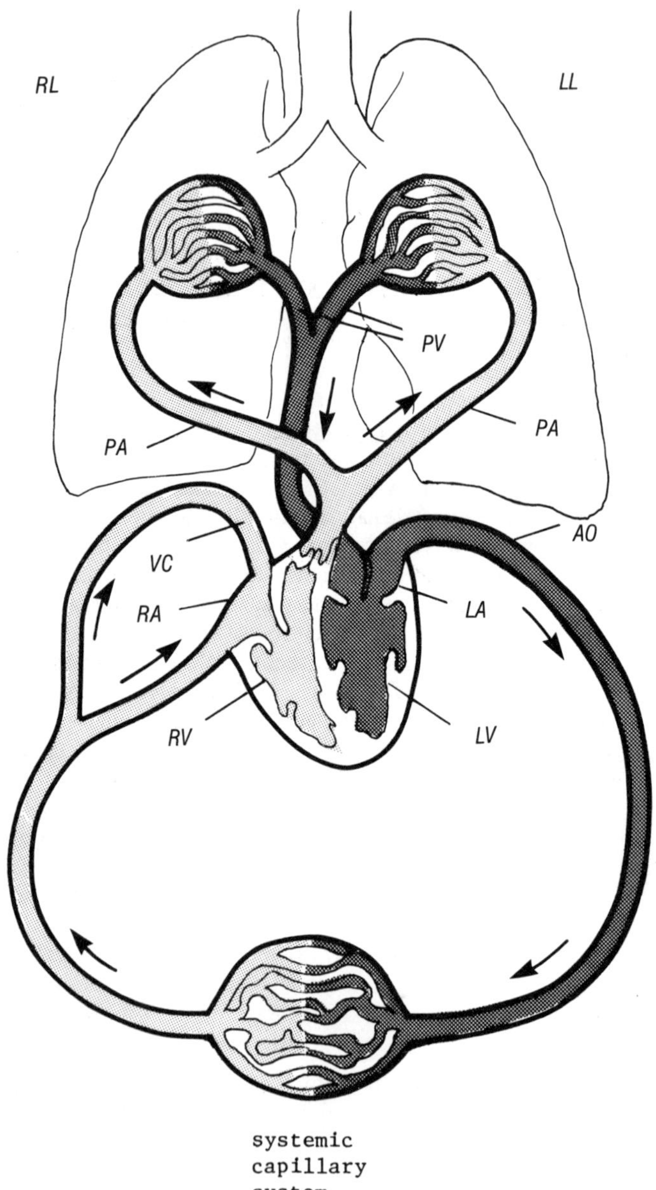

FIGURE 1-4 Pulmonary and systemic blood circulation.

RL = right lung
RV = right ventricle
RA = right atrium
VC = vena cava
PA = pulmonary arteries
LL = left lung
LV = left ventricle
LA = left atrium
PV = pulmonary veins
AO = aorta

right ventricle. Blood that enters the right ventricle has given up much of its oxygen to the tissues, and so is oxygen poor (de-oxygenated or venous blood). It returns first to the right atrium, then to the right ventricle where it is ready to be pumped to the lungs and receive a fresh supply of oxygen.

Right ventricular blood begins its journey to the lungs via one large blood vessel, the main pulmonary artery. This soon divides into two pulmonary arteries, one going to each lung. Each of these gives rise to many divisions, and in short order the blood is divided among millions of tiny pulmonary capillaries, the smallest unit of circulation. These capillaries are in contact with millions of alveoli, the tiny sacs where fresh air is delivered. Because the distance between the air sac and the capillary is very short, oxygen from the air can diffuse into capillary blood at the same time that CO_2 diffuses out of the capillary to enter the air sac. The stale air is then exhaled, and fresh air is brought in with the next breath.

Oxygenated blood leaving the millions of pulmonary capillaries enters a series of chambers in the other side of the heart, the left atrium and the left ventricle. From the left ventricle this oxygenated blood is pumped, via the body's arterial system, to all the muscles, tissues and organs (kidneys, brain, liver, heart, bones, and so forth). (When an arterial blood gas analysis is performed, the arterial blood is usually obtained by inserting a small needle into the radial artery of the wrist. Unlike venous blood, arterial blood reflects the status of gas exchange in the lungs and is therefore useful to examine in patients with various forms of lung disease.)

The pulmonary and systemic circulatory systems are demonstrated in Figure 1-4. The heart, normally between our two lungs (Figure 1-3), is here removed and drawn to show its four chambers and the vessels leading to and from them. Each pulmonary artery branches into millions of tiny capillaries before picking up oxygen and giving off CO_2 (gas exchange). After the process of gas exchange the millions of capillaries merge to become the pulmonary veins. The pulmonary veins carry oxygenated blood back to the left heart, from where it is pumped, via the systemic arterial circulation, to the organs and tissues of the body. From these organs and tissues it then returns via the systemic venous system back to the right heart.

In this figure light stipple represents venous blood and dark stipple represents arterial or oxygenated blood. Arrows show the direction of blood flow. Note that pulmonary *arteries* carry venous or de-oxygenated blood, pulmonary *veins* carry oxygenated or arterial blood. The role of veins and arteries is reversed in the systemic circulation.

After entering the tissue, organ, or muscle, each systemic artery divides into smaller and smaller vessels, the smallest of which is the systemic capillary. These capillaries are structurally similar to the ones in the lung (pulmonary capillaries) and have the same function: to allow gas exchange to occur. In the lung, oxygen diffuses into the capillaries and CO_2 diffuses out. In all other capillaries (non-pulmonary or systemic capillaries) oxygen diffuses out of the capillary into the cells of the organ, and CO_2 diffuses into the capillary from the cells of the organ. In this way oxygen is delivered for cellular metabolism and CO_2, a waste product of metabolism, is removed.

Gas exchange is a vital process; it occurs not only in the lungs but in all other tissues as well. It requires both ventilation, provided by breathing adequate amounts of fresh air, and circulation, provided by the heart pumping blood to the lungs and then out to all other parts of the body.

Blood entering the systemic (nonpulmonary) capillary is oxygenated. When the blood leaves it is de-oxygenated and called venous. Venous blood, what you see in the veins of your arm, is blue under the skin but is actually dark red in a test tube, whereas arterial blood is normally bright red.

The systemic capillaries, after delivering their oxygenated blood to the tissues, merge and form the veins that carry the venous blood; eventually all the systemic veins in the body come together to form the two great vena cavae, the superior, that carries blood leaving the head and neck, and the inferior, that carries blood leaving the rest of the body. Both vena cavae enter the heart at the level of the right atrium. Blood from the right atrium enters the right ventricle and then is pumped to the lungs to once again begin the process of oxygenation.

The circle is completed.

DOES THE RESPIRATORY SYSTEM HAVE OTHER FUNCTIONS BESIDES GAS EXCHANGE?

Yes. A particularly important respiratory system function is body defense. A healthy respiratory system prevents many airborne particles from damaging the alveoli or from entering the blood stream. The nose filters large airborne particles out of the air we inhale. This efficient filtering mechanism is bypassed, however, during mouth breathing.

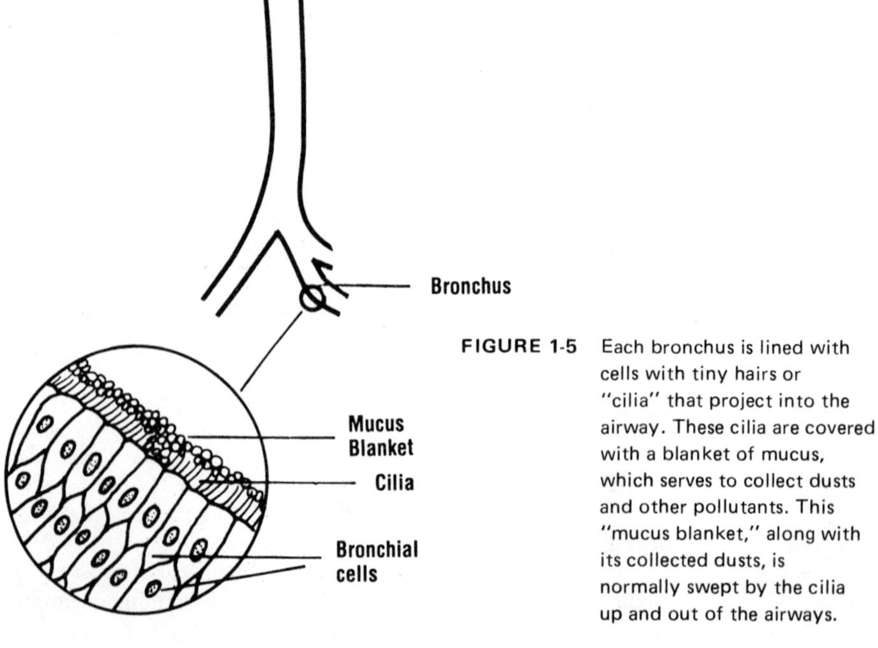

FIGURE 1-5 Each bronchus is lined with cells with tiny hairs or "cilia" that project into the airway. These cilia are covered with a blanket of mucus, which serves to collect dusts and other pollutants. This "mucus blanket," along with its collected dusts, is normally swept by the cilia up and out of the airways.

The trachea and main bronchi are also effective in keeping dusts and other large particles from reaching the alveoli. Coughing is one way we attempt to clear the large airways of noxious material.

Even when our nose and normal cough response are not helping keep out dusts, our bronchi function silently to move out any unwanted material. This is accomplished by a blanket of mucus that covers the bronchi, and tiny hairs (cilia) which sweep the mucus out of the airways (Figure 1-5). When this dust-laden mucus reaches the top of the trachea, it is usually swallowed.

Even if particles get past all of these defenses, special alveolar cells (called macrophages) are mobilized to help digest any foreign substances such as bacteria or tiny particles of dust.

All of these normal defense mechanisms may be damaged from chronic cigarette smoke, making smokers much more vulnerable to inhaled dusts. This is one reason why diseases such as asbestosis, silicosis, and coal workers' pneumoconiosis are much more severe in cigarette smokers (see Chapter 4).

CHAPTER TWO
Smoking and Your Health

HOW DO WE REALLY KNOW SMOKING IS HARMFUL?

Evidence has been accumulating for years relating cigarette smoking to disease. As cigarette consumption in the first half of this century increased, many began to suspect a connection with lung cancer. Several pioneering studies published in the 1940s and 1950s established this link. However, the evidence was not universally accepted and was challenged especially by tobacco companies during this period. In the 1950s, to help resolve the issue, the U.S. Public Health Service reviewed the published evidence from all parts of the world. Based on evidence accumulated up until 1957, Surgeon General Leroy E. Burney stated ". . . excessive smoking is one of the causative factors in lung cancer." An official "Public Health Statement" reinforcing this position was published in the *Journal of the American Medical Association*, November 28, 1959. This official government position formed the basis for further developments in the 1960s.

In 1962 the British Government issued its own report, concluding: "Cigarette smoking is a cause of lung cancer and bronchitis, and probably contributes to the development of coronary heart disease . . ." About this time other studies linked cigarettes to various diseases. As a result many people, including U.S. congressmen, called for further investigation.

On June 7, 1962 Surgeon General Luther L. Terry announced the establishment of an expert committee to undertake a comprehensive review of all data on smoking and health. The result was the first Surgeon General's report on *Smoking and Health*, published in January 1964. This report proved pivotal for all subsequent government action toward cigarettes. No new research had been done for this report, only an objective and critical analysis of all the research done in the world up to that time. Results of this study were conclusive: based on epidemiologic, clinical, and basic research, cigarettes were found to be causally related to human diseases including lung cancer, chronic bronchitis and heart disease.

WHAT HAS BEEN LEARNED SINCE THE 1964 SURGEON GENERAL'S REPORT?

Since 1964 the government has periodically updated its reports on smoking and health to include all new evidence accumulated each year. In 1979 the Public Health Service published a totally new Suregon General's report, including all the evidence on smoking and health accumulated between 1964 and 1979. The 1979 report confirms an ever wider range of human diseases caused by cigarette smoking, and states that cigarettes are "far more dangeous than was supposed in 1964."

The 15-year interval between reports had established dangers to women smokers (most of the evidence prior to 1964 dealt with men only). We now know, for example, that lung cancer deaths among women increase as more women smoke longer. "Women who smoke like men die like men who smoke." We also know that smoking during pregnancy adversely affects the fetus and increases the risk of birth defects. Women who smoke during pregnancy are more apt to have low birth weight babies, increasing the risk to the neonate.

In addition, we have learned that smoking greatly increases the risk of workers exposed to certain occupational hazards, such as asbestos fibers. The 1979 report documents also the rather shocking increase in smoking among teenage girls: The percentage of girls age 12 to 14 who smoke increased eight-fold between 1968 and 1978!

Perhaps most importantly, the 1979 Report puts to rest any possible objection that the evidence against cigarettes is sketchy and circumstantial. This document–a review of 15 years of solid research–deals a final blow to those who doubt the dangers of cigarette smoking.

WHAT PERCENTAGE OF THE POPULATION SMOKES?

The total percentage of the adult population that smokes cigarettes has declined, from 42 percent in 1965 to 33 percent in 1980. There are estimated 30 million *ex-smokers* in this country.

Although the percentage of smokers fell, the population increased enough during this period to keep the *number* of smoking adults about the same–53.3 million in 1965 and 52.4 million in 1980. Partly as a result, the number of cigarettes sold has gone up, from 529 billion in 1965 to 615 billion (in 1978); this represents an increase in the number of cigarettes sold per active smoker.

Despite the increases in number of cigarettes smoked, the percentage decline of adult smokers indicates definite progress. Indeed, without the massive educational effort launched since the 1964 Surgeon General's Report, probably almost half of the adult population would be smoking cigarettes today.

Table 2-1 gives the percentage of adult smokers in 1965, 1978, and 1980.

TABLE 2-1 Percentage of Adult U.S. Population Classified as Active Cigarette Smokers*

	1965	1978	1980
TOTAL	42	33.7	32.6
Male	52.4	37.4	36.7
Female	34.1	30.4	28.9

*Source: National Center for Health Statistics.

WHAT ARE THE DISEASES CAUSED BY CIGARETTES?

Based on the 1964 and 1979 Surgeon General reports, the diseases or conditions shown in Table 2-2 are now known to be related to cigarette smoking.

In addition, cerebrovascular disease (stroke) is thought possibly related to cigarette smoking, but the evidence is yet inconclusive.

It should be emphasized that the above conditions would still occur in the population if there were no cigarette smoking, but much less frequently. Thus, cigarettes are estimated to cause 90 percent of lung cancer, 65 percent of laryngeal cancer, 25 percent of coronary artery disease, and so forth. For the individual, not smoking considerably lessens the chances of contracting any of these illnesses.

WHAT IS THE WORST EFFECT OF CIGARETTE SMOKING?

Considering the number of people affected, the worst effect of smoking is not lung cancer, bronchitis, or emphysema. It is coronary artery heart disease (CHD), a disease involving the vessels (coronary arteries) supplying blood to the heart. Smoking is one of three major independent risk factors for CHD; the others are high blood pressure and elevated serum cholesterol. The risk of CHD increases both with the number of cigarettes smoked and with the presence of other risk factors.

Hardening of these arteries (coronary arteriosclerosis) and resultant heart attacks (coronary thrombosis) killed over 640,000 Americans in 1978. Through

TABLE 2-2 Diseases or conditions related to cigarettes

Lung cancer
Other cancers—larynx (voice box)
oral cavity
esophagus
bladder
pancreas
kidney
Bronchitis
Emphysema
Coronary artery heart disease
Stomach ulcers
Peripheral vascular disease
Low birth weight pregnancies

careful statistical analysis of patients who smoke and patients who get heart disease, it has been concluded that about 25 percent of these deaths would have not occurred if patients had not smoked cigarettes. Over 160,000 of these deaths were directly attributable to cigarette smoking.

HOW MANY DEATHS FROM LUNG CANCER, BRONCHITIS AND EMPHYSEMA ARE ATTRIBUTABLE TO CIGARETTES?

In the United States, lung cancer accounts for over 100,000 deaths per year, over 90 percent of these directly due to cigarette smoking. Chronic obstructive pulmonary diseases (bronchitis and emphysema)–diseases almost exclusively due to cigarettes–cause another 50 to 60 thousand deaths each year. Over 300,000 smoking–related deaths (cancer, COPD, and heart disease) occur each year. This makes cigarette smoking the number one known cause of death in the United States.

This statistic makes an interesting contrast to the number of Americans who died:

- During Battle in World War II (1941-1945) 292,131
- During Battle in Viet Nam (1964-1972) 45,926
- In Motor Vehicle Accidents (1978) 53,600

The mortality ratio for all smokers of cigarettes is about 1.7 when compared to nonsmokers. This means life expectancy is shortened by cigarette smoking–a 30-year-old, 2-pack-per-day smoker has a life expectancy 8.1 years *less* than his nonsmoking counterpart.

There is a dose-response relationship between smoking and mortality. The risk of dying from a cigarette-related illness (lung cancer, coronary heart disease, and so forth) increases the more one smokes.

HOW DOES CIGARETTE SMOKE RESULT IN HEART DAMAGE?

Cigarette smoke is actually made up of many compounds and gases, divided into three main groups.

"Tar" — represents all of the particulate matter left over from the smoke after removal of moisture and nicotine; tar is the smoke's residue, and is the main cause of pulmonary disease, particularly lung cancer.

Nicotine — a chemical present in all cigarettes and responsible for giving one a 'flushed' feeling.

Carbon monoxide (CO) — a colorless, odorless gas present in all cigarette smoke. (In addition, CO is a component of automobile exhaust, and can be found whenever incomplete combustion takes place.)

Nicotine and carbon monoxide can have damaging effects on the heart. Nicotine can constrict or narrow the coronary arteries that supply blood to the heart. When this occurs in patients who have hardening of the coronary arteries, the result may be decreased oxygen delivery to the heart muscle. The patient may experience severe chest pain, known as angina. If oxygen delivery is severely impaired, part of the heart muscle dies and the patient experiences a heart attack.

Carbon monoxide can contribute to this process. CO binds avidly with hemoglobin in the red blood cells. Hemoglobin bound with CO can no longer carry oxygen—the more carbon monoxide in the blood, the less oxygen is available. Inhaling two packages of cigarettes a day may remove up to 15 percent of the blood's oxygen. In other words, people who smoke this much may be walking around with up to 15 percent less oxygen in their blood than if they didn't smoke. An otherwise normal person has ways of compensating for this oxygen deficit; however, when combined with the damaging effects of nicotine and already hardened coronary arteries, the result can be devastating.

Heart attacks do kill nonsmokers, although other risk factors, such as high blood pressure and elevated blood cholesterol, are usually present. If you have never smoked, you may still get coronary artery disease, but the chances are less likely. Smoking *doubles* the risk of dying from coronary artery disease for men and increases the risk for women, but not to the same level as for male smokers.

WHAT ABOUT PIPE AND CIGAR SMOKING?

Cancers of the mouth and throat occur much more commonly in pipe and cigar smokers than in nonsmokers; also, pipe smoking is a major cause of lip cancer. However, lip and mouth cancers are relatively less common diseases than the major killers—lung cancer, heart disease, bronchitis, and emphysema.

Death rates from lung cancer are close to those for nonsmokers if the smoke is not inhaled. The more pipe or cigar smoke is inhaled, the more death rates and medical problems rise. Thus, pipes and cigars are not inherently 'safe' to use, but the overall habits of pipe and cigar smokers (less is smoked, less is inhaled, compared to cigarette smokers) do tend to minimize the overall risks.

IS CIGARETTE SMOKE ADDICTING?

The original 1964 Surgeon General's Report stated that smoking was not an addiction since there were no withdrawal symptoms on quitting. Research in the intervening years has clearly shown the opposite to be true. Nicotine in cigarette smoke is addictive, and smokers can and often do get withdrawal symptoms when they quit. Symptoms include restlessness, irritability, intense craving for a cigarette, and trouble in concentration. The ability to measure nicotine levels in the blood has enabled researchers to closely study nicotine's addicting aspects.

In the preface to the 1979 Surgeon General's Report nicotine is blamed for the apparent paradox of an educated smoking public wanting to quit the habit but unable to ". . . perhaps because nicotine is a powerful addictive drug." Without nicotine in tobacco, cigarette smokers would not have the intense desire to continue smoking and would be no more inclined to smoke than, say, eat a candy bar. Gratifying perhaps, but not addicting.

HOW CAN ONE OVERCOME THE NICOTINE ADDICTION AND STOP SMOKING?

It is fair to say there is no proven or widely accepted method of stopping smoking. Table 2-3 broadly categorizes the many methods advocated today. Within each category are dozens of variations, many advertised and promoted for profit. The philosophical differences in approach, as well as the sheer number of methods advocated, attest to the lack of any simple, acceptable method that will help a majority of smokers. Although various stop-smoking methods have been advocated as long as cigarettes have been a recognized problem, the relatively recent appreciation of nicotine's addicting property has provided a rationale for a host of methods, old and new. These are discussed later in this chapter.

IF NICOTINE IS ADDICTING, WHY ARE SOME PEOPLE ABLE TO QUIT "COLD"?

Different people respond differently to habituating substances. Nicotine's addicting properties are mild compared to the opiates such as heroin. Abrupt withdrawal does give some people unpleasant effects, such as a gnawing sensation in the stomach, a headache, and, not least, an intense craving for cigarettes (actually for nicotine). It is likely that the intensity of symptoms ranges widely in any group of smokers and that many people can either ignore or overcome them in their desire to quit. There may be an attenuation of symptoms with age so that older people, who have also smoked longer, are better able to quit than younger people smoking the same number of cigarettes a day. Whatever the explanation, the fact remains that millions have been able to kick the habit without much, if any, ill effect.

TABLE 2-3 Methods advocated to quit smoking*

1. *Quitting Cold*
2. *Weaning* (Includes methods designed around smoking less and less each day, either by number of cigarettes, use of various filters, or smoking cigarettes with progressively lower tar and nicotine content)
3. *Nicotine Substitution* (Includes methods with and without tobacco)
4. *Behavioral* (Includes hypnosis, aversion therapy, and group reinforcement)
5. *Miscellaneous* (Includes acupuncture, procaine injections in the ears, and so on)

*Many commercial methods employ more than one technique, such as weaning plus behavior modification.

Contract To Stop Smoking

I ______________________________ hereby promise
(your name)

to stop smoking by completing the American Lung Association's self-help program, *Freedom from Smoking in 20 Days*. I promise

to start this program on ______________________________ and
(date you plan to start program)

to finish this program on ______________________________.
(date you plan to finish program)

Date______________ Signed______________________________
(date you sign contract) (your signature)

AMERICAN LUNG ASSOCIATION
The Christmas Seal People ®

FIGURE 2-1 Contract to stop smoking. (Reproduced by permission, American Lung Association.)

WHAT IS THE BEST METHOD TO QUIT SMOKING?

If by this question one means what is the most healthful method, quitting "cold turkey" is the obvious answer. The effects of nicotine withdrawal are not medically significant, continued smoking is.

As to which method is likely to be most successful, there is no single answer. The many different approaches and individual methods, with none the clear winner, mean each smoker has to find what works best for him or her.

The categories in Table 2-3 are based on methods the smoker might seek out. Also discussed are methods used by physicians when patients are not seeking help but must quit nonetheless. The single most effective method of getting a patient to quit is constant reinforcement by his or her physician, done in an intelligent, persistent manner, using the physician's own nonsmoking behavior as example.

1. Quitting Cold

Quitting cold means stopping smoking suddenly without substituting any other potentially harmful tobacco product. This is also the method chosen, consciously or not, by most people who have kicked the habit. For unknown reasons many people are able to just stop, period. The impetus may come from years of no-smoking propaganda, a personal or family illness, or some sudden insight into their problem. This is certainly the most economical of all methods.

2. Weaning

Weaning means slowly decreasing the amount smoked each day, either by decreasing the number of cigarettes, their potency, or the amount of smoke inhaled from each cigarette.

There are an enormous number of weaning variations. One popular type uses a series of four filters and advertises "one day at a time"; each filter, used for two weeks, is designed to eliminate more of the toxic smoke than the one preceding it. At the end of the eight week period about 90 percent of the tar, nicotine, and carbon monoxide is said to be removed from the smoke. Like all weaning methods it may work for some but carries no unique advantages.

There are many books that advocate specific programs based on some form of weaning. They are all essentially self-help and teach the smoker how to quit on his or her own. Techniques advocated include: smoking only at certain times of the day regardless of location or activity; listing important trigger activities and then, one at a time, gradually eliminating cigarettes associated with them; keeping cigarettes in inaccessible areas or locking them up; and restricting smoking to an uncomfortable place.

Aspects of the weaning technique have been carefully incorporated into the American Lung Association's "Freedom From Smoking In 20 Days" program. This is a self-help program, completely contained and explained in one booklet, designed and scientifically tested over a two year period by a panel of physicians. The program begins by asking the smoker to sign a contract before embarking on the 20 days (Figure 2-1). In the first few days of the program the smoker assesses why, where, and how much he or she smokes. A detailed log (incorporated in the booklet) is kept. On day 7 opportunity is given to quit cold, although this is not the program's main focus.

Starting on day 8 and progressing through day 16 the smoker changes to lower tar and nicotine brands (a list is provided) and also smokes fewer cigarettes. Helpful advice is given about weight, exercise, and activities to occupy the mind and replace the smoking urge. On day 17 the smoker is off cigarettes. Although the entire program takes 20 days, a companion booklet teaches the new nonsmoker how to maintain a "Lifetime Of Freedom From Smoking." Both the "20 Day" and "Lifetime" programs are available for a nominal charge from your local branch of the American Lung Association.

Even with highly motivated people, weaning is not always successful. Unfortunately for some, weaning may reinforce the need to smoke. If you have the will to make a choice between quitting cold and weaning off cigarettes, choose the former.

3. Nicotine Substitution

The idea behind methods based on nicotine addiction is to maintain a high blood nicotine level without inhaling harmful tar and carbon monoxide in cigarette smoke. Most of these methods are designed to provide nicotine in a form other than inhaled tobacco smoke; among these the most popular consist of using tobacco without smoking it—chewing or snuffing. Less popular are tobaccoless aids, such as nicotine chewing gum and nicotine lozenges, and nicotine substitutes, drugs and similar properties.

Tobacco Without Smoking. Snuff is pulverized chewing tobacco; a pinch of snuff can be placed in the nose or in the cheek. An article in the medical journal *Lancet* showed that nicotine from snuff is readily absorbed into the bloodstream.

Chewing tobacco is nonpulverized and is chewed slowly in the mouth. Like snuff, it also provides nicotine without the harmful effects of cigarette smoke.

Nicotine Without Tobacco. Nicotine-containing chewing gum and nicotine lozenges have also been developed as an aid to satisfy the nicotine craving without inhaling tobacco smoke. Experience with these aids has been limited so far.

Drugs Similar to Nicotine. Tobacco substitutes contain lobeline, a natural substance obtained from dried leaves and herbs that has similar effects as nicotine. However, controlled studies have not found lobeline any better than a placebo (inert drug). There is also no evidence that tranquilizers such as Valium offer any benefit for people who wish to quit smoking.

4. Behavioral

Many programs attempt to alter the behavior of the smoker in a way that discourages or eliminates all smoking. Fear is the simplest technique employed, often used by physicians on their patients. By detailing possible consequences such as lung cancer and emphysema, doctors hope that patients will quit smoking out of fear of the consequences. Often, however, this backfires because some patients may smoke even more to relieve anxiety.

Adverse conditioning is a form of behavioral therapy that seeks to make the smoking experience very unpleasant. There are drugs on the market that claim to make cigarette smoke taste unpleasant; these have not found widespread acceptance. Other adverse methods are electro-shock, blowing smoke at the smoker, and rapid smoking. The rapid smoking technique has received much attention recently and has been presented in reputable medical journals. Here the patient smokes very rapidly until he or she becomes sick with dizziness or nausea. Because their carbon monoxide level is increased, patients with heart disease may be at some risk from this procedure, though it appears safe for otherwise healthy people. This technique is still under investigation and is obviously limited to only a small number of people in a controlled setting.

Clinics and organized groups, profit and nonprofit, usually employ some form of behavior modification. They may help some people to stop smoking, at least temporarily. The problem in evaluating their effectiveness is that the programs begin with people who have already decided to quit and just need a slight push; they are not as successful with the less motivated. A number of organizations sponsor such groups, including:

Seventh Day Adventists—Five-day plan; lectures offered by physicians and clergymen.

Shick Laboratories—Program for one hour on five consecutive days. This program relies mainly on aversion therapy, including rapid smoking and electro-shocks, over eight weeks of reinforcement in weekly one hour sessions.

Smokenders—A very popular course offering eight weekly meetings with a highly structured program emphasizing self-awareness, behavior modification, positive conditioning, and periodic reunions for a year afterward.

Some programs, particularly in industry, reward people monetarily if they stop smoking. These programs can be very effective.

In conclusion, there is a plethora of anti-smoking drugs, devices, educational programs, and other methods advertised to help people stop smoking. As may be expected, no single program is widely accepted.

CAN HARM COME FROM INHALING SECOND-HAND SMOKE?

"Second-hand smoke" refers to smoke given into the atmosphere from a lighted cigarette. It comes from two sources. The first is sidestream smoke, which enters the air directly from the burning end of a cigarette. The second source is mainstream smoke, which is the smoke inhaled by the smoker and then exhaled into the atmosphere. An average cigarette burns for 12 minutes, polluting the air continuously with sidestream smoke, while mainstream smoke is exhaled by the smoker for part of this time.

Sidestream smoke has higher concentrations of noxious compounds than mainstream smoke. For example, about twice as much tar and nicotine, three times as much carcinogenic 3-4 benzpyrene (a component of "tar"), and five times as much carbon monoxide are in sidestream smoke as compared to mainstream smoke. Thus, exposure to other people's cigarettes (passive smoking) means exposure to the same harmful chemicals and gases that cause cancer, heart disease, and other cigarette-related illnesses.

Passive Smoking by Healthy People

Based on epidemiologic studies similar to those in smokers, several harmful effects of passive smoking have been shown in groups of healthy people, incuding:

Newborns—Children born of smoking mothers have lower birth weights and more medical problems, on the average, than children from nonsmoking mothers.

Children—Asthma symptoms are much more frequent, common colds more prolonged and pneumonia more common, in children of smoking parents compared with children brought up in a nonsmoking environment.

Adults—Several studies point to the potential adverse effects of inhaling other people's cigarette smoke. However, the evidence so far indicates, at most, minor respiratory impairment from passive smoking.

The evidence for serious disease from passive smoking is unclear. Although at least one study purported to show an increased risk of lung cancer in passive smokers, this has not been substantiated.

Passive Smoking by Patients with Medical Problems

Common sense tells us that diseased hearts and lungs can only get worse from a continued assault of cigarette smoke, even when passively inhaled. Several studies have scientifically confirmed this, at least in patients who suffer from angina pectoris, or heart pains that come from lack of oxygen to the heart muscle. In the early 1970s Dr. Wilbert Aronow and colleagues at Long Beach Veterans Hospital in California studied groups of patients with angina. In one study, they did tests of heart and lung function before and after patients were driven for 90 minutes in heavy freeway traffic with the car windows open. These patients were tested to see how long it took for heart pains to occur. Dr. Aronow repeated the tests with the patients breathing compressed air from a tank while driving through the traffic. The results: Exposure to freeway traffic air increased carbon monoxide levels in the blood and caused heart pain to occur sooner than when the patients breathed nonpolluted air.

It is probable that second-hand smoke is very dangerous to some people, but not by itself a major cause of alarm for healthy people exposed infrequently. There is as yet no conclusive evidence that long-term exposure in otherwise healthy people will have the same devastating effects as occur in regular smokers. However, prudence dictates that one should avoid cigarette smoke as much as possible.

ARE THE NEWER LOW TAR AND NICOTINE CIGARETTES SAFER THAN THE OLDER BRANDS?

This is a complex question and the topic of the 1981 Surgeon General's report on *Smoking and Health.* As with prior reports, many contributing scientists and physicians reviewed all the relevant evidence. Among the conclusions of the report were:

> There is no safe cigarette and no safe level of consumption . . . Smoking cigarettes with lower yields of 'tar' and nicotine reduces the risk of lung

cancer and, to some extent, improves the smoker's chance for longer life, provided there is no compensatory increase in the amount smoked. However, the benefits are minimal in comparison with giving up cigarettes entirely. The single most effective way to reduce hazards of smoking continues to be that of quitting entirely . . . A final question is unresolved, whether the new cigarettes being produced today introduce new risks through their design, filtering mechanisms, tobacco ingredients, or additives. The chief concern is additives. The Public Health Service has been unable to assess the relative risks of cigarette additives because information was not available from manufacturers as to what these additives are.

DOES QUITTING SMOKING IMPROVE SURVIVAL?

No matter how long one has smoked, quitters can expect to live longer than those who continue the habit. Dr. G. D. Friedman and colleagues studied 25,917 people who answered detailed health questionnaires over a ten year period at Kaiser-Permanente Medical Centers in Oakland and San Francisco. Based on the results of multiple questionnaires during this period, the subjects were grouped according to their smoking habits as persistant smokers, persistant quitters, temporary quitters, and never smokers. Cause of death was determined from California death certificates for several diseases, including lung cancer and coronary artery heart disease.

Quitting and Coronary Artery Heart Disease (CHD)

A major purpose was to determine if quitting smoking improved survival from CHD. It had been suggested that people who quit live longer because they are healthier to begin with, and that during their smoking years those who will later quit smoke less, have less pre-existing heart disease, are thinner, or possess other characteristics that distinguish them as a group from those who will persist in smoking. Not so. When all other factors were accounted for, the study found persistent quitters have less than half the chance of dying from CHD as do persistent smokers! *Quitting smoking is an independent factor that substantially lessens the risk of dying from CHD.* In fact, the risk for quitters is about the same as for those who've never smoked.

Quitting and Lung Cancer

Dr. Friedman's study is also interesting for its results about lung cancer. Compared to never smokers, persistent smokers had a 45 times greater chance of dying from lung cancer; in contrast to CHD, they found that persistent quitters still had a 15-fold greater chance of dying from lung cancer.

These are group statistics. Other studies have shown that the longer one has quit smoking, the less the chances of developing (and dying from) lung cancer.

HOW LONG AFTER QUITTING DOES ONE ACHIEVE THE SAME LUNG CANCER RISK AS A NONSMOKER?

The answer to this depends on how long and how much one has smoked. Heavy smokers maintain a definite increased risk of developing lung cancer years after quitting, although after ten years this risk approaches that of nonsmokers. For people with fewer years of smoking behind them (for example, pack/day for three years) the increased risk of developing lung cancer or another serious disease (if one is not already present) is probably negligible.

Fortunately, other benefits of quitting become more immediately obvious. Within one to two days the new nonsmoker has more oxygen carrying capacity than when he or she smoked, since the blood is no longer being polluted with carbon monoxide. Consequently, his or her exercise tolerance improves. Symptoms such as coughing and sputum production also begin to improve within days to weeks after quitting. And, not to be dismissed, money spent on cigarettes becomes available for other things.

IS MARIJUANA HARMFUL TO THE LUNGS?

There is a striking parallel between attitudes toward marijuana today and toward cigarettes 50 years ago. In the 1920s cigarettes were generally regarded as harmless, even relaxing. We now know unequivocally that they are a cause of most lung cancer and disabling chronic lung disease, plus a large proportion of coronary artery disease. Each year hundreds of thousands of Americans die from the effects of cigarette smoking. Despite the enormity of the statistics, it has taken decades of increasing cigarette consumption, first among men, then women, plus countless scientific studies along the way, to appreciate fully tobacco's harmful effects.

Widespread marijuana use is a relatively new phenomenon, largely limited to people under 35. There is simply not the cumulative experience with marijuana that there is with cigarettes; for this reason less is known about its long-term effects.

One of the short-term effects of marijuana (occurring within minutes to hours after inhaling) is an opening up of the airways in asthmatic patients. This 'bronchodilating' effect of marijuana smoke has been confirmed in several studies done in the early and mid-1970s. Thus, along with whatever high one obtains, an asthmatic may also notice easier breathing after a few puffs. However, because of the other active (and potentially harmful) ingredients in marijuana smoke, this must be considered the worst imaginable treatment for asthma.

More recent studies suggest that the potential harm from long-term marijuana smoking is similar to that from smoking tobacco. Both are plants whose smoke is inhaled deeply into the lungs. Many chemicals and products of combustion are inhaled when either is smoked (acrolein, formaldehyde, and NO_2, among others). One major difference is that marijuana contains no nicotine. Instead it contains THC (delta-9-tetrahydrocannabinol). THC, the major psychoactive ingredient, is responsible for the high experienced when marijuana is smoked Along with THC hundreds of other compounds, similar to the "tar" of cigarettes, are also inhaled. For this reason marijuana smoke has the potential for causing the same lung diseases caused by cigarettes.

It is thus not surprising that scientific studies show chronically-smoked marijuana has an irritating effect. The respiratory effects have been demonstrated by Dr. Donald P. Tashkin and associates at UCLA, using volunteers solicited through newspaper advertisements. In one study, daily smoking of an average of five marijuana joints over a period of 47 to 59 days caused mild but statistically significant decreases in several measurements of lung function. This study involved 28 young men.

A more recent study from UCLA included 74 young, habitual marijuana smokers (frequency of smoking ranged from three times a week to several joints every day), with most having a smoking history of over five years. All were white, between the ages of 21 and 33. Their lung function was compared to control groups of non-marijuana-smoking subjects. Results of sophisticated lung function tests showed that marijuana smokers were found to have subtle changes in airflow, mainly in the larger airways of the lungs. In addition, these changes were more pronounced than those found in cigarette-smoking subjects who did not use marijuana! As a possible explanation, Dr. Tashkin postulates that there may be "a greater irritant effect of constituents in marijuana smoke than of those in tobacco smoke."

Studies such as these must be considered preliminary. Most marijuana smokers are asymptomatic, and the observed lung function changes in the studied subjects may not predict future respiratory difficulties. But since marijuana smoke contains the same or similar respiratory irritants as cigarette smoke, one must logically expect long-term detrimental changes. The current state of knowledge can be summarized by a quote from Dr. Robert L. DuPont, president of the National Institute on Drug Abuse: "Smoke is bad for the lungs, whether it's industrial smoke, tobacco smoke or marijuana smoke."

Those interested in a summary of all the health effects of marijuana should read *Marijuana and Health*, a comprehensive review published by the Institute of Medicine (see References).

CHAPTER THREE
Air Pollution

WHAT IS AIR POLLUTION?

Most respiratory diseases are caused by airborne agents. These may be bacteria, viruses, chemicals in cigarette smoke, allergens, various gases, or dusts. Our lungs are uniquely vulnerable to contamination from the air we breathe. To this extent most lung disease is caused by air pollution or air contamination. However, the term air pollution is usually used in a narrower sense to mean contamination of the air with noxious material given off by machines (factories, automobiles, and so forth). This type of air pollution can affect people in a large general area such as a city or valley. Of course one can also define air pollution in the context of inhaling your own or someone else's cigarette smoke (see Chapter 2) or of inhaling contaminated air unique to your work area (See Chapter 4). In this chapter air pollution refers to the general or community air pollution that affects a general population.

WHAT MAKES UP GENERAL AIR POLLUTION?

Many different particles and gases make up what we commonly refer to as air pollution. For convenience they can be divided into six major groups:

1. *Carbon Monoxide*. This is a colorless, odorless, invisible gas, the product of internal combustion engines. It combines with hemoglobin in red blood cells and displaces oxygen. In small amounts carbon monoxide can cause headaches and fatigue. Large amounts can be lethal. (See Chapter 5 for discussion of carbon monoxide toxicity.)

2. *Particulates.* This is a general term for a mixture of solid and liquid particles in the air, usually produced by stationary fuel combustion and industrial processes. Particulates include small bits of soot and ashes that emanate from incinerators and smokestacks.
3. *Sulfur oxides.* These are acrid, corrosive, poisonous gases that come from burning sulfur-containing fuel such as coal and oil. They are produced mainly by industrial plants that burn fuel containing sulfur as an impurity.
4. *Hydrocarbons.* So named because they contain both hydrogen and carbon, these compounds come from the incomplete burning of fuel, mainly gasoline. Although hydrocarbons are not very harmful themselves, they can react with sunlight to form smog, which is irritative. In industrial areas most hydrocarbons are from automobiles.
5. *Nitrogen oxides.* These include nitric oxide and nitrogen dioxide (NO_2), produced when fuel is burned at very high temperatures; this occurs mainly in automobiles, electric utilities, metal-fabricating plants, and chemical plants. NO_2 is a yellow-brown gas that can combine with hydrocarbons and sunlight to form smog and ozone. Ozone is a specific photochemical oxidant that can be irritative to the lungs and eyes.
6. *Miscellaneous.* A host of other pollutants, including lead, arsenic, asbestos, mercury, beryllium, plutonium, cadmium fluoride, and organic pesticides, may enter the atmosphere from various sources. Airborne lead, mainly from leaded gasoline, has decreased considerably since the conversion by many cars to unleaded gasoline.

WHAT IS SMOG?

There are actually two kinds of smog: photochemical smog due to the action of sunlight on air pollutants, and a combination of smoke and fog (hence smog) that has nothing to do with sunlight. This combination, the original smog, used to be common in London when coal was widely used to heat homes. The term smog has since been adopted to describe the haze that occurs when sunlight reacts with the hydrocarbons and nitrogen dioxide that are part of automobile exhaust.

The reaction of sunlight with hydrocarbons and NO_2 results in a variety of chemical products. One of these is ozone. Ozone is a molecule made up of three atoms of oxygen, abbreviated O_3. Regular oxygen, which of course is vital to life, is a molecule of 2 oxygen atoms, abbreviated O_2. Adding an extra oxygen atom to form ozone results in an irritative, noxious gas. Other undesirable chemicals, such as aldehydes, also result from this photochemical reaction and account for the harmful effects of smog: eye irritation, cough, and, for some, trouble in breathing. Because sunlight is essential to this type of smog, the concentration of ozone and other measurable chemicals is maximum around noon and falls off considerably at night. (See Chapter 2 for a discussion of the harmful effects of Los Angeles smog on patients with heart disease).

WHAT RESPIRATORY DISEASE IS CAUSED BY COMMUNITY AIR POLLUTION?

The effects of air pollution should be viewed in two different groups: healthy people and people with chronic heart or lung disease. Most studies demonstrating harmful air pollution effects have been done on chronic disease patients and the very elderly, two groups more susceptible to air pollution than the general population.

The most notorious example of air pollution in the United States occurred in 1948 in Donora, Pennsylvania. Weather conditions caused the already heavily polluted air to stagnate for several days. Out of a population of 14,000, 20 died and over 6,000 became ill. All of the deaths and most of the serious illness occurred in people with underlying heart or lung disease.

Various epidemiologic studies in the United States, Canada, and England have associated increased levels of air pollution with:

- an increase in the hospitalization rate of children with pre-existing asthma
- diminished lung function tests in children when compared with tests in unpolluted areas
- an increase in the hospitalization rate for acute respiratory illness in the general population
- an increase in deaths when compared to less polluted areas of the same city
- an increase in the incidence of severe emphysema in cigarette smokers when compared with smokers in unpolluted areas

In London, attacks of bronchitis associated with air pollution led to the British Clean Air Act of 1956. Subsequently, there was a marked decrease in mortality and morbidity from bronchitis.

On a year to year basis there is no doubt that air pollution, as exists in and around our cities and industrial plants, makes the lives of chronic heart and lung disease patients more difficult. Various local governments now publicize a "pollution standard index" or PSI to warn such patients to stay indoors when the air is unsafe (Table 3-1). The PSI scale ranges from 0 to 500 and is based on the air pollutant with the highest concentration at the time the test is done. Five major pollutants are measured at various points throughout the area: nitrogen dioxide, sulfur dioxide, carbon monoxide, photochemical oxidants (mainly ozone), and particulate matter. The PSI was originally developed by the U. S. Environmental Protection Agency to provide consistency in reporting on air quality. The PSI is published every morning in large city newspapers or is available from your local pollution control agency.

TABLE 3-1 Pollution standard index (PSI)

0-50	The air is clean and does not pose a serious health hazard.
50-100	Moderate air pollution.
100-200	Unhealthy level; the amount of air pollution may aggravate symptoms in people with underlying heart or lung disease.
200-299	*First Stage Alert:* "Very unhealthful"—elderly people and those with chronic heart or lung disease should stay indoors. Everyone may experience symptoms of lung or eye irritation.
300-399	*Second Stage Alert:* Anything above 300 is considered very hazardous. All people should avoid outdoor activity.
400-500	*Third Stage Alert:* A level of air pollution that may cause premature death in elderly people and those with chronic heart of lung disease.

Common sense dictates that anyone suffering chronic cardiac or pulmonary disease—asthma, bronchitis, emphysema, cystic fibrosis, coronary artery disease, heart failure, and so forth—should avoid air pollution to the maximum extent possible, including altering lifestyle, residence, or occupation if necessary and economically feasible.

DOES GENERAL AIR POLLUTION LEAD TO SPECIFIC DISEASE IN HEALTHY PEOPLE?

It is difficult to pin down specific examples of cause and effect between general air pollution and diseases such as asthma, chronic bronchitis, emphysema, and lung cancer. This question, although studied for many years, remains largely unanswered. Data have been published from England linking chronic bronchitis to heavy sulfur oxide and particulate exposure, and most investigators seem to accept that severe air pollution of this type can cause chronic bronchitis.

Apart from this link, there is no body of data, analogous to the data for cigarette smoke, proving cause and effect between current levels of air pollution and specific diseases.

Many of the compounds listed above (in concentrated form) have been shown to cause skin cancer in laboratory animals. Although lung cancer is definitely more prevalent in urban than in rural populations, there are many differences between urban and rural populations besides levels of air pollution that might cause differences in lung cancer rates. These differences include total smoking history, exposure to passive smoke (see Chapter 2), population density, and work environ-

TABLE 3-2 Effects of community or general air pollution

Known Effects	See Chapter
A cause of chronic bronchitis	12
Exacerbation of chronic bronchitis	12
Exacerbation of asthma	12
Exacerbation of emphysema	12
Impairment of pulmonary function	8
A cause of cough and other symptoms of respiratory irritation	6
Contributing factor to excess respiratory deaths in "air pollution disasters"	3
Possible Effects	
A possible cause of emphysema	12
Weakening defense mechanisms against infection	19
A cause of lung disease in people who live for many years in the vicinity of manufacturing plants that produce certain products, such as asbestos	4
A contributing factor to the excess lung cancer in cities, compared to rural areas	21

ment. At present there is no accepted epidemiologic proof that lung cancer is caused by general or community air pollution.

We do know that air pollution is definitely irritative, particularly to the eyes and bronchial tubes. The watery eyes and coughs experienced by many otherwise healthy people during heavy bouts of smog are but two examples. There is no reason to doubt that repeated exposure to heavy concentrations of air pollution can cause major pulmonary disease. Factors such as cigarette smoking and work-related exposure are known causes of specific illnesses (see Chapters 2 and 4). It is likely that general air pollution, if severe enough, can also lead to specific diseases in otherwise healthy people.

A summary of effects of community air pollution is given in Table 3-2. Next to each effect is the chapter in this book where the reader will find a more general discussion of the specific condition or disease.

CHAPTER FOUR

Trouble Breathing in the Workplace: Occupational Lung Disease

WHAT IS OCCUPATIONAL LUNG DISEASE?

Most respiratory disease is caused by breathing in some potentially noxious agent, such as bacteria, viruses, cigarette smoke, allergens and dusts. Nowhere is our respiratory vulnerability more evident than with the constant air pollution that occurs in some jobs. Although information about occupational hazards goes back to antiquity (for instance, mining), we have only recently accumulated evidence proving specific occupations hazardous.

Occupation-related disease is now a widely studied and reported field of medicine with its own journals and specialty training programs. Occupational lung disease, a major aspect of this field, is caused by inhaling noxious agents in the workplace, mainly dusts, fumes, gases, and vapors.

There are two broad categories of occupational lung disease:

1. *Diseases that are not occupation-specific.* This group includes people suffering from common conditions such as emphysema, bronchitis, asthma, and interstitial lung disease. These all may be caused by workplace exposure, but may also be due to factors unrelated to the job, such as cigarette smoking and general air pollution. They may also be due to causes that can't be pinpointed. Although not occupation-specific, these conditions can definitely be aggravated, if not caused, by exposure at work; they are discussed in the chapters dealing with the individual diseases. This chapter will concentrate on the next category, occupation-specific illnesses.

2. *Diseases related to a specific occupation,* such as asbestosis in asbestos workers (pipe fitters), silicosis in people exposed to silica dust (sandblasters) and coal workers' pneumoconiosis in coal miners. These diseases and many others like them have a specific cause and effect relationship with the inhaled material and would not occur if the workers did not have the specific exposures.

HOW COMMON IS OCCUPATIONAL LUNG DISEASE?

Surprisingly common. Although there are no exact figures, thousands of Americans are adversely affected by their workplace, the majority from lung damage. The Department of Health and Human Services estimates that every year 400,000 people develop a disease caused by their jobs. An estimated 100,000 deaths each year are caused by occupational diseases. More than half of these diseases and deaths are due to lung disease.

Many occupations are associated with some form of illness. Liver cancer in vinyl chloride workers, lung cancer in asbestos workers, deafness in jackhammer operators, bronchitis in toll-booth workers—these are but a few examples. The economic costs are staggering. Some $5 billion is paid out in workers' compensation annually for job-related illness and injuries.

The sad fact is that much of the human misery behind these statistics is preventable. Unfortunately, the connection between the patient's illness and the job is often not made until too late. This delay in recognition is related to several factors, one of which is the slow and insidious progress of most occupational diseases.

WHAT ARE THE SPECIFIC OCCUPATIONAL LUNG DISEASES?

The list of all known occupational lung diseases would fill several volumes and be incomplete anyway since new ones are frequently being discovered. This reflects the amazing number of new compounds and industrial methods introduced yearly, as well as improved detection methods. For simplicity we can divide occupational lung disease into three main groups based on the type of material inhaled: mineral dusts, organic dusts, and a third group that includes smoke, fumes, vapors, mists, and sprays.

Mineral dusts come from rocks, stones, and ores in the earth's crust. Diseases arising from inhalation of mineral dusts are called *pneumonconioses.* The most common are coal workers' pneumoconiosis (black lung), silicosis, and asbestosis.

Organic dusts come from living materials such as plants, animals, and microorganisms. A common example is farmer's lung.

Smoke comes from burning organic material such as cigarettes, wood, trash, and so forth. *Fumes* are formed when very hot vapors cool rapidly and condense into very fine solid particles; this occurs in welding, smelting, and furnace work. *Gases* are found apart from liquids and can be defined as a liquid that will expand to fill any size space. *Vapors* are essentially the same as gases except that they are encountered only in the presence of the parent liquid. *Mists* and *sprays* are terms used interchangeably; they are fine suspensions of liquid droplets in air or some other propellant gas.

WHAT IS BLACK LUNG DISEASE?

Black lung refers to lung disease caused by inhaling coal dust. The medical term is coal workers pneumoconiosis (CWP). Black lung comes from the fact that the lungs of deceased coal miners often appear black from the heavy deposits of coal. The normal human lung has a healthy pink appearance. Although people living in and around cities will have some black deposits in their lungs, coal workers may have much more extensive involvement.

The disease is diagnosed by two simple criteria:

1. History of working in coal mines, and
2. Abnormal chest X-ray showing the characteristic spots in the lungs caused by coal dust deposits.

Only a small percentage of ex-coal miners, perhaps fewer than 10 percent, have any X-ray evidence of coal dust deposits; when present, they usually show up as small spots, less than one centimeter in diameter. Such a chest X-ray pattern, in an ex-coal miner, is called simple CWP (see Figure 4-1).

Simple CWP causes no symptoms and does not lead to respiratory disability. In fact epidemiologic studies show that coal miners who have breathing impairment, but have only simple CWP on chest X-rays, are invariably heavy cigarette smokers; smoking, not coal dust, is responsible for the breathing problem.

Although coal dust can certainly infiltrate the lungs and make them black, it

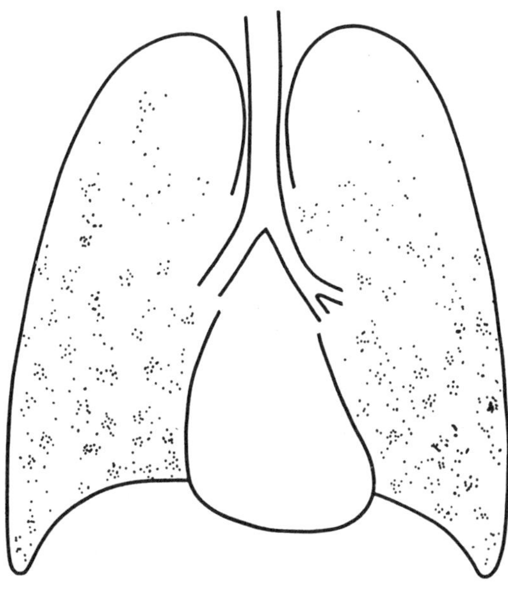

FIGURE 4-1 Drawing of chest x-ray picture showing simple coal worker's pneumoconiosis ("black lung"). Dust deposits, represented by black dots, are scattered throughout both lungs. See Chapter 8 for further discussion of chest x-ray drawings.

is doubtful whether coal dust by itself ever causes major breathing impairment. How then to account for severe black lung disease, which has claimed many victims in the past? This more virulent form of black lung disease is manifested by progressive fibrosis (scarring) of the lungs and shows a very different X-ray picture from simple CWP. It is not due to cigarette smoking, but also doesn't seem due to coal dust per se. Some investigators think it is due to silica dust mixed in with the coal in the particular mine that was worked. Silica is much more fibrogenic (likely to lead to scarring) than coal. The cause for progressive fibrosis seen in coal miners is not known with certainty, but fortunately it is much less common than simple CWP.

A far greater threat to the health of most miners is cigarette smoking. Added to the inhaled coal dust, the smoking miner is at much greater risk for bronchitis, emphysema and lung cancer than his nonsmoking co-worker (see Figure 4-2).

WHAT IS SILICOSIS?

Inhalation of silica dust (which is sometimes inhaled in pure form during sandblasting*) causes much more severe disease than inhalation of pure coal dust. This type of pneumoconiosis is called silicosis. Silica may also be responsible for the severe cases of black lung disease seen in coal workers. Pure silica dust can lead to widespread scarring of the lungs and can be extremely disabling. In addition, silicosis makes the patient more susceptible to tuberculosis and lung cancer.

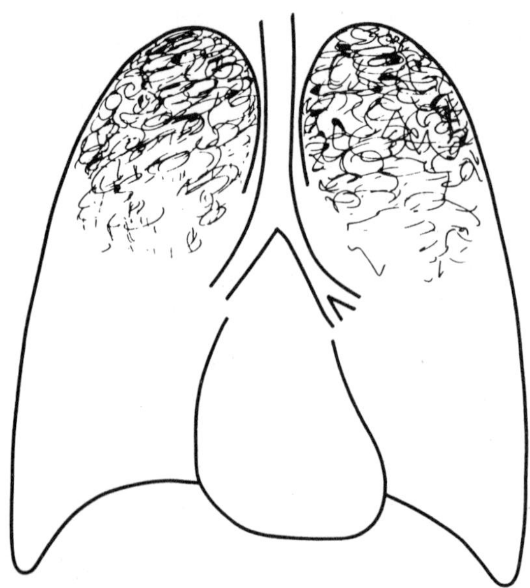

FIGURE 4-2 Chest x-ray appearance of silicosis. Silicosis, caused by inhaling silica dust, affects mainly the upper parts of the lungs.

*A form of abrasive cleaning in which a stream of sand is projected by compressed air under high pressure. Sandblasting is used to clean metal surfaces in shipyards and steel fabrication plants, as well as facades of buildings.

Given the presence of pneumoconiosis on the chest X-ray, silicosis can usually be separated from coal workers' pneumoconiosis by work history and appearance of the chest X-ray (see Figure 4-2). If the patient worked in coal mines, he may have silicosis along with CWP, but he most certainly has CWP. Patients who have never worked in coal mines, but have worked as sandblasters or in other silica dust areas have characteristic findings on their chest X-rays—usually widespread scarring in the upper parts of the lungs.

Not everyone who works around silica and coal dust gets silicosis or coal worker's pneumoconiosis. Contraction of either disease is related to the intensity and duration of dust exposure; the longer one works with these dusts and the more dense the air concentration, the better the chance that the disease will occur. Cigarette smoking also contributes to any impairment that results from dust inhalation.

WHAT ARE THE HEALTH HAZARDS FROM ASBESTOS?

Asbestos is a family of naturally occurring minerals that are widely used as insulating material. Asbestos has over 3,000 uses, including insulation for boilers and pipes, automobile brake linings, and, until recently, insulating hair dryers. An estimated 30 million tons has been used in the United States since 1900.

Asbestos can cause serious disease when inhaled over a period of time. Minute asbestos fibers are taken up by the lung cells; unlike many ordinary dust particles, these fibers cannot be removed by the lung defenses. The physical property of the fibers (small size, thin, and narrow) allows them to penetrate the deepest lung tissues where they reside throughout life. Many years later, even two to three decades after exposure, one of several diseases can show up, including asbestosis, lung cancer, mesothelioma, and some less common conditions.

Asbestosis

Asbestosis is the most common form of asbestos-related lung disease. It occurs in only a small number of people who have worked with asbestos, and is diagnosed by a typical apppearance on the chest X-ray plus a history of occupational exposure (see Figure 4-3). Asbestosis is really a lung tissue reaction to the inhaled asbestos dust and is, therefore, a type of pneumoconiosis, comparable to silicosis or other mineral dust diseases. Asbestosis is not cancer (though it may lead to cancer) and is not invariably fatal, although patients can die from severe forms of the disease. The usual picture is scarring and fibrosis of the lung tissue. The reason why only some of the people exposed to asbestos dust get asbestosis is not known. There is no effective treatment for asbestosis. Complications, such as pneumonia or lung cancer, can be fatal in patients with asbestosis. If the patient smokes, he or she should quit forever; smoking tremendously increases the risk of developing lung cancer in people with underlying asbestosis.

Lung Cancer

This is the most dreaded result of chronic asbestos inhalation. It is usually found in patients who also smoke; the combination of smoking and asbestos exposure sharply increases the risk of lung cancer over that of people who only smoke

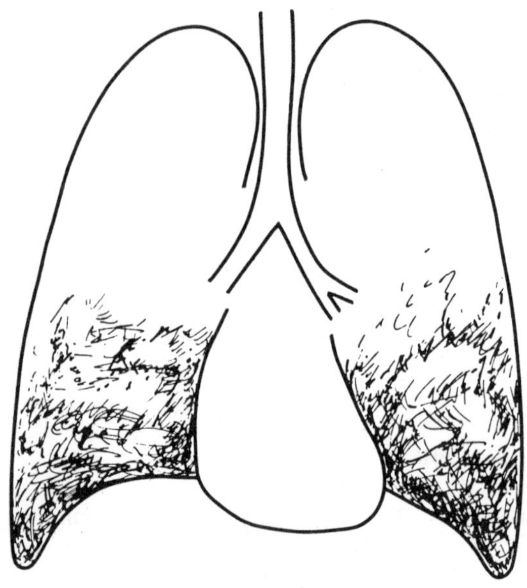

FIGURE 4-3 Typical x-ray appearance of asbestosis. The disease affects mainly the lower parts of the lungs.

or only have chronic asbestos exposure. Smoking and asbestos exposure are synergistic for the development of lung cancer. X-ray findings of asbestosis don't have to be present to develop asbestos-related lung cancer; the cancer can begin growing in a patient whose chest X-ray has been negative for years following exposure to asbestos dust. The cure rates for any lung cancer are dismal and asbestos-related lung cancer is no exception.

Mesothelioma

This is a tumor of tissues that cover either the lungs (the pleural membranes) or the contents of the abdominal cavity (the peritoneal membranes) and is related to asbestos exposure. Although occasionally these tumors can be benign, when they occur due to asbestos exposure they are usually malignant. Unlike lung cancer, their occurrence is not related to cigarette smoking. There is no effective treatment for malignant mesothelioma.

Other Conditions

Other diseases have been linked to asbestos exposure, including cancer of the larynx (voice box) and cancer of the stomach, colon, and rectum. The association of asbestos exposure with these tumors is not as strong as with lung cancer, but asbestos workers contract these tumors more often than the general public.

HOW WAS ASBESTOS FOUND TO BE DANGEROUS?

Asbestos has been mined since the late 1800s, with industrial uses expanding greatly after the turn of the century. In the 1930s and 40s several investigators made the association between asbestos exposure and an increased incidence of lung cancer. Further recognition of this association occurred in the 1960s when

Dr. Irving Selikoff and colleagues at New York City's Mt. Sinai Hospital published data on 632 members of the International Association of Heat and Frost Insulators and Asbestos Workers. They found a much higher than average number of deaths from lung cancer in these workers as well as a much larger than expected number of mesotheliomas. This and other studies have also demonstrated that cigarette smoke adds a synergistic effect to asbestos exposure so that the rate of lung cancer is far greater than with either exposure alone. People who smoke *and* work with asbestos are in a potentially very dangerous situation.

More recently Dr. Selikoff published data on asbestos insulation workers who had been at their job for at least 20 years. This large group (12,051 workers) was compared with another large group of men followed by the American Cancer Society and in whom smoking habits were known. They reported the following risks for developing lung cancer:

NS = Nonsmokers NA = Non-asbestos workers
S = Smokers A = Asbestos workers

	NS/NA	NS/A	S/NA	S/A
Relative risk of developing lung cancer	1	5.2	10.8	53.2

The nonsmoker not exposed to asbestos has a very low risk of ever getting lung cancer. This risk is arbitrarily assigned a value of 1. Work with asbestos increases the risk of lung cancer 5-fold. People who smoke but are not exposed to asbestos have an almost 11-fold greater chance of getting lung cancer than non-smokers. Add smoking to the asbestos exposure and the risk is enormous. Asbestos exposure increases the risk of lung cancer 5-fold over the already large risk from smoking alone.

Anyone who smokes is inviting lung cancer; any asbestos worker who smokes is making sure the invitation is answered. According to Dr. Selikoff, among asbestos workers *one in every five deaths is due to lung cancer*!

IS THERE ASBESTOS EXPOSURE APART FROM THE WORKPLACE?

Yes. If carefully searched for under the microscope, asbestos fibers are often found in lungs of non-asbestos workers. This is considered a normal finding in most people, and differs from the disease asbestosis mainly in the small numbers of fibers present. Thus, healthy lungs may have a few fibers in lung tissue whereas people with asbestosis have tremendously more fibers, enough to form scar tissue. If it is absolutely unavoidable that you work with asbestos, then a special mask and filter should be worn at all times to avoid inhaling these fibers.

WHAT OTHER DUSTS CAN CAUSE PNEUMOCONIOSIS?

Actually the list is long. Virtually any mineral dust inhaled to excess over a long period of time can cause some pulmonary reaction and a resulting abnormal chest X-ray. For unknown reasons some dusts tend to be relatively inert and almost never cause severe lung scarring. Examples of the more benign mineral dusts are tin, iron, and aluminum. Exposed workers can show extensive X-ray evidence of inhaled tin, for example, yet have no pulmonary impairment or symptoms. The more commonly inhaled dusts such as coal, asbestos, and silica can be very damaging, especially the latter two, although exposure usually has to be prolonged (years). It is likely that a one-time exposure will have little if any harmful effect in most individuals.

WHAT IS ORGANIC DUST DISEASE?

We have just discussed lung diseases that may occur from inhaling mineral dusts; these are the pneumoconioses. Lung disease may also occur from inhaling living or organic dusts. Such dusts include spores, fungi, and other tiny organisms that may be inhaled in occupations dealing with plants, trees, animals, crops, and so forth. Aside from the material inhaled, this group differs from the pneumoconioses in one important aspect: patient symptoms.

Patients suffering from organic dust disease generally manifest one of two acute syndromes: a diffuse pneumonia accompanied by shortness of breath and fever (so-called hypersensitivity pneumonitis) or an acute asthma-bronchitis problem. With chronic exposure the patient may end up with chronic obstructive or restrictive lung disease.

There is a diversity of occupations and materials that may lead to organic dust disease. Table 4-1 lists many of the jobs and associated conditions that have

TABLE 4-1 Occupational lung disorders caused by exposure to organic dust

Disease	Inhaled Material
Bagassosis	Moldy bagasse (sugar cane)
Bird fancier's, breeder's, or handler's lung	Avian droppings or feathers (including parakeets, chickens, turkeys, and pigeons)
Byssinosis	Cotton dust
Cheese washer's lung	Moldy cheese
Coffee worker's lung	Coffee beans
Farmer's lung	Moldy hay, grain, silage
Fish meal worker's lung	Fish meal
Furrier's lung	Animal pelts and hair
Humidifier or air-conditioner lung	Contaminated water in humidification and air-conditioning systems
Malt worker's lung	Moldy barley
Maple bark disease	Maple bark
Maple bark stripper's disease	Maple tree logs or bark
Mummy disease	Cloth wrappings or mummies
Mushroom worker's lung	Mushroom compost
Paper mill worker's and puplwood handler's disease	Moldy wood pulp
Paprika slicer's disease	Moldy paprika pods
Sauna taker's disease	Contaminated sauna bathwater
Sequoiosis	Redwood sawdust
Suberosis	Moldy cork dust
Wheat thresher's lung	Wheat flour containing weevils
Woodworker's lung	Oak, cedar, and mahogany

been reported. Only a minority of workers in each occupation suffer from inhalational lung disease; why this is so is not known.

When patients present with an asthma-bronchitis picture, the chest X-ray is usually clear and the patient complaints are coughing, wheezing, and shortness of breath. This is also known as occupational asthma (see Chapter 10). Classically, the symptoms are worse on returning to work after a weekend off and abate after stopping work at the end of the week. One of the best studied of such diseases is found in cotton workers; it is called byssinosis or brown lung.

The second major manifestation of organic dust exposure is called hypersensitivity pneumonitis (HP). In HP the patients are clinically sick with pneumonia and the X-ray shows an infiltrate. In contrast to infectious pneumonia, HP is not an infection and is not treated with antibiotics. HP is caused by an allergic reaction to the inhaled dust. One of the best studied examples of HP is farmer's lung. Farmers who work around moldy hay may inhale the fungal spores that make the hay moldy. They may become sick within a few hours of inhaling the fungal dust and develop fever, cough, and shortness of breath. The chest X-ray shows a stringy infiltrate. Hypersensitivity pneumonitis usually responds to treatment with corticosteroids.

There is still much to learn about all of the various occupational diseases, and active research is underway on many of them. Over a period of time repeated exposure and reaction to organic dusts can definitely lead to chronic lung disease and chronic airway obstruction. Anyone suspected of suffering from occupational dust exposure should be thoroughly evaluated and, if necessary, undergo a change in job or alter his or her work pattern to avoid dust exposure.

It should be noted that not everyone exposed to organic dusts becomes ill. Many organic dust reactions are allergic in nature and only affect a small percentage of the exposed population. Other reactions are perhaps due to the bulk load of inhaled dust and may affect a greater percentage of people. Unless large scale screening studies are done on all exposed workers, the only way these diseases can be identified is by patient symptoms. For this reason, it is imperative for any worker to report symptoms that could possibly be related to dust exposure.

WHAT IS BYSSINOSIS?

Byssinosis is the medical term for brown lung, the lung disease that comes from inhaling cotton dust. Byssinosis occurs mainly in people who work with hemp, flax, or cotton dust and thus is prevalent in the textile industry.

In the early stages byssinosis can lead to shortness of breath and cough while at work (so-called acute byssinosis). When the worker is removed from the dusty environment, as at home or on vacation, these symptoms improve or disappear. After about five years or longer of constant exposure, the worker may develop chronic byssinosis, leading to permanent breathing trouble.

Byssinosis differs from other occupational dust diseases in that there are no characteristic chest X-ray findings and a lung biopsy does not reveal any evidence of the cotton dust. Except for the work history, chronic byssinosis is indistinguishable from chronic obstructive pulmonary disease. Byssinosis is diagnosed by the work history and the presence of breathing impairment. If clear worsening of symptoms or airflow obstruction can be demonstrated after arriving at work, the diagnosis is more secure.

No one knows for sure how cotton dust leads to lung disease. The term brown lung comes from the brown dust of the leaves surrounding the cotton balls. But what in the cotton dust is responsible for byssinosis? Is it a chemical? bacteria? fungus? The answer is not known.

Like all occupational diseases the symptoms attributable to byssinosis are worse and more prevalent in cotton workers who smoke, compared to nonsmoking workers. This is particularly true of chronic byssinosis with irreversible airways obstruction. Perhaps something in cotton dust hastens the damaging effects of cigarettes, or vice versa.

Regardless of the cause of byssinosis, the advice is the same for anyone potentially exposed to dust at work. Avoid dusty areas as much as possible. Wear whatever protective devices or masks are available. And above all, don't smoke—on or off the job.

WHAT DISEASES OCCUR FROM INHALING SMOKE, FUMES, GASES, VAPORS, MISTS, AND SPRAYS?

These gaseous-type products are given off in many industrial processes; some of the better characterized diseases, and their causes, are given in Table 4-2.

TABLE 4-2 Some common gases, fumes, and vapors that can be inhaled on the job

Chemical	Occupations at Risk	Medical Problem
Ammonia	Fertilizer; refrigeration workers	Lung irritation
Chlorine	Bleaching; disinfectants; plastics	Lung irritation
CO (Carbon Monoxide)	Coal miners; coal field workers; firefighters	Fatigue, dizziness, headache (low c.*); coma (high c.)
CO_2 (Carbon dioxide)	Foundry work; mining	Same as CO
NO_2 (Nitrogen dioxide)	Silo workers; farming; dye & fertilizer industries	Lung irritation, bronchitis, cough, dyspnea (low c.); pulmonary edema (high c.)
SO_2 (Sulfur dioxide)	Coal, oil-burning plants	Same as NO_2
H_2S (Hydrogen sulfide)	Sewage treatment plants	Same as NO_2
Ozone	Aircraft personnel; arc welding	Lung irritation
Phosgene	Paint & chemical industry	Lung irritation; pulmonary edema
Cadmium fumes	Welding & smelting industries	Emphysema (low c.); pulmonary edema (high c.)
TDI—(toluene diisocyanate)	Paint, varnish industries	Asthma-like symptoms
Zinc oxide fumes	Welding	Metal fume fever; pulmonary edema
Polyvinyl chloride vapor	Meat wrappers	Asthma
Formalin vapors	Insulation workers; embalmers	Asthma; lung irritation
Radioactive gases	Uranium mines; power plants	Lung cancer

*c = concentration

Inhaling these noxious materials can lead to a wide variety of clinical reactions. For example, metal fume fever, which comes from inhaling fumes of hot, burning metal, can lead to nausea, vomiting, headaches, and general malaise. TDI, an industrial solvent, can cause asthma in some individuals. Meat wrappers' asthma occurs from inhaling the fumes given off when the plastic used to wrap meat is cut with a hot wire. Arc welders can get a form of chronic lung scarring.

There are many examples and the list grows longer with the addition of new or exotic industrial processes. The advice given in the previous section holds here as well. Anyone suffering symptoms suspected from inhaling industrial products should be evaluated medically and, if necessary, change his or her job or the workplace situation.

CHAPTER FIVE

Common Respiratory Emergencies: What You Can Do

WHAT IS CARDIOPULMONARY RESUSCITATION?

Cardiopulmonary resuscitation, or CPR, is a universally accepted way for anyone to revive a patient whose heart or breathing has suddenly stopped. The steps outlined below are those developed over the years as effective. They are adapted from the American Heart Association's Standards and Guidelines for Cardio-Pulmonary Resuscitation (CPR), which are based on a 1979 conference co-sponsored by the American Heart Association and the National Academy of Sciences-National Research Council.

The key to CPR is *A B C.*

*A*irway
*B*reathing
*C*irculation

A. *Airway.* In order to restore breathing, first clear and open the victim's airway. To do this:
   1. Lay victim on his back on a firm rigid surface such as the floor or the ground.
   2. Quickly clear the mouth and airway of foreign material with your fingers.
   3. If there does not appear to be any neck injury, gently tilt the victim's head backward by placing one hand beneath his neck and lift upward. Place the heel of the other hand on his forehead and press downward as the chin is elevated (Figure 5-1).

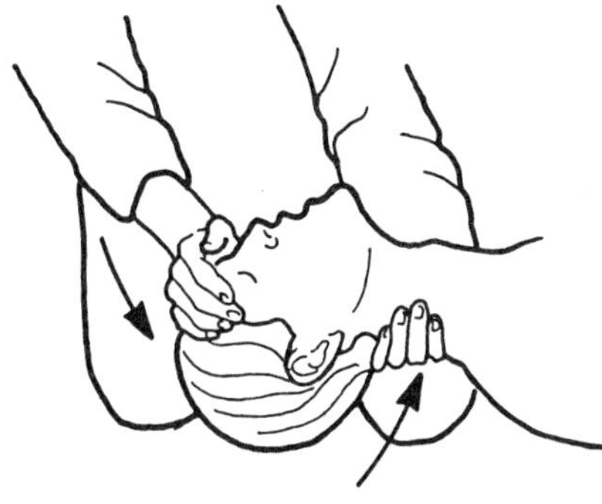

FIGURE 5-1 Airway maintenance in CPR.

B. *Breathing.* To restore breathing:
   1. Keep victim's head tilted backward.
   2. With the hand that is placed on his forehead, pinch the nostrils using your thumb and index finger (Figure 5-2).

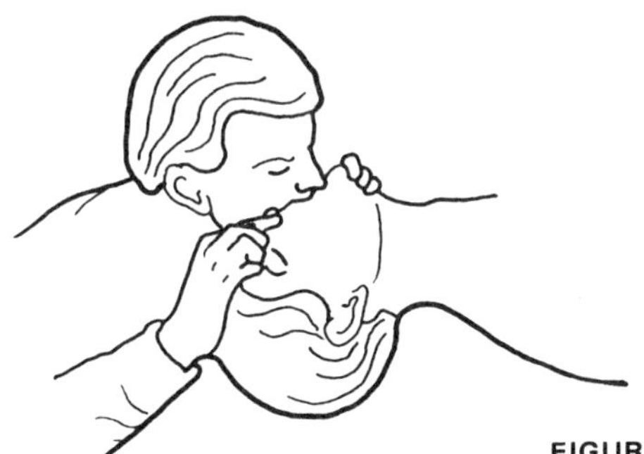

FIGURE 5-2 Mouth-to-mouth resuscitation.

   3. Open your mouth widely and take a deep breath.
   4. Place your open mouth tightly around the victim's mouth and give four quick breaths. TAKE A DEEP BREATH BETWEEN EACH BLOW. Continue blowing into his mouth at approximately *12 breaths per minute.* Quantity is important, so provide plenty of air—one breath every five seconds until you see the chest rise. (Seconds may be counted "one-one thousand, two-one thousand, three-one thousand," and so forth.)
   5. Stop blowing when the victim's chest is expanded. Remove your mouth from his and turn your head toward his chest so that your ear is over the victim's mouth. Listen for air leaving his lungs and watch his chest fall. Repeat breathing procedure approximately 12 times/minute.
   6. Continue mouth-to-mouth breathing until victim is breathing well on his own or until medical assistance arrives.

      Note: If the victim's mouth cannot be used due to an injury, remove your hand from under his neck and close his mouth, then place your hand over his mouth. Open your mouth widely and take a deep breath. Place your mouth tightly around the victim's nose and blow into it. After you exhale, remove your hand from the victim's mouth to allow air to escape.

Moderate resistance will be felt with blowing. If the chest does not rise, the airway is not clear and more airway opening is needed. Place hands under the victim's lower jaw and thrust lower jaw forward so that it juts out.

To Restore Breathing in Infants and Children

Mouth-to-mouth or mouth-to-nose artificial breathing is basically the same for infants and small children as for adults. However, the head should not be tilted as far back for infants and small children as for adults and large children. Place your mouth tightly over both the mouth and nose of the infant or small child (Figure 5-3). Breathe small puffs of air into the child's mouth and nose every three seconds (20 breaths per minute); each breath should be sufficient to make the chest rise.

C. *Circulation. The American Heart Association recommends circulation support only be given by those trained in the procedure; when performed it must be in conjunction with artificial breathing.*
To restore circulation:
1. Check neck artery for pulse. (Check for heartbeat below left nipple in infants.)
2. If no pulse is felt, begin cardiac compression. For one rescuer, give 15 compressions (80 per minute), followed by two quick, mouth-to-mouth breaths. For two rescuers, give 5 compressions (60 per minute) for every one breath. Repeat until medical assistance arrives. Figure 5-4 shows the correct position for two-rescuer CPR.

Call paramedics or ambulance immediately. If this is not possible, take the victim to the nearest hospital emergency room. Have someone else drive so that you can continue artificial breathing and cardiac compression if necessary.

The American Heart Association distributes a free wallet card which briefly summarizes CPR (Figure 5-5). The back blows and abdominal thrusts mentioned on the card are discussed in conjunction with the next question.

WHAT SHOULD I DO IF SOMEONE IS CHOKING?

First immediately decide if the person is only partially or completely choking. A person completely choking is unable to talk or breathe—he or she is choking to death! If the person is able to talk and cough, breathing is taking place—leave him

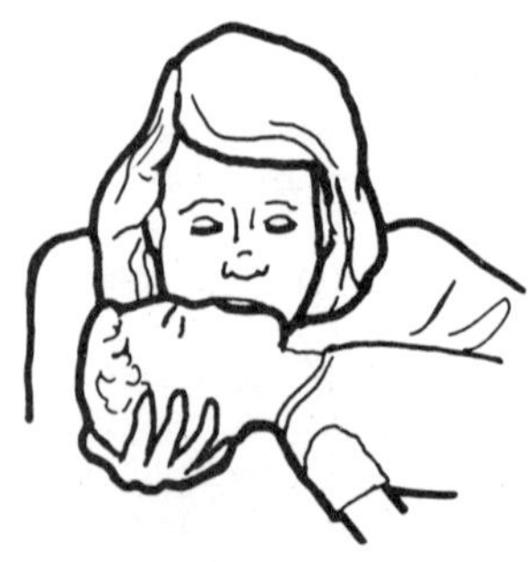

FIGURE 5-3 Infant resuscitation.

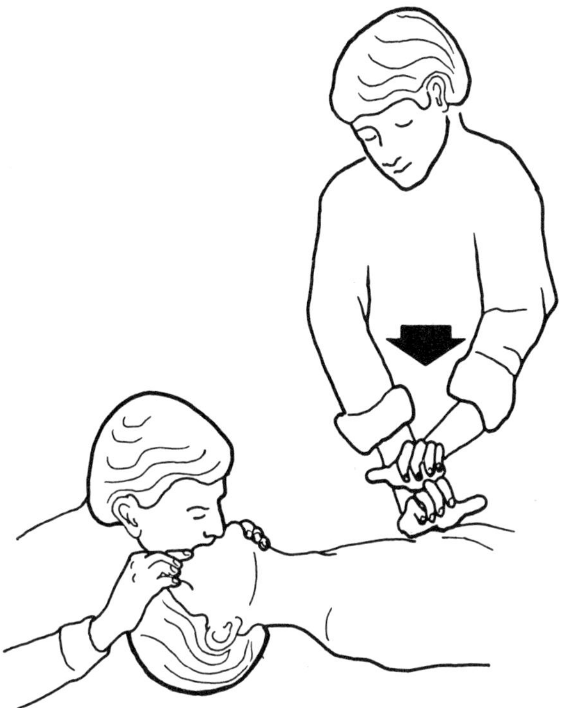

FIGURE 5-4 Two-peson cardiopulmonary resuscitation.

alone! The natural coughing mechanisms are better than anything artificially applied. Continue to observe until the choking spell has passed.

Major concern is with the victim who has completely obstructed his airway with food or other material–this person is *unable to talk or breathe.* Note that management of the choking victim is very different from CPR. Also, unlike the CPR procedure, there is considerable controversy regarding the preferred method to use in the choking victim. This controversy will be discussed before listing the steps you should take to save the life of a choking victim.

Historical Background of the Heimlich Maneuver

For many years it was noted that some people died suddenly while eating. Until the 1960s such deaths were attributed to heart attacks (the most common cause of sudden death) and each event was called a "cafe coronary." Then autopsy studies revealed many of the deaths were *not* from heart attacks, but from acute asphyxiation when a food bolus lodged in the victim's windpipe! This revelation was followed by the recommendation to "try and remove the food bolus" in choking victims, either with one's fingers or by using a curved appliance designed to grasp the food and extract it. Although such an appliance was marketed it did not sell widely.

HEART ATTACK

Signals and Actions for Survival

Know the signals: an uncomfortable pressure, squeezing, fullness or pain in the center of the chest, behind the breastbone, which may spread to the shoulder, neck or arms (the pain may not be severe); other signals may include sweating, nausea, shortness of breath and a feeling of weakness.

Action

1. Recognize the "signals",
2. Stop activity and sit or lie down,
3. Act at once if pain lasts for two (2) minutes or more — call the emergency rescue service or go to the nearest hospital emergency room, with 24 hour service.

American Heart Association 7320 Greenville Ave. Dallas, Texas 75231

78-001-C (REV 81) 77-80-5.5MM 6-81-2MM

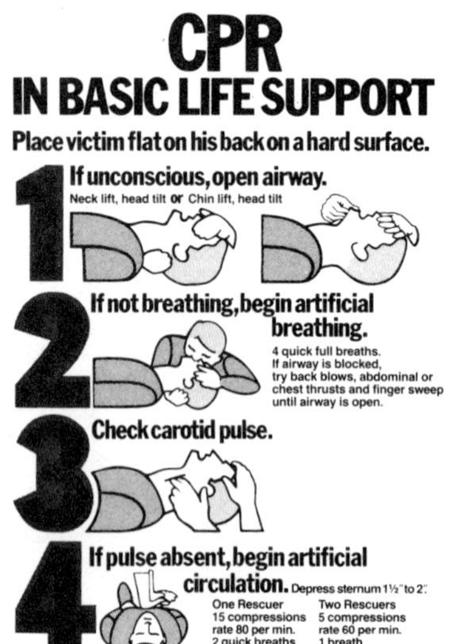

FIGURE 5-5 CPR in Basic Life Support. (Reproduced with permission, American Heart Association.)

In the early 1970s Dr. Henry Heimlich, then a professor of surgery at the University of Cincinnati, published an altogether different technique for removing the food bolus. It has since become known as the Heimlich Maneuver. In this maneuver the rescuer stands behind the choking victim and places his fists below the xiphoid (lower breast bone) area. Once in position, a series of quick, sharp, upward and inward manual thrusts are given to compress the air in the thorax. This pressure is transferred to the obstructed upper airway and the lodged food bolus; the result is a dislodged bolus that is projected out of the throat.

Because it is impossible to conduct a controlled trial (where some victims receive the Heimlich Maneuver and others do not), only anecdotal information has been collected about this (or any other) technique. By Dr. Heimlich's own account, in the first few years after he introduced the method hundreds of patients worldwide were saved from dying because his maneuver was used.

Dr. Heimlich feels strongly that other maneuvers applied first to the choking victim, such as back slapping, may worsen the patient. He is thus at odds with the American Medical Association (and other major medical groups), who have recommended back slapping as well as abdominal thrusts. (Both Dr. Heimlich and officials of these organizations feel that any attempt to remove the obstructing bolus with one's fingers or an appliance should be the last resort.)

HOW DOES THE HEIMLICH MANEUVER WORK?

The foreign object obstructs the airway so that below it are two lungs full of air. By pushing up on the lungs—by the abdominal thrusts—the air in them is compressed; this creates a positive pressure that acts against the obstructing object to eject it out of the airway. The principle is to create a sudden surge in air pressure below the obstructing object.

WHAT ARE THE OFFICIAL RECOMMENDATIONS FOR THE CHOKING VICTIM?

The official recommendations are to use both back blows and abdominal thrusts, since both together are purported to be better than either alone. To quote from the Standards and Guidelines article: "Thus, either back blows followed by thrusts or thrusts followed by back blows was found to be acceptable, as long as the two techniques are employed. The 1979 Conference recognizes and recommends that because more information is needed before a definitive recommendation can be made, controlled prospective studies be conducted to study this difficult problem." Dr. Heimlich does not agree with this and states that back blows can actually worsen the situation by dislodging the food bolus and allowing it to travel further down into the windpipe.

Since the case for either back blows or manual abdominal thrusts (Dr. Heimlich's maneuver) as the first step in the choking situation is unproved, both steps are given here. In the sequence of steps below the officially recommended back blows is listed first, followed by Dr. Heimlich's maneuver. Dr. Heimlich–and many other physicians–would omit the back blows completely and begin with step 2–abdominal thrusts–for the reason given above. If back blows are tried first and fail, no time should be wasted in applying the Heimlich Maneuver.

HOW CAN I RECOGNIZE THE CHOKING VICTIM?

The universal sign is the victim's hand to his throat; he cannot speak or breathe and rapidly becomes pale and blue (Figure 5-6). The setting is usually while eating or in an area where food has recently been swallowed.

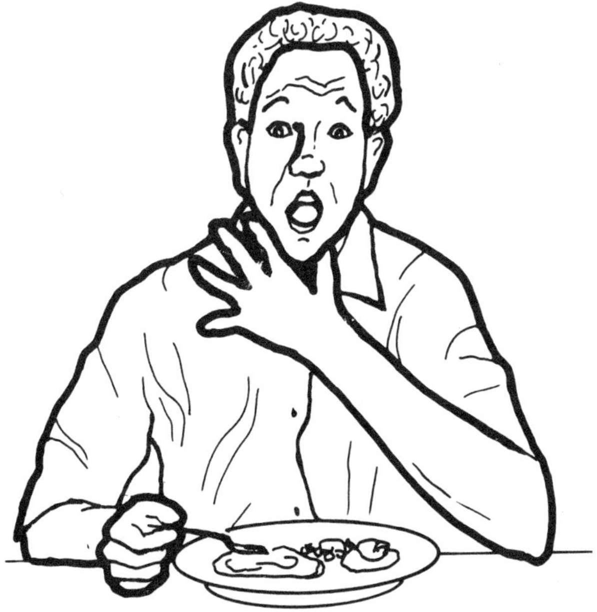

FIGURE 5-6 Choking victim.

HOW CAN I HELP THE CHOKING VICTIM?

If the choking victim can speak, cough, or breathe, do not interfere in any way with his efforts to cough out a swallowed object.

1. *Backblows.* If the victim cannot breathe and is standing or sitting, stand behind and slightly to one side of him and support his chest with one hand. With the heel of the other hand give four quick, very forceful blows on the back between the shoulder blades. If he is lying down, kneel beside him and roll him onto his side so that he is facing you. Place his chest against your knees for support. With the heel of your hand give four quick, very forceful blows on the victim's back between the shoulder blades.

2. *Abdominal Thrusts (Heimlich Maneuver).* If backblows do not dislodge the object and the victim is sitting or sitting, stand behind him with your arms around his waist. (Figure 5-7). Place your fist with the thumb side against his stomach slightly above the navel and below the ribs and breastbone. Hold your fist with your other hand and give four quick, very forceful upward thrusts. This maneuver increases pressure in the abdomen that pushes up the diaphragm. This, in turn, increases the air pressure in the lungs to force out the object. Do not squeeze with your arms, just use your fists. If the victim is lying down, turn him on his back (Figure 5-8). Kneel astride him and put the heel of one hand on the victim's stomach slightly above the navel and below the ribs. Keep your elbows straight. Put your free hand on top of the other to provide additional force. Give four quick, very forceful downward and forward thrusts toward the head in an attempt to dislodge the object. If this gives no results, repeat the back blows and/or the upward abdominal thrusts until the victim coughs up the object or becomes unconscious. Look to see if the object appears in the victim's mouth or top of his throat. Use your fingers to pull it out.

If the choking victim becomes unconscious:

1. Give four quick, very forceful *back blows* between the shoulder blades.

2. If unsuccessful, give four quick, very forceful upward *abdominal thrusts* IN ANY POSITION. IF THESE PROCEDURES FAIL, grab the victim's lower jaw and tongue with one hand and lift up to remove the tongue from the back of the throat. Place the index finger of the other hand inside the victim's mouth alongside the cheek. Slide your fingers down into the throat to the base of the victim's tongue. Carefully sweep your fingers along the back of the throat to dislodge the object. Bring your fingers out along the inside of the other cheek. Be careful not to push the object further down the victim's throat. Do not attempt to remove the foreign object with any type of instrument or forceps. REPEAT ALL OF THE ABOVE STEPS UNIL THE OBJECT IS DISLODGED OR MEDICAL ASSISTANCE ARRIVES. DO NOT GIVE UP!

If the victim is an infant or small child: Place the infant or small child across your forearm or lap with his head low and his face down.

1. *Back blows* (not recommended by Dr. Heimlich). Give four quick blows with the heel of your hand on the child's back between his shoulder blades. Blows should be more gentle than those for an adult.

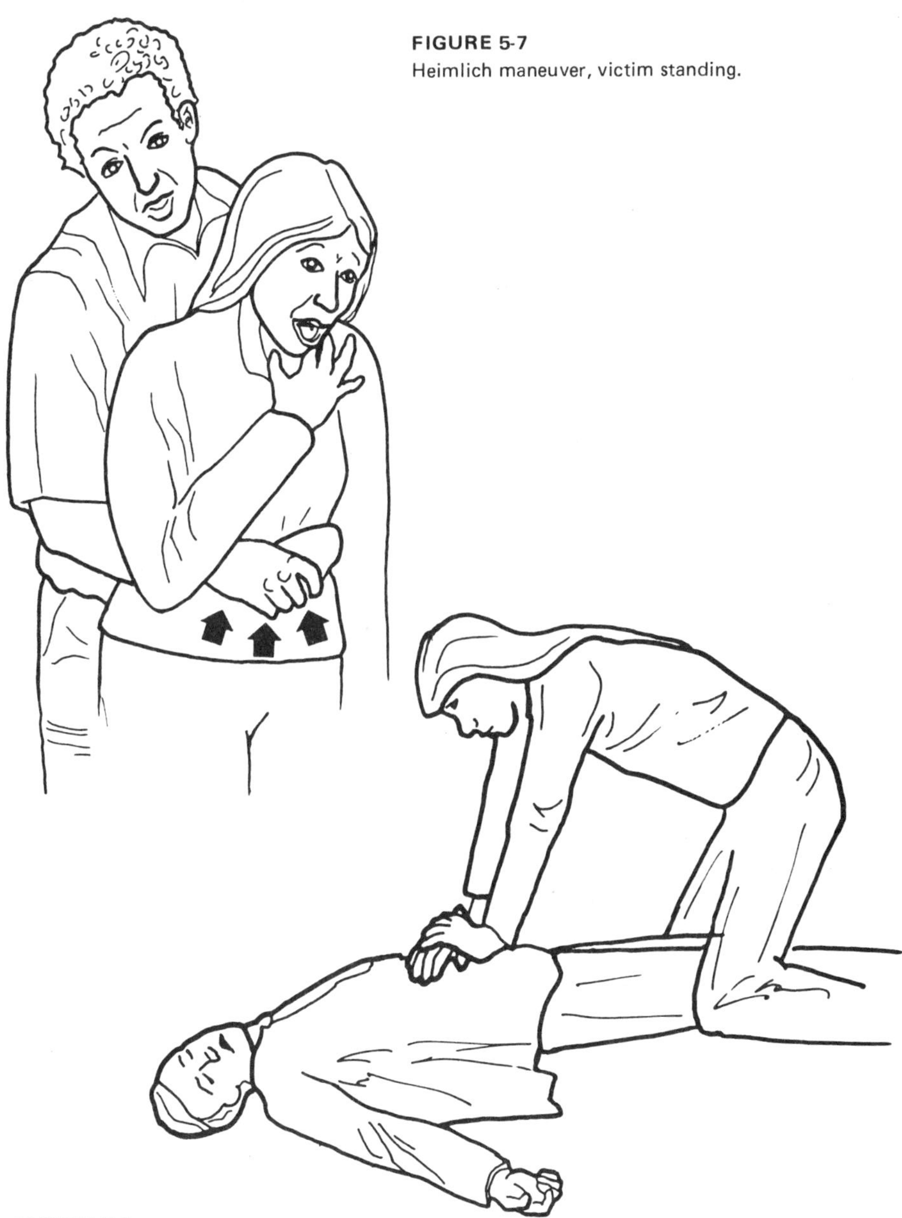

FIGURE 5-7
Heimlich maneuver, victim standing.

FIGURE 5-8
Heimlich maneuver, victim supine.

2. *Abdominal thrusts* (Figure 5-9) If unsuccessful, turn child over onto his back and give four quick abdominal thrusts. Thrusts should be more gentle than those for an adult. In contrast to adult abdominal thrusts, rescuer should place index and middle fingers of both hands on child's abdomen, above navel and below rib cage. The rescuer presses into abdomen with a quick, upward thrust. Repeat thrusts may be necessary to expel the swallowed object.

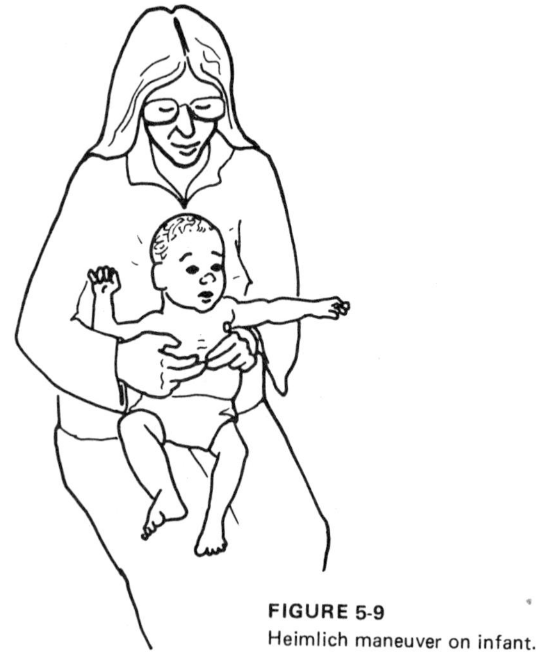

FIGURE 5-9
Heimlich maneuver on infant.

If the victim is very fat or pregnant:

1. *BACK BLOWS:* Apply four quick back blows as described earlier.

2. *ABDOMINAL THRUSTS:* Place your fist and your other hand up the middle of the breastbone in the chest (not over the ribs) and give four quick, forceful movements. These are chest thrusts and vary slightly from the abdominal thrusts used in other victims, principally in location of the hands. Do not squeeze with your arms. Use your fists.

If you are alone and choking and cannot speak or breathe, only abdominal thrusts will save your life! Place your fist and other hand into your abdomen slightly above your navel and below your ribs. Give yourself four quick, very forceful upward abdominal thrusts. Pressing your abdomen forcefully over a chair, table, sink, or railing may also be helpful (Figure 5-10).

To summarize, the official (AMA, AHA) sequences are listed below (from *Journal of the American Medical Association*, August 1, 1980, page 466, by permission). In addition, the American Heart Association distributes a convenient wallet card (Figure 5-11) outlining what to do for the choking victim who is either conscious, or who becomes unconscious.

1. *For the conscious choking victim:*
   a. Identify complete airway obstruction (ask victim if he is able to speak).
   b. Apply four back blows in rapid succession.
   c. Apply four manual abdominal thrusts.
   d. Repeat four back blows and four manual abdominal thrusts until they are effective or until the victim becomes unconscious.

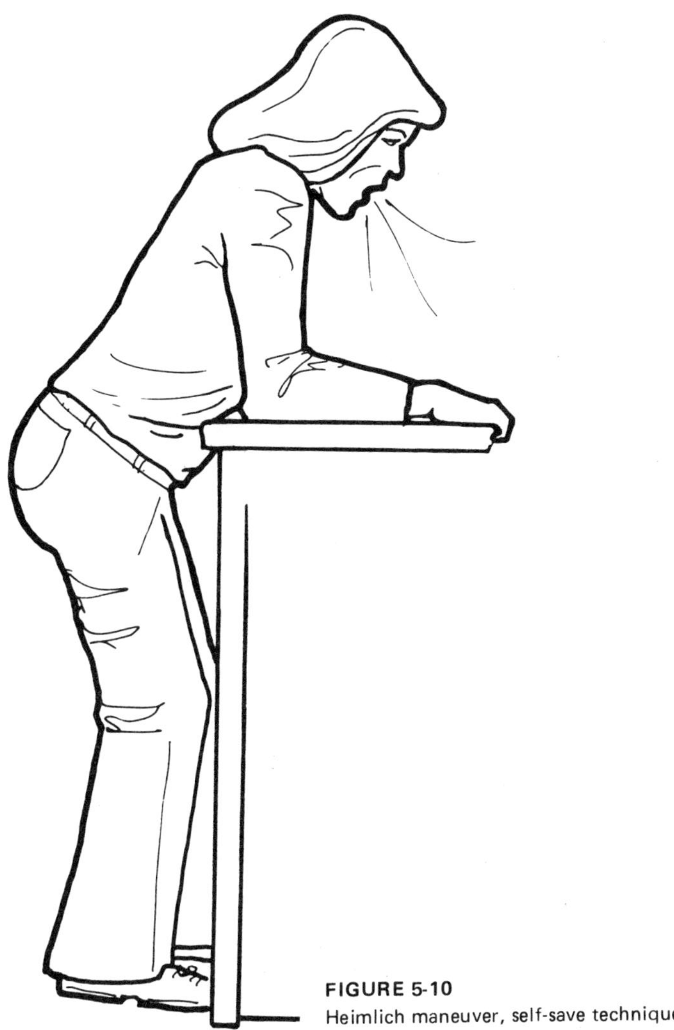

FIGURE 5-10
Heimlich maneuver, self-save technique.

2. *For the choking victim who becomes unconscious:*
The rescuer should call for help, open the airway, and attempt to ventilate. If he is unsuccessful at ventilation, he should quickly perform the following:
   a. If a second person is available, he should activate the EMS (emergency medical service) system.
   b. Apply four back blows in rapid succession.
   c. Apply four manual abdominal thrusts.
   d. Apply the finger sweep. Dentures may need to be removed to improve the finger sweep.
   e. Reposition the head, open the airway, and attempt to ventilate. If the victim cannot be ventilated,
   f. Repeat steps b, c, and d.

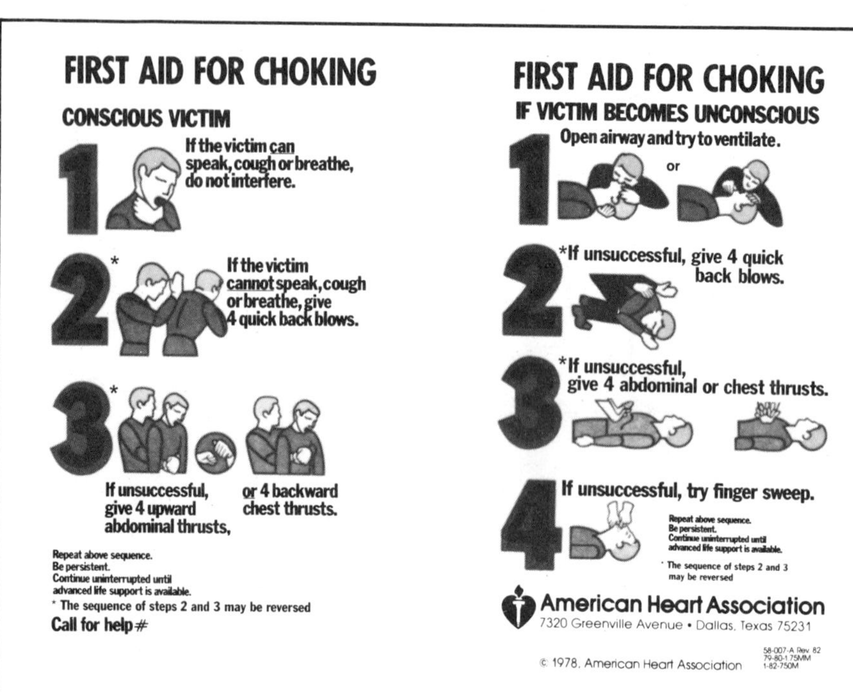

FIGURE 5-11 First aid for choking. (Reproduced with permission, American Heart Association.)

HOW CAN I DETECT CARBON MONOXIDE POISONING?

Carbon monoxide (CO), a colorless, odorless gas that is a product of combustion, is given off in all cigarette smoke, fires, automobile exhaust, and furnaces that burn solid or liquid fuels. When products of combustion are adequately ventilated into the atmosphere no buildup of carbon monoxide occurs and there is no danger. The problem of CO intoxication comes with inadequate ventilation.

CO is poisonous because it combines avidly with hemoglobin in our red blood cells, displacing oxygen. CO combines with hemoglobin 200 times stronger than does oxygen! For this reason even relatively little buildup of CO in the air can be fatal.

Many deaths occur each year from CO inhalation. While this is also a form of suicide, most deaths are from unintentionally inhaling faulty exhaust of combustion products. Proof of CO poisoning requires measuring the gas in the blood of poisoned individuals. Chronic CO poisoning (from a low level of CO in the air) can lead to a variety of non-specific symptoms often attributed to other causes, including psychosomatic. If CO poisoning is not considered, it will be missed; continued exposure may be fatal.

Common symptoms of CO intoxication include headache, sore throat, dizziness, nausea, and ringing in the ears. Unexplained symptoms should at least raise the suspicion of CO poisoning, especially if there is any possibility of exposure to faulty heating systems or automobile exhaust. Once suspected the level of CO can be measured in the blood. It is a simple test that may prevent needless deaths.

Annie C.—A Case of CO Intoxication

Emergency medical service (EMS) was called to the home of a 72-year-old woman who had been found unresponsive by a neighbor. Arriving within 10 minutes, the EMS medics found her comatose, lying in bed. Although she was breathing and did not appear blue, she responded only to painful stimuli. EMS began oxygen therapy and brought her to the hospital, five minutes away.

In the emergency room physicians confirmed the coma and assessed her breathing as very shallow and her pulse quick and faint. Because of this, four steps were taken simultaneously by the doctors and nurses.

1. endotracheal intubation to secure an airway and to provide artificial ventilation and oxygen therapy;
2. treatment with intravenous glucose to counteract the possibility of very low blood sugar as a cause of her coma;
3. electrocardiogram (EKG) to look for a heart attack or other cardiac problem;
4. arterial blood gas to assess ventilation and oxygenation (See Chapter 8).

The EKG was normal. A few minutes later the arterial blood gas results gave the reason for her coma. Forty percent of her hemoglobin was saturated with carbon monoxide—she was the victim of acute CO poisoning.

With artificial ventilation and continuous supplemental oxygen she slowly improved over the next 36 hours. By this time the level of CO in her blood was down to eight percent and she was waking up. After 48 hours she could safely breathe on her own, and the endotracheal tube was removed. Two days later she was improved sufficiently to be discharged. (A city inspector had gone to her home and found a faulty space heater that was easily repaired.)

Mrs. C. was fortunate. Another few hours delay in finding her and she would probably have died of acute CO poisoning. When her neighbors were questioned in the hospital, they remembered her complaining of headaches and dizziness and saying that she had planned to see a physician soon. Alertness to the possibility of CO intoxication could have prevented this near tragedy. People living in old homes with faulty heaters run a particular risk of CO poisoning.

Above all, one has to be suspicious of the possibility of CO poisoning.

The early signs and symptoms are:	HEADACHE CONFUSION DIZZINESS LASSITUDE
The late signs are:	COMA CARDIOVASCULAR COLLAPSE DEATH
The common causes are:	FAULTY HEATERS FAULTY EXHAUST OF COMBUSTION PRODUCTS INCOMPLETE VENTILATION OF AUTOMOBILE EXHAUST

Remember! CO poisoning is preventable.

CHAPTER SIX

Symptoms and Signs of Lung Disease

WHAT ARE THE SIGNS AND SYMPTOMS OF LUNG DISEASE?

First I should clarify the difference between signs and symptoms. *Symptoms* are what bother the patient; they are whatever abnormalities the patient notices, such as chest pain, shortness of breath, or cough. Signs are what the physician sees or observes about the patient, such as blue nailbeds, fast breathing, abnormal sounds heard with the stethoscope, or a temperature of 103°. Signs may also include abnormal chest X-rays and other laboratory findings. We can think of symptoms as the subjective aspect of illness and signs as the objective aspect. Both are important in diagnosing and treating any illness, especially lung disease.

The most common *symptoms* of lung disease are:

- cough
- shortness of breath (either at rest or on exertion), also known as dyspnea
- chest tightness or chest pain
- hemoptysis (coughing up blood, as observed by the patient)
- chills
- noisy breathing (as heard by the patient)

The most common *signs* of lung disease are:

- dyspnea—although as classically defined dyspnea is a symptom, physicians often say a patient looks "dyspneic" when there is noticeable tachypnea, hyperpnea and/or use of accessory muscles. Thus, the term dyspnea may be used as a sign or symptom.
- tachypnea (breathing faster than normal)
- hyperpnea (taking deeper breaths than normal)
- using accessory muscles of respiration (neck muscles to help in breathing)
- hemoptysis (coughing up blood, as observed by the physician)
- using pursed lip breathing (narrowing mouth by pursing lips to aid in exhalation)
- cyanosis (blue color of skin from low oxygen in the blood)
- noisy breath sounds (as heard with a stethoscope)
- fever
- confusion, combativeness, lethargy (may result from oxygen lack)

DO THESE SIGNS AND SYMPTOMS ALWAYS MEAN LUNG DISEASE?

Definitely not. These signs and symptoms are non-specific; they may indicate lung disease, disease in other organs, or *no* disease. For example, shortness of breath may occur due to anemia (low blood count), heart disease, or even pregnancy, to name a few non-respiratory causes. Cough could be due to a simple cold and be of no consequence, or could be the first symptom of lung cancer. Hemoptysis, always a frightening symptom, could be from a bleeding nose or tooth; more commonly it is due to lung disease, but patients with some types of heart disease can also cough up blood. Chest pain could of course be cardiac in origin, but many times chest pain is due to indigestion or even muscle spasm of the chest cage.

Signs are also non-specific. Tachypnea and hyperpnea are present in every healthy person who exercises vigorously. When present in a resting individual they may be related to heart or lung disease, or less commonly to disease elsewhere. Finally, an abnormal chest X-ray (a spot or mass in the lung; fluid in or around the lungs) could be from a benign condition or from something serious, such as lung cancer.

Because of this non-specificity of signs and symptoms, each patient must be evaluated in view of the entire clinical picture. Given the presence of a bothersome symptom or abnormal sign, there is simply no substitute for a good clinical evaluation by an interested, competent physician.

WHEN SHOULD I BE WORRIED ABOUT SYMPTOMS OF RESPIRATORY DISEASE?

Most symptoms of benign respiratory disease are self-limiting, that is, they last no more than a few days and then go away. (See also Chapter 18 on flu and the common cold.)

Symptoms lasting longer than a few days should probably be investigated, especially if they limit you in any way. Certain symptoms should be investigated immediately. These include:

- Severe or crushing chest pain. This may reflect a heart attack or other serious problem.
- Gross hemoptysis. This is more than simple blood-streaking of sputum; it means coughing up at least a teaspoon of bright red blood.
- Sudden shortness of breath at rest. This may be due to sudden development, or worsening, of heart or lung failure.
- Sudden deterioration of mental status. Although this is usually not due to respiratory causes, it may be from changes in O_2 or CO_2 tension, and demands immediate evaluation.
- Any symptom accompanied by incapacitating apprehension. This is another way of saying that if a symptom bothers you to the point you cannot function from worrying about it, you should probably have it investigated immediately. Your apprehension may be warranted.

WHAT CAUSES COUGH?

We all cough at times. It is a natural and normal protective mechanism to clear our airways of particulate matter that doesn't belong there. Cough is due to irritation of the airway lining by something, usually mucus, dust, secretions, or blood. The underlying condition may range from a simple cold or a mild asthma attack to heart failure or lung cancer.

When a cough lasts only a few minutes we think no more about it. However, many times, particularly after a cold or virus infection, the cough persists. Because it is so commonly associated with colds and upper respiratory infections, coughing is one of the most frequent respiratory complaints. Whenever a cough is associated with high fever, shortness of breath, production of foul smelling sputum, or severe chest pain, it should be evaluated by a physician. These all point to potentially serious but treatable causes. Beyond these associated symptoms, it is convenient to discuss the symptom of cough based on its time span.

Acute Cough Lasts only a few minutes; it is a universal experience and is a normal protective mechanism.

Cough of Short Duration This is a self-limited cough lasting less than three weeks, usually due to colds or upper respiratory infections. It may also be due to asthma, bacterial infections, or limited exposure to noxious material.

Chronic Cough Lasts longer than three weeks; this is a time beyond which a cough can no longer be simply attributed to colds or viral infections.

MOST COMMON CAUSES OF A CHRONIC COUGH
Cigarette smoking
Chronic bronchitis
Emphysema
Asthma

Lung cancer
Chronic post-nasal drip due to sinusitis or allergy
Tuberculosis
Chronic viral infection of the airways

WHAT IS HEMOPTYSIS?

Hemoptysis is the coughing up of blood. Many physicians distinguish between blood streaking and gross hemoptysis. In the former a few streaks of blood can be seen in a sea of otherwise whitish or grayish mucus; it is a common (but not to be ignored) finding in chronic bronchitis and in protracted coughs from any reason. Gross hemoptysis is when the majority of what is coughed up is blood. Although this may also be found in patients with chronic bronchitis, it usually demands a thorough evaluation for lung cancer or other serious illnesses.

MAJOR CAUSES OF HEMOPTYSIS

Bronchiectasis (chronic infection of the airways that leads to weak and dilated bronchial tubes)
Tuberculosis
Lung cancer
Pulmonary embolism
Pneumonia
Some forms of heart disease
Blood arising from anywhere in the mouth or nose
Chronic bronchitis (chronic inflammation of the airways associated with chronic cough)

WHAT IS THE BEST TREATMENT FOR A COUGH?

For a cough of short duration the best treatment is no treatment. Most cough medicines are really expectorants, designed to help you mobilize secretions, not prevent the cough. Although many times it may be helpful to give an expectorant, this cannot be considered "treating the cough." True cough suppressants, such as codeine, are related to narcotics and potentially harmful if they suppress the coughing of mucus or other irritating material. If a cough is truly non-productive of mucus and suppression is desired, one of the many codeine-containing compounds may be tried for a short period of time.

When a cough is due to a limited condition such as a cold, it will disappear when the patient improves. A chronic cough demands investigation for the underlying cause that, if found and treated, will also do away with the cough. If a thorough investigation does not reveal a specific cause, a trial of bronchodilators and/or corticosteroids may be helpful (see Chapter 11). However, it cannot be overemphasized that treatment of a chronic cough is not the same as treating the underlying condition. *Cough is a symptom and not a disease: treating only the symptom may miss the disease.*

WHAT CAUSES SHORTNESS OF BREATH?

"Shortness of breath" is perhaps the most common respiratory complaint. Other phrases used by patients to explain the sensation are: "I can't catch my breath"; "my chest is tight"; "I can't get all the air in (or out.)" The medical term used for all such cases is *dyspnea*, which means difficult breathing.

Dyspnea may occur at rest or with exertion, the latter being more common. Dyspnea at rest is a serious symptom, deserving full evaluation. Such patients are usually incapacitated with the slightest exertion.

The most common causes of dyspnea are heart and respiratory disease. Because dyspnea is a symptom and therefore subjective (what the patient feels), it is difficult to predict which patients will have dyspnea even though their disease is well characterized. For example, two patients the same age and with identical respiratory impairment can have varying complaints of dypsnea. This may be because of different degrees of body conditioning, body weight, lifestyles (one sedentary, one active), amount of blood cells, and a host of other factors.

Another common cause of dyspnea is psychological. So-called psychogenic dyspnea is present when a patient has a consistent complaint of dyspnea but careful testing and examination reveal no physical reason. Such patients often breathe with frequent, deep sighs. Another clue to the diagnosis of psychogenic dyspnea is its presence only on rest and disappearance on exercise. This confirms the lack of significant heart or lung disease.

WHAT IS THE HYPERVENTILATION SYNDROME?

This is a condition of "over-breathing" due to psychological or anxiety-related factors. Patients with hyperventilation frequently (but not necessarily) complain of dyspnea. They also report numbness and tingling around the mouth, in the fingers and toes. This sensation is due to "blowing off" excess carbon dioxide (CO_2), making the blood too alkaline.

In severe, acute situations the excess alkali in the blood can lead to tetany, a drawing up of the hands and feet. Acute hyperventilation syndrome can be treated by having the patient re-breathe from a paper bag placed over the face. This allows re-breathing of exhaled CO_2 and helps establish normal acidity to the blood.

Hyperventilation syndrome is most commonly found in young people, both men and women. Reproducing the symptoms by having the patient take deep breaths helps establish the diagnosis. Psychotherapy may occasionally be indicated for recurring episodes or when the problem interferes with normal lifestyle.

WHAT CAUSES CHEST PAIN?

After coughing and dyspnea, chest pain is the next most common symptom of respiratory disease. Since chest pain is also the most common complaint of patients with coronary artery disease (hardening of the arteries supplying blood to the heart, the cause of most heart attacks), the symptom is frequently a serious diagnostic challenge. Certain characteristics of the pain may help separate a respiratory from a cardiac condition or point to some other cause.

Crushing chest pain is sometimes also described as the squeezing of the chest as if it were in a vise, or as if an elephant were standing on the chest. This type of pain is usually cardiac in origin, often the first symptom of a heart attack, and demands immediate evaluation.

Sharp chest pain made worse on inspiration is called pleuritic chest pain and is usually respiratory in origin since it arises from inflammation of the pleural membranes surrounding the lungs. Many conditions can cause this including pneumonia, pulmonary embolism (blood clots in the lungs), and pleurodynia (viral infection of the pleural membranes).

Chest pain that occurs with eating may be cardiac or gastrointestinal in origin; pain that occurs mainly on recumbency is usually related to the stomach and digestive system; this type of pain represents a form of indigestion.

Pain and tenderness to touch of some area of the chest is usually due to inflammation of the bones, joints or muscles of the chest wall and not to lung or heart disease.

There may be many atypical manifestations of chest pain as well as overlap of symptoms when more than one condition is present. Although diagnosing the cause of pain usually requires some laboratory tests, these may be no more complicated than a chest X-ray and electrocardiogram. Chest pain should be investigated if it is severe enough to limit your activities or to cause apprehension and worry.

WHAT ARE UPPER RESPIRATORY SYMPTOMS?

These are symptoms usually found in patients with infection of the upper respiratory system. From a practical standpoint respiratory infections can be divided into those predominantly affecting either the upper respiratory or lower respiratory tract. The upper respiratory tract includes the trachea (windpipe in the neck) and all respiratory passages above; the lower respiratory tract includes all respiratory passages below the trachea, i.e. airways within both lungs.

Upper respiratory infection (URI) symptoms can usually be distinguished from lower respiratory ones. URI symptoms include one or more of the following: cough, runny nose, runny eyes, sore throat, laryngitis, headache, sinus tenderness, and post-nasal drip. Most URI's are viral in origin and therefore self-limiting. Any sputum (phlegm) expectorated in these infections is usually white and not foul smelling.

In contrast, lower respiratory tract infections—the most common of which are bronchitis and pneumonia—may be manifested by cough, chest pain, shortness of breath, and expectoration of dark and/or foul smelling sputum, occasionally blood-tinged. Lower tract infections may also be viral in origin but are commonly caused by bacteria and therefore amenable to antibiotic treatment.

WHAT ARE SOME COMMON SIGNS OF RESPIRATORY DISEASE?

Physicians usually have no trouble recognizing patients in respiratory distress. This is because certain signs point to difficult breathing, although they may not reveal the specific cause. Tachypnea (rapid breathing) and breathing with the aid of one's neck muscles are the most frequently observed signs of dyspnea.

Other signs that patients indicate may be in respiratory distress include sweating, blue discoloration to the skin, nails, and/or lips (cyanosis), and mental changes such as confusion. Patients with severe asthma or bronchitis may breathe so nosily they can be heard from across the room. Of course with a stethoscope physicians can hear many abnormal breath sounds not otherwise audible.

WHAT IS FLUID IN THE LUNGS?

"Fluid in (or around) the lungs" is a frequently used explanation given to patients manifesting a variety of different respiratory conditions. This fluid can be seen on chest X-ray, and may be within the lung alveoli or surrounding the lungs (in which case it is actually outside the lungs, between them and the chest wall). Some patients may have fluid in both places.

When fluid builds up in the alveolar spaces it is called pulmonary edema (see Chapter 17). When it builds up around the lungs it is called a pleural effusion, because the pleura are the thin membranes surrounding the lungs (see Chapter 14).

The most common cause for fluid *in* (pulmonary edema) or *around* (pleural effusion) the lungs is congestive heart failure (CHF). Congestive is a good term, because that is just what the lungs become–congested, or backed up with fluid. The cause is a weak and therefore failing heart. Treatment with medication to remove the fluid (diuretics, digitalis) is often beneficial and can relieve the accompanying dyspnea. Another sign of congestive heart failure is swollen ankles and legs (but not all swollen feet are due to CHF).

There are many other causes for fluid in or around the lungs, some of which are discussed in other parts of the book (see Index).

WHAT IS A SPOT IN THE LUNGS?

A spot in the lung usually refers to a small, discrete, rounded nodule visible on a routine chest X-ray. Spots may range in size from that of a dime to a silver dollar; because their shape is rounded they are often referred to as coin nodules. Coin nodules are never a normal finding, although they may be benign or malignant.

Benign *lesions* (another word for abnormal spots or coin nodules) are usually due to old infections that have healed to form a scar. Malignant lesions are usually due to lung cancer or cancer that has spread from elsewhere in the body to the lungs. Utilizing only the routine chest X-ray it is seldom possible to differentiate between benign and malignant lesions. This difference is critical since a malignancy (cancer) may be in its early stages and amenable to surgery. Conversely, a benign lesion usually warrants no treatment and will not affect the patient's life. What to do after finding a coin nodule on chest X-ray depends on the patient's age, smoking history, availability of old X-rays, and a host of other factors.

A lung *infiltrate* is an abnormality on chest X-ray larger than a coin lesion or spot. It is also non-specific and may be due to a variety of causes: pneumonia, partial lung collapse, cancer, tuberculosis, and pulmonary blood clots are common examples. The X-ray appearance of these terms is shown in Chapter 8.

CHAPTER SEVEN

How to Find a Doctor and Choose a Hospital

WHAT TYPE OF PHYSICIAN SHOULD I LOOK FOR?

An estimated 65 percent of all Americans have a personal physician, someone who knows their medical history and can be called on for medical care if the need arises. This section will be of particular interest to the large minority who have no such physician as well as those who, for whatever reason, need or wish to change doctors.

When seeing a doctor for general medical purposes you should look for a primary care physician. This is someone able and willing to give primary (first) care for your medical problem, follow you if the problem is within the scope of his or her practice, and refer you if necessary to a competent specialist.

In the United States four large groups are recognized as primary care physicians: general internists, general pediatricians, family and general practitioners, and obstetricians/gynecologists. They all have the M.D. (Doctor of Medicine) or D.O. (Doctor of Osteopathy) degree and, with one exception, two or more years of training after medical school. The older group of general practitioners has been superseded by a new medical specialty, Family Practice. The requirement to become a GP had been only one year of post-graduate training, now considered an unacceptable length of time for training new physicians; hence GP's are the only primary care group whose numbers are declining. With the exception of GP's, each primary care group is considered a specialty area of medical practice and is thus covered by a separate certification board. In each instance becoming board certified requires both a minimal amount of formal training after medical school plus a passing score on a rigorous written examination.

General Internists

This is the largest group of primary care physicians. Internal medicine training emphasizes diagnosis and treatment of adult, non-surgical diseases. General internists are concentrated mainly in urban and metropolitan areas; relatively few practice in rural areas. Their specialty board is the American Board of Internal Medicine and the minimum requirement for taking the exam is three years of hospital training in internal medicine after graduation from medical school; at least two of these years must be in the United States.

In addition to the general internists there are over 20,000 *subspecialists* in internal medicine, including those trained in heart disease, pulmonary disease, allergy, gastroenterology, kidney disease, and so forth. Subspecialty training is generally two years following general internal medicine training, so each subspecialist is, in effect, a general internist first. Certification boards for each subspecialty require not only the requisite subspecialty training but prior certification in General Internal Medicine.

After subspecialty training many physicians concentrate on their relatively narrow subspecialty area. However, many of these doctors also render primary care for patients whose major problem is in their area (for example, a patient with chronic heart disease may receive his primary care from a fully trained cardiologist). Some subspecialists (the percentage is not known) choose to practice their subspecialty *plus general internal medicine.* Subspecialists generally state their interests and limitations in the phone book or in official announcements ("practice limited to . . .").

Although the array of specialists and subspecialists may seem bewildering (other specialty areas besides general internal medicine also have recognized subspecialties) it is mainly important for you to know that your physician is willing and able to render primary care—be responsible for problems as they arise, treat when possible, and refer when necessary.

General Pediatricians

This group of doctors has training similar to the internists except for the age of their patients. Pediatricians usually do not follow patients past the 21st birthday nor accept new patients past adolescence. Like internists they practice mainly in urban and metropolitan areas. There are recognized pediatric subspecialty areas analogous to internal medicine, but the total number of such physicians in relation to the general pediatric group is far less than for internal medicine. Thus, in seeking a pediatrician you are less likely to encounter one whose practice is limited to a narrow area of pediatrics.

Family Practitioners

This is a relatively new speciality group that has replaced the older general practitioners in name and concept. FP's have their own specialty board and require a minimum of three years post-graduate training. In contrast to pediatrics and internal medicine, FP training includes a combination of internal medicine, pediatrics, obstetrics, gynecology, and surgery. FP's tend to practice in smaller cities and rural areas where they render primary care for people of all ages, do uncomplicated obstetrics, and perhaps assist in some surgery. FP's are not trained to do major surgery.

Obstetricians/Gynecologists

This large group has training in both obstetrics and gynecology—hence, they are physicians for women only. Many women have only an OB-GYN doctor as a primary physician, and many of these physicians recognize themselves as primary care providers for their patients, particularly women of child-bearing age. Generally, the older a woman becomes, the more likely a general internist will be called on to render primary care.

HOW CAN I FIND THE NAMES OF SPECIFIC DOCTORS?

There are at least four resources you can use to find names of physicians:

1. *Friends and relatives.* Perhaps the most common referral source is someone you know who has used and been satisfied with a particular physician. Sometimes these physicians are too busy to accept new patients, but if you call they may recommend a new partner in their practice.
2. *Referral from another physician.* In many instances one physician you know, perhaps a specialist, will refer you to a primary care physician. Physician referral may also occur when you move from one city to another, when your physician is retiring or moving, or when you know a physician on a social or family basis. Referral from another physician helps to assure an appointment.
3. *Call to your local medical society.* This will usually elicit the names of doctors willing to take on new patients. Many of these physicians are relatively new in practice, but nonetheless should be fully trained and eager to see you.
4. *Look up the names yourself.* There are two sources of information available in general medical and large public libraries:

   The *AMA Directory of Physicians* publishes the name, age, practice pattern, and address of every living physician who graduated from an accredited medical school (including foreign); its several volumes lists physicians by state and city as well as alphabetically.

   The *Directory of Medical Specialists* publishes the name of every living physician who has passed one of the recognized American Specialty Boards (such as the American Board of Internal Medicine), and lists the training background of each physician. There are 23 such boards, and this directory lists over 20,000 doctors by geographic location and alphabetically. You can look up the names of physicians practicing in your area, picking out those who are close to where you live and are of an age acceptable to you (some patients prefer older, some prefer younger, physicians).

SHOULD ONE SEE A PULMONARY SUBSPECIALIST FOR PROBLEMS DISCUSSED IN THIS BOOK?

There are an estimated 3,000 internal medicine physicians in the United States who are certified as pulmonary disease subspecialists. Although all should be competent to diagnose and manage any of the problems discussed in this book (excluding those requiring surgery), it is not necessary nor desirable for respiratory patients to seek out only a subspecialist for care.

From a purely practical standpoint this is not possible. Millions of people in this country suffer from acute and chronic respiratory disorders (an estimated eight to nine million with chronic obstructive lung disease alone). There is no way this large group could receive ongoing care from only pulmonary subspecialists.

In fact general internal medicine and family practitioners are trained to take care of common respiratory problems such as bronchitis, emphysema, asthma, pneumonia, and influenza. They are also trained to manage heart disease, arthritis, gastrointestinal disorders, and a host of other common conditions–in short, to take care of the entire patient, not just one organ system. Generally, when a patient's problem is severe or intractable, or presents a diagnostic puzzle, a subspecialist might be called in. However, this is also true for pulmonary and other subspecialists who practice some general internal medicine and encounter an unfamiliar problem. In summary, a pulmonary subspecialist is not necessary for primary care of most respiratory problems.

WHAT CRITERIA SHOULD I USE IN CHOOSING A PHYSICIAN?

Finding a physician right for you can be one of your most important moves, and the time to do it is when you are healthy or have only a minor problem, not when you are very sick. By then the selection process is rushed and you may be desperate. Although choosing a physician can be frustrating and time consuming (especially when your initial choice is not a good one), the United States fortunately has the greatest concentration of well-trained doctors in the world.

Obviously finding a physician is not as difficult as finding the right one for you (except in some rural areas where there may be no doctor for miles). The actual choice will in many cases depend on proximity to a medical building or hospital, practice patterns in your community, social and economic preference, and family recommendations. When you do have a choice to make, or want guidelines in choosing a physician, I recommend you pay particular attention to five characteristics: competence, availability, affiliation, concern, and compatibility.

Competence

Your state assures that each physician has a minimal level of competence merely by issuing a license to practice medicine. Until recently this license meant only that the physician graduated from an accredited medical school and was not a convicted felon or known drug addict when the license was granted. Now many states are requiring proof of Continuing Medical Education (CME) as a requirement for license renewal (every two or three years). However, these credits are easily obtained by attending a variety of medical conferences, the quality and learning value of which vary widely. Thus, since a license is held by every legally practicing physician, it can only serve to eliminate fraud, not guarantee competence.

Three aspects of an individual physician may help assure competence: board certification, academic affiliation, and reputation.

Physicians certified by their specialty board have achieved a minimal level of knowledge and training in that area (such as Internal Medicine, Pediatrics, Ophthalmology, and so forth) . As a group these individuals have a higher level of competence (as defined by knowledge and training) than those practicing the same field without board certification. Even so, it cannot be overemphasized that there are many highly competent physicians, practicing in all fields, who for one reason or another are not board certified.

A physician who has an academic affiliation with a major teaching hospital or medical school is likely competent in the area he practices. This is because he or she has gone through a screening process and peer review to obtain the affiliation.

Finally, a physician known for being competent or skilled in a particular area likely deserves this reputation.

Competence is only one of five characteristics you should look for. Some highly competent physicians may be bad for you.

Availability

This is the second important characteristic you should consider. It is of little help if your physician is the most competent in the city if he or she is unavailable. At least one book *(The Best Doctors in the U.S.)* contains a list of physicians considered best by their peers, in all fields and in all sections of the country. While this is certainly an exemplary list, many of these physicians are so involved with teaching, research, or academic pursuits that they may not satisfy the availability requirement. For a one-time consultation or procedure it would be hard to improve upon this list. However the best doctor may not be right for you if he or she is not available when you need help.

You need a physician who sees patients, who has an active practice, or is otherwise available most of the time. Such an actively involved physician, when not available, will arrange for adequate coverage of his or her patients.

Affiliation

This refers to the hospital where your physician has admitting privileges and where you will be hospitalized if the need arises. You want to make sure this hospital is one to which you will go if necessary, that it is convenient to your home and family, and that you won't wish you were hospitalized elsewhere once you arrive. Emergencies can necessitate immediate hospitalization, and that is not the time to second guess the institution you are entering. Because the hospital is so important for many patients with serious lung disease, this aspect will be dealt with later in the book.

Concern and Compatability

The above three characteristics can, to some extent, be quantified. The physician's compatibility and concern are something only you can determine. They encompass the bedside manner so often said to be lacking in today's modern medicine. Do you feel comfortable with your physician? Does he take an interest in your problem, talk to you intelligently, and answer your questions honestly? Or does he lack empathy, talk down to you, and give only perfunctory answers? You can have the most competent, available, and well-affiliated doctor, but if he doesn't care about you or if you and he are not compatible, it can adversely affect your illness. *Concern* and *compatibility,* although highly subjective, are every bit as important as all the objective aspects.

WHAT ABOUT HEALTH MAINTENANCE ORGANIZATIONS?

Health maintenance organizations (HMO's) provide medical care to millions of Americans. They are essentially prepaid group plans, the largest and best known of which is the Kaiser Permanente plan based in California.

Physicians in HMO's are usually salaried and do not send bills for services rendered. They have the same skills and training, on average, as physicians not in HMO's. The principal differences for the patient are: 1. pre-payment of a fixed charge for all subsequent medical care, and 2. not having a single "private" physician responsible for primary care. In essence the patient must decide on joining or not joining an HMO (and if so, which one), with choice of physician then limited to those practicing within the HMO.

Even in HMO's, however, patients can usually choose or change physicians, especially in larger organizations. For this reason, the previous discussion of what to look for in a physician is equally relevant if you choose your care with an HMO, a solo private physician, or any other plan.

WHAT TYPES OF HOSPITALS ARE THERE?

There are 6,933 hospitals in the United States (based on the 1981 American Hospital Association Annual Survey), ranking in size from fewer than 25 beds to over 1,000 beds. Most are accredited by the Joint Commission on Accreditation of Hospitals (JCAH). This accreditation assures a minimal standard that often has more to do with building codes and medical record keeping than with quality of patient care. This is not because JCAH is uninterested in patient care, but because patient care is difficult or impossible to assess in the limited time JCAH has to review each hospital. Although hospitals are categorized in several ways, one major distinction is between *teaching* and *non-teaching* hospitals.

A teaching hospital is one that trains post-graduate M.D.'s and D.O.'s (called residents) in the various medical specialties (internal medicine, pediatrics, surgery, obstetrics-gynecology, radiology, pathology, anesthesiology, and psychiatry are the most common). Not all teaching hospitals train in all areas, but most classified as such have at least programs in internal medicine and surgery. These hospitals tend to be larger than non-teaching hospitals and offer a wider range of medical and non-medical services.

Almost all teaching hospitals are affiliated with one of the nation's 126 medical schools.

In 1979 there were 968 hospitals with approved residencies, 792 of which had medical school affiliations. The care of indigent patients, especially in urban areas, is almost exclusively done in teaching hospitals. Finally, most hospital-based research is done in these institutions.

The bulk of hospitals in this country are non-teaching. They have no training program for medical residents, although many have programs for training nurses and various paramedical personnel such as respiratory technicians. Generally, non-teaching hospitals are not affiliated with medical schools.

WHICH TYPE OF HOSPITAL OFFERS BETTER CARE?

Contrary to opinion held by many academic health professionals, you do not necessarily receive better care in a teaching hospital. The care for a given patient may be excellent, in all aspects, in many non-teaching hospitals. People who are steadfast in their bias against all non-teaching hospitals do not understand the nature and variety of human illness nor the workings of a modern hospital.

Quality of patient care, except from a strict medical standpoint, is highly subjective and difficult (if not impossible) to assess. It is common knowledge among physicians that patients can receive topflight medical care yet complain bitterly about the unresponsiveness of nurses, the poor quality of food, the noise in the halls, and the rudeness of one or two overworked technicians. Such patients may perceive their care as bad although an audit of their hospital record could reveal superb medical care. Which is correct? Conversely some patients can receive a totally bungled medical workup, with all the wrong tests ordered and medication given, yet possibly perceive their care as good because of the sensitivity of their doctor, and the quality of ancillary services.

Thus there are two major aspects of hospital care. The first is strictly medical (or surgical) and involves the scientific application of modern knowledge to the patient's problem. Although many aspects of modern medical care are subject to some controversy, such care is still quantifiable and assessable. There is a definite body of knowledge about what to do for many common conditions; in fact certification boards test for this type of knowledge with written examinations.

The second aspect of hospital care is less objective; it involves the manner in which you are taken care of while hospitalized, how your needs are met, how you are treated as a person, and so forth. The physician obviously plays a major role in this area, as he or she is the one person to whom the patient looks for answers and help. Nurses occupy a critical role as well, since in carrying out physician's orders they have more contact with the patient than any other group. However, not to be underestimated are the important roles of housecleaning and dietary personnel, X-ray and blood-drawing technicians, and a host of other people who daily interact with patients.

In a very general way, it is my opinion that the sicker you are the bettter off you will be in a teaching hospital. By sicker I mean the more you need or are likely to need sophisticated treatment, special diagnostic procedures, consultation by other physicians, ventilator support, long term-oxygen therapy, or long-term intravenous fluids. Teaching hospitals are simply better equipped to provide more sophisticated care and to have available the ready expertise needed for many acute and complicated medical problems.

However, it is also true that many non-teaching hospitals have developed a high level of sophisticated care by attracting to their staffs well-trained specialists who prefer non-teaching hospitals (or prefer practicing in areas that do not happen to have teaching hospitals). In such situations you may receive excellent care for a complicated problem, though of course you are more dependent on well-trained nurses to alert your physician to problems since there may be no resident doctors available. (Some non-teaching hospitals have fully qualified "house doctors" on their staffs; these physicians are employed by the hospital, do not have private patients, and are available for any emergencies that may arise).

In the final analysis the single most important component of good medical care, the one you should be most concerned about, is that you come under the care of a competent physician who is interested in you. The quality, reputation and size of the hospital should come second. A concerned, available, and competent physician will more than compensate for whatever institutional inadequacies exist, and will even transfer you to another hospital if necessary.

CHAPTER EIGHT

Diagnostic Tests and Procedures

SHOULD I HAVE A YEARLY CHEST X-RAY?

There is no simple answer to this question. Until 1980 the recommendation of the American Cancer Society was "yes" in smokers or anyone over age 40. Now the recommendation is "no"; only if you have symptoms (or your physician suspects a problem) is a chest X-ray recommended. The change in recommendation results from many studies, all of which failed to prove the benefit of yearly chest X-rays in any group of people.

Detecting lung cancer in its early stages using currently available techniques does not improve long-term survival for most patients. By the time cancer shows up it is simply too late to be cured in most people. If you smoke you are at increased risk for cancer and yearly X-rays will not protect you. The best protection is to quit smoking, period.

Tuberculosis (TB) is very unusual in asymptomatic patients, so routine chest X-rays are no longer performed for TB. However, the chest X-ray remains invaluable for diagnosing TB in patients who have symptoms. Cough, fever, and weight loss may be due to many diseases besides TB, and a chest X-ray is the surest way to rule out pulmonary tuberculosis.

WHO SHOULD HAVE A CHEST X-RAY?

Any patient who seeks medical care for an acute or chronic pulmonary condition deserves at least one diagnostic chest X-ray. If an X-ray has been recently taken, another may not be necessary, but this should be left to the physician's discretion.

A chest X-ray can uncover many lung diseases such as cancer, pneumonia, tuberculosis, and pneumothorax. The chest X-ray is also important in diseases that don't show up on X-ray—such as bronchitis, asthma, and emphysema—to rule out a complicating lung condition. Thus, a normal X-ray is often reassuring and an abnormal one helpful in diagnosing a patient's condition.

One final note. If you see a doctor because of an upper respiratory problem (such as a cold or sinus condition), not strictly a pulmonary condition, a chest X-ray may not be indicated.

HOW IS A CHEST X-RAY TAKEN?

Figure 8-1a shows a standard "posterior-anterior" chest X-ray from a normal young woman: she is standing erect and her position in relation to the X-ray camera is shown in Figure 8-2. Note that the X-rays penetrate from back to front and the X-ray film is flush against her chest. The resulting X-ray is viewed as if she were facing you so that her right side is on the viewer's left, and vice versa. This is the convention for reading chest X-rays in the United States. It does sometimes confuse patients when a doctor talks about something on the patient's right side and then points to the left side of the film.

The standard front view is technically known as a "PA" view because the X-rays travel from posterior to anterior. Along with this a lateral or side view is usually taken as well.

FIGURE 8-1a Standard "posterior-anterior" chest x-ray of a young, normal woman.

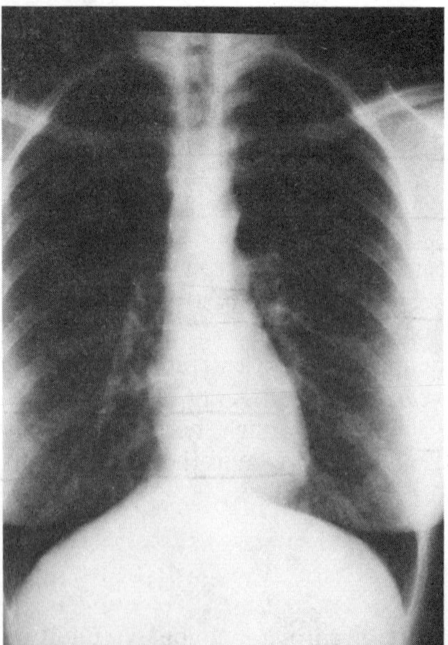

FIGURE 8-1b Schematic outline of the chest x-ray. Note that the subject's "right" is to the reader's left, and vice-versa.

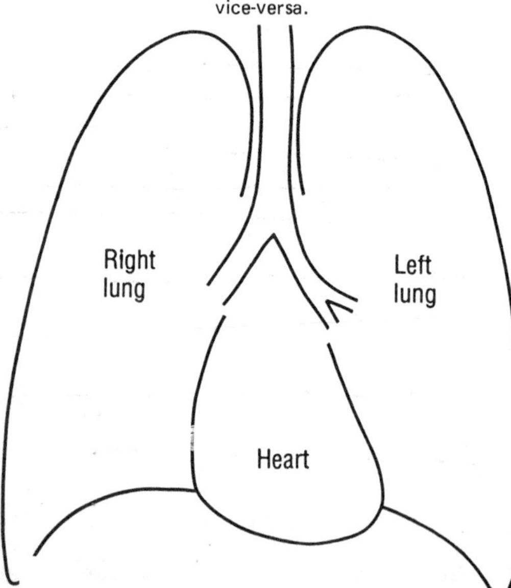

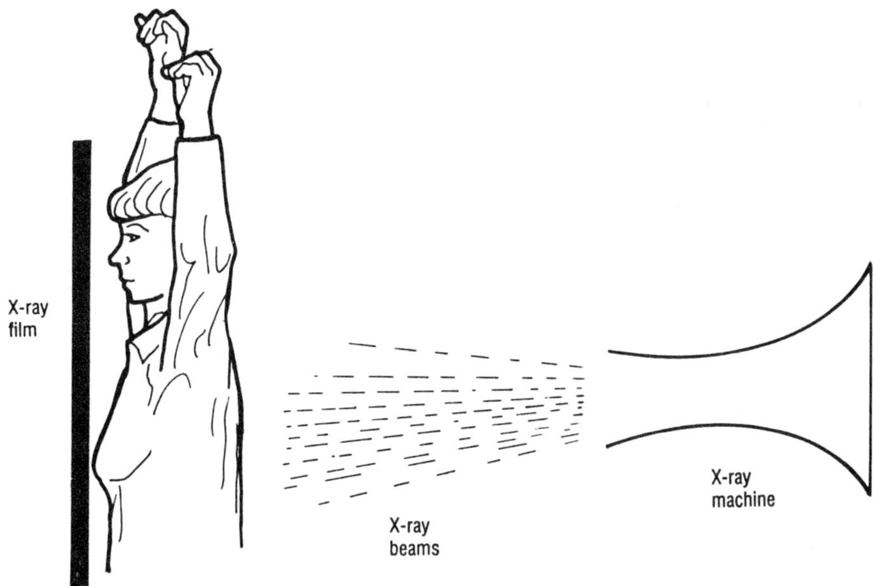

FIGURE 8-2 Schematic diagram of subject having a routine "posterior-anterior" (PA) chest x-ray. She stands facing the x-ray film with arms above her head; the x-ray beams (represented by drawn lines, but actually invisible) enter from the back and travel through the chest to hit the film. When the film is developed, the result is a standard PA view of the lungs and surrounding structures, shown in Figure 8-1a. (For a lateral chest x-ray, the subject would place one side of her chest against the film plate; a routine chest x-ray usually consists of both a PA and lateral view).

Throughout this book a simple schematic diagram will be used to display abnormalities as they might show up on the PA chest X-ray. This schematic, shown in Figure 8-1b, omits the bones, blood vessels and other structures normally visible, and outlines only the major bronchi, lungs and heart. Although greatly simplified, this diagram will be useful to convey an idea of what a physician might see in each of the diseases illustrated.

Several abnormal X-ray signs are also discussed throughout this book, including coin nodule, infiltrate, and fluid around the lungs. These are drawn in Figure 8-3, using the schematic of the PA chest X-ray.

WHAT ABOUT OTHER RADIOLOGIC TESTS?

The Radiology Department of today's hospital is vastly different from that of a generation ago. So many new tests have become available, all in the province of the radiologist, that it is impossible for any one physician to be knowledgeable of them all. Many of these tests have particular relevance to diagnosis of chest diseases and will be discussed here. It is also likely that new ones will appear by the time you read this, such is the pace of radiologic diagnosis.

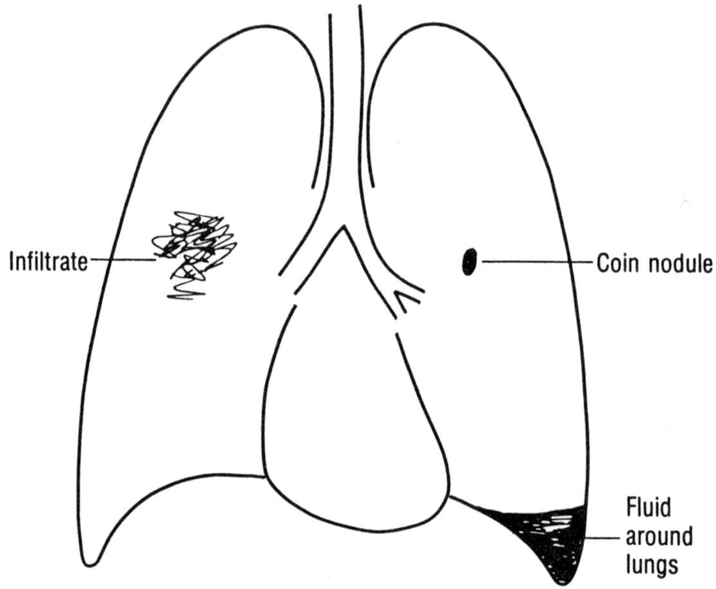

FIGURE 8-3 A few abnormal chest x-ray findings or "signs": inflitrate, "coin" nodule, and fluid.

Tomograms

This test involves multiple X-rays taken at different angles to show up a lesion or spot that doesn't appear well on the conventional chest X-ray. Tomograms, also called laminograms, are ordered less often now that the CAT scan (see below) has become available, though on occasion they are still very useful.

Fluoroscopy

Fluoroscopy is a technique that allows X-ray viewing on a continuous basis. If the regular chest X-ray is thought of as a "snapshot," fluoroscopy is like a movie. This is especially helpful to see if the diaphragms are moving. Because of newer techniques fluoroscopy is ordered relatively little today as an isolated test; however it is used quite frequently during other procedures such as bronchoscopy, needle aspiration, and cardiac catheterization (see below). Fluoroscopy allows the physician to see, via X-ray, the location of the bronchoscope, needle, or catheter in the patient's chest.

CAT Scan

"CAT" stand for "computerized axial tomography." The CAT scanner is a sophisticated machine that can "slice" virtually any area of the body with X-rays, then via the computer reconstruct the various X-ray penetrations into a series of pictures. The thoracic CAT scan, for example, takes a series of slices of the chest cavity and its contents, from the neck to the diaphragm. Each slice shows all the structures through that level, including the lungs, heart, bones, blood vessels, and so forth. Moreover, since the data used for each reconstruction are stored in the computer, the radiologist can order the picture in any contrast desired and determine if a particular shadow is fat, blood, bone, or whatever. The CAT scan has often proven valuable in diagnosing lesions obscure or invisible on a conventional chest X-ray.

Although CAT scans are superb for delineating structures, and even for revealing if the structure is fat, bone, or other tissue, they cannot tell if any abnormal tissue is malignant (cancer). So although an abnormal tissue may presumptively be malignant, definitive diagnosis still requires obtaining a piece of the tissue (biopsy) and examination under the microscope.

WHAT ARE ISOTOPE SCANS?

Isotope scans are obtained when the patient is injected with a radioactive substance and scanned by a machine that picks up the radioactive emissions. There are many types of isotope scans available; the ones most useful for patients with lung disease include:

Lung Scan

This looks at both the *perfusion* and *ventilation* aspects of lung function. For the perfusion lung scan radioactive material, usually the protein albumin, is injected into the arm and travels to the lungs where it is captured in the pulmonary capillaries. Only a small fraction of the blood vessels trap this material so the test is safe. The distribution of radioactive material tells if the blood flow throughout the lung is even or uneven. If uneven it may indicate pulmonary embolism or more commonly, some other type of lung disease.

When pulmonary embolism is suspected the ventilation lung scan is often performed. In this test the patient inhales a different radioactive substance, usually xenon, which in normal lungs is distributed evenly to all the airspaces. Analogous to the perfusion lung scan, the ventilation lung scan reveals if ventilation is even or uneven. By comparing the ventilation and perfusion lung scans (they can be done at the same time) doctors can achieve a good idea about the likelihood of pulmonary embolism.

Gallium Scan

This is a relatively new test that has proven useful in recent years. Radioactive gallium is injected into the patient's arm and 24 to 48 hours later the body (or a portion of the body) is scanned to find out where the gallium has accumulated. Gallium normally accumulates in the liver and bowels. In other areas however, accumulation is abnormal and usually related to inflammation (as from an infection) or tumor. The gallium scan does not discriminate between these two possibilities, so like most scans it is non-diagnostic. However, in conjunction with the overall clinical picture the gallium scan may point to an abnormal area for possible tissue biopsy.

The gallium scan may be very helpful in confirming a suspected diagnosis of sarcoidosis. There is a characteristic pattern of gallium uptake peculiar to this disease. This sarcoid pattern, plus a compatible clinical and chest X-ray picture, may be suffiicient for making the diagnosis of sarcoidosis even without a tissue biopsy (see Chapter 16).

WHAT ARE PULMONARY FUNCTION TESTS?

Pulmonary function tests are helpful in determining how well the lungs and respiratory system are working. There are two broad categories: tests of lung mechanics and tests of gas exchange.

Lung Mechanics

Tests of lung mechanics tell how well the lungs and chest cage move air in and out—the mechanical function of the respiratory system. In these tests the technician will ask you to perform some sort of breathing maneuver, usually a forced expiration after a deep inhalation. How much air you breathe out and how fast you exhale it are measured by collecting the air in a special device called a spirometer; hence the basic test of lung mechanics is called spirometry.

Spirometry is a very simple test, in routine use for many years. It measures the vital capacity, or amount of air you can blow out after a deep inhalation. Since the patient is asked to force the air out, the test is called forced vital capacity (FVC). During an FVC maneuver, you should be able to blow most of the air out of your lungs in less than five seconds. Both the total amount of exhaled air and its rate of flow will determine if any serious mechanical impairment is present.

Before spirometry equipment became widely available, doctors often used the match test. The patient was asked to blow out a lighted match held 6 inches from the mouth. Inability to do this correlates with severe airway obstruction. The match test is no longer used since spirometry is much more accurate and reproducible.

Figure 8-4 shows the setting for spirometry. To perform this test, the subject breathes normally through a hose attached to the spirometer (there are many types and models of spirometer). The subject is then asked to take in a deep breath and blow all the air out, as hard and fast as possible. During exhalation the air is collected by the spirometer, displacing a movable "bell"; this displacement is recorded by a needle marker on a piece of rotating graph paper. The result is a plot of the total air displaced (the forced vital capacity) versus seconds (the length of time for total expiration).

A representation of the normal forced vital capacity is also shown in the first panel of Figure 9-1. Point A represents the end of a regular, quiet breath. Point B represents maximum inhalation. After holding the breath for about a second, the subject exhales as forcibly and rapidly as possible (beginning at point C), until all the air is exhaled (point D).

One component of this test is called the peak flow. Just as its name implies, peak flow represents that part of the forced vital capacity where the air flows fastest out of the mouth. You can see this for yourself. Take in a deep breath and place a finger in front of your mouth. Now blow out as hard and as fast as you can. The entire amount of air you blew out is the forced vital capacity (point C to D in Figure 9-1). However, note that the *speed* of the air flowing past your finger decreased over time, and was fastest just after you began blowing out. The air

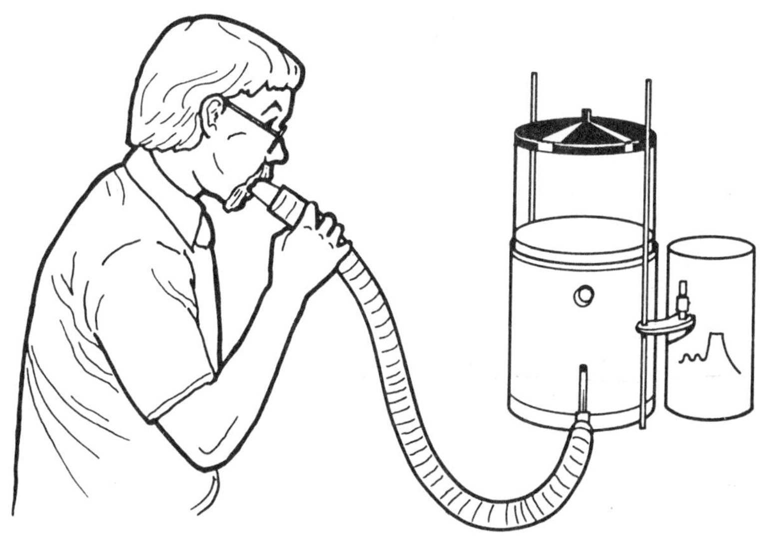

FIGURE 8-4 To perform spirometery, the subject takes in a full, deep breath, then exhales forcefully and rapidly into the tube. The tube is connected to the spirometer, which records a tracing of the effort on a rotating drum. Representations of these "spirometric" curves are shown in Figure 9-1.

speed at this fastest point (always within the first second after beginning) is the "peak flow." The normal peak flow varies according to age, sex, and height, but for most adults it falls somewhere between 400 and 700 liters/minute. Peak flow is reduced during asthma attacks. With the aid of easily portable apparatus designed to measure just peak flow, physicians now routinely use this test to determine both severity and degree of improvement from an asthma attack. (See case of Cheryl L. in Chapter 10).

Gas Exchange

Tests of gas exchange tell how well your lungs and respiratory system are bringing in oxygen and getting rid of CO_2. This is best assessed by measuring the O_2 and CO_2 tension (the amount of pressure exerted by the gas; it reflects the quantity of gas in the blood) in arterial blood since this part of the circulation reflects what happens in the lungs. The basic test of gas exchange is called an arterial blood gas (ABG).

Venous blood fills the blue veins of your arm and is easily obtained by syringe and needle. Except for blood gas analysis, all routine blood tests are done on venous blood. Venous blood is not useful for an ABG since it does not tell how much oxygen is being delivered to the tissues. Arterial blood is somewhat more difficult to obtain than venous blood, since arteries cannot be seen. However, their pulse can be felt. Arterial blood is under higher pressure than venous blood, and arterial pressure pulsates or varies with each heart beat.

An ABG test will also give the amount of acidity in the blood, called the pH. Hence, an ABG is ordered when your physician is worried about the amount of oxygen, carbon dioxide, or pH in your blood. It is a routine test in patients with serious lung disease because there is no other way to obtain this information so quickly and accurately.

One can get very sophisticated in ordering various lung mechanics and gas exchange tests. However, spirometry and arterial blood gas analysis together are sufficient to diagnose and manage most respiratory diseases. At times other tests of pulmonary function will be done, especially in patients scheduled for major surgery of who have complex or unusual problems. Even those patients, however, will have as a minimum spirometry and ABG analysis.

WHAT CAN BE FOUND ON A SPUTUM EXAMINATION?

Patients with a wide variety of lung diseases will often be asked to provide a sample of sputum or phlegm for examination. A wealth of information can be obtained by looking at sputum under the microscope, especially when it is stained and examined by experienced personnel.

Lung cancer can often be diagnosed by examining the cells in sputum; this technique is called sputum cytology. Experienced pathologists may not only be able to diagnose a lung cancer, but also to tell what cell type it is (see Chapter 21). Careful sputum exam in a patient suspected of lung cancer may obviate more invasive procedures including lung biopsy.

The type of pneumonia a patient has is often determined by staining sputum for bacteria. Absence of bacteria in a patient who has pneumonia by chest X-ray also points to certain causes, such as a virus or some types of bacteria that don't routinely take up the stain.

Pulmonary tuberculosis is commonly diagnosed by performing special acid-fast stains on sputum and looking for the characteristic red-staining tubercle bacilli.

Patients with asthma also have a characteristic sputum, usually full of pink-staining cells called eosinophils. Finding eosinophils may help to rule out other causes of wheezing such as heart failure.

PROCEDURES

Lung Surgery

On March 30, 1981, President Ronald Reagan was struck by a bullet and began hemorrhaging into his chest cavity. Within 90 minutes he was undergoing successful surgery to remove the bullet and repair the damaged lung. While the whole world waited for the outcome, his physicians were calmly and competently performing what for them had become a routine surgical procedure.

There is no better illustration of the long way lung surgery has come since the first pneumonectomy in 1933. Today, in trauma cases such as the President's, lung surgery is often immediate and life saving.

Lung surgery involves an incision in the thoracic cavity so the lung on that side can be visualized and operated on. The surgical procedure of opening the thoracic cavity is called a *thoracotomy*. Except in extreme cases of severe trauma, a thoracotomy is only done on one side at a time.

Aside from trauma the other major indication for thoracotomy and lung surgery today is for diagnosing and treating lung cancer. However, since most lung cancer can be diagnosed without thoracotomy, most non-emergency lung surgery ends up being done for treatment (removal) of lung cancer. In such cases there is always ample time to discuss the surgery thoroughly and obtain a clear understanding of the risks and benefits. Lung surgery is a major procedure not be taken lightly. There must be clear indications and potential benefits to the patient, and no other way to obtain them.

WHAT IS CHEST TUBE DRAINAGE?

A chest tube is a large, plastic tube that can be inserted into a patient's chest cavity in order to drain abnormal collections of fluid or air. Once inserted, it is generally left in place for two to four days, or until full drainage has occurred. Indications for chest tube drainage are massive collections of pleural fluid, infected pleural fluid, or a large pneumothorax. In addition, one or more chest tubes are always left in a patient's chest cavity after thoractomy. This is to help drain air and any fluid that accumulate during and after the procedure.

WHAT IS BRONCHOSCOPY?

This is a very useful technique done with the aid of a flexible tube about two feet long, called the flexible fiberoptic bronchoscope (Figure 8-5). (It has largely supplanted the older rigid bronchoscopes–long, rigid pipes that are distinctly uncomfortable for any patient and usually require general anesthesia for insertion.)

The flexible fiberoptic bronchoscope was introduced by Japanese physicians in 1968 and has been in widespread use in this country since the early 1970s. With-

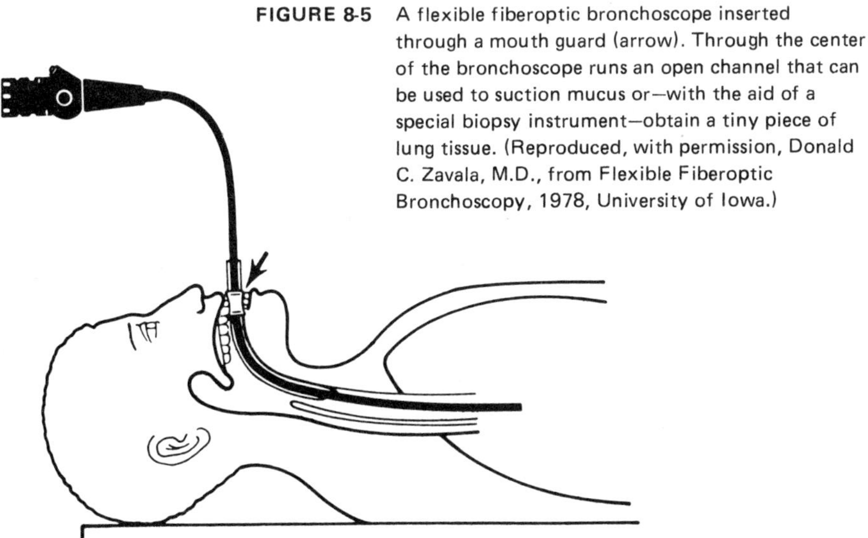

FIGURE 8-5 A flexible fiberoptic bronchoscope inserted through a mouth guard (arrow). Through the center of the bronchoscope runs an open channel that can be used to suction mucus or—with the aid of a special biopsy instrument—obtain a tiny piece of lung tissue. (Reproduced, with permission, Donald C. Zavala, M.D., from Flexible Fiberoptic Bronchoscopy, 1978, University of Iowa.)

in its five millimeter diameter are a narrow channel through which secretions can be suctioned and a fiberoptic bundle that carries light from a machine into the patient's lungs. Standing at the patient's head, the operator can insert the tip of the scope into any of the large airways and literally see inside the patient's lungs. Then, depending on the condition, a tiny biopsy of tissue can be done, secretions suctioned, or medication instilled. Not only is the instrument flexible, but so are its uses. Flexible fiberoptic bronchoscopy is frequently employed in the modern practice of pulmonary medicine.

WHAT IS A BIOPSY?

A biopsy is removal of a piece of tissue for purposes of diagnosis. "Biopsy" is used as a verb (to biopsy) or a noun (a tissue biopsy). Some biopsies involve general anesthesia, some can be done at the bedside. Following is an alphabetical list of routine biopsy procedures used in respiratory medicine.

Biopsy, Bronchoscopic A tiny piece of tissue is obtained using a bronchoscope inserted into the patient's lungs through the mouth or nose. This is now most commonly done with the fiberoptic bronchoscope, a technique that can be done out of the operating room and without general anesthesia.

Biopsy, Mediastinal Tissue is obtained during a procedure known as *mediastinoscopy.* It involves an incision above the breastbone and requires general anesthesia. For this reason, it should be considered *major surgery* even though it is only done for diagnostic purposes–to obtain pieces of tissue in the area between the two lungs. This tissue–usually one or more lymph nodes–is often valuable for diagnosing lung cancer, sarcoidosis, and other pulmonary diseases. However, since there are usually simpler methods of making these diagnoses, mediastinoscopy is generally a diagnostic procedure of last resort.

Biopsy, Needle Aspiration This technique involves inserting a thin needle through the skin of the chest and directly into the abnormal area in the patient's lung. Although only a small amount of tissue is obtained in this way, it may be diagnostic for many cases of lung cancer. This technique is most useful for abnormal areas in the periphery of the lung, near the chest wall. It is less useful for lesions near the center of the chest cavity.

Biopsy, Open Lung This requires a thoracotomy and is the procedure described under lung surgery. In many instances this is the only way to make a diagnosis. Although major surgery, it is a relatively safe procedure and as sure as any to give a diagnostic result.

Biopsy, Pleural The pleural membranes that line both the lungs and the inside of the chest cavity may be involved by many disease processes. Using a specially designed pleural biopsy needle, several tiny fragments of pleural membrane can be safely removed at the bedside. This test is most useful for diagnosing tuberculosis or cancer.

Biopsy, Scalene and/or Supraclavicular Node There are lymph nodes throughout the body. Lymph nodes in the neck region (near the scalene muscle) and above the clavicle (supraclavicular) are often biopsied since they may be involved with disease originating in the lungs. General anesthesia is not required for these biopsies.

WHAT IS CARDIAC CATHETERIZATION?

The idea of putting a long, thin wire or tube (a catheter) into someone's heart seems commonplace today. However, it was so radical an idea initially that the first person to try it had to do it on himself—and in secret! The year was 1929 and the subject was a German physician named Werner Forssmann. For his pioneering effort in cardiac catheterization. Dr. Forssmann shared in the Nobel prize for physiology and medicine in 1956.

The 1950s and 60s saw widespread use of this technique in diagnosing and managing heart problems. Since the 1970s this technique has also become useful in treating lung problems. The procedure is a variation of "right heart" catheterization, and can be done at the bedside in intensive care units. From portal of entry at an arm or neck vein, a specially designed catheter is threaded into the right side of the heart and then into the pulmonary artery. This allows measurement of pulmonary vascular pressures and cardiac function, providing much useful information about the patient's status. The technique is commonly referred to as Swan-Ganz catheterization, after the two co-inventors of this specially designed right heart catheter.

WHAT IS A PULMONARY ANGIOGRAM?

A pulmonary angiogram (or arteriogram) is a special study that uses dye to outline the pulmonary blood vessels. The procedure is called pulmonary angiography (or arteriography) and incorporates cardiac catheterization (see previous section). A specially-designed catheter is inserted into a vein of the arm or leg and threaded through the right side of the heart and into the main pulmonary artery. Once in place (as determined by fluoroscopy) dye is injected into the catheter and out into the pulmonary circulation. By carefully manipulating the tip of the catheter, the dye can be aimed to outline the entire pulmonary circulation or only one small part of it.

Pulmonary angiography is most commonly employed to diagnose clots in the pulmonary circulation (see Chapter 22), especially when the diagnosis is equivocal by lung scans.

WHAT ARE INTUBATION AND ARTIFICIAL VENTILATION?

Intubation is placing a plastic or rubber tube into a patient's trachea (windpipe) for purposes of securing an airway. The procedure is called endotracheal intubation. The tube, ranging between seven and nine millimeters in internal diameter, can be placed either through the nose or through the mouth. An endotracheal tube helps guarantee an open airway between the atmosphere and the patient's trachea.

By far the most common reason for intubation is so the patient can receive *artificial* ventilation. The artificial ventilator (also called respirator) is a machine attached via hoses to one end of the endotracheal tube. A circular cuff on the other end of the tube (the end within the patient's trachea) is inflated with air to seal the tube. In this way all the air pushed through the tube by the venilator will not escape prematurely. This cuff also helps prevent patients from aspirating secretions into their lungs.

Only when the patient is unable to maintain adequate oxygenation or ventilation on his own is artificial ventilation required. The ventilator not only can provide more air, but can also distribute oxygen to the lungs much more effectively than can a face mask or nasal tubing.

WHAT IS TRACHEOSTOMY?

Tracheostomy is a surgical procedure that places a hole into the trachea, below the Adam's apple. Through this hole is placed a breathing tube that has the same function as the endotracheal tube discussed above. Tracheostomy is usually done after prolonged endotracheal intubation when patients still require an artificial airway or artificial ventilation. The vast majority of patients who ever receive oral or nasal endotracheal intubation have the tube removed within a week or so. Beyond a week problems of discomfort and inability to eat become major factors, so tracheostomy is usually performed. Tracheostomy allows removal of the endotracheal tube from the patient's mouth or nose and transfers the origin of the artificial airway to the neck. For awake patients this allows eating and swallowing. There is no set rule on when to perform tracheostomy after prior endotracheal intubation. There is some morbidity with tracheostomy just as there is with prolonged endotracheal intubation.

Examples of many of the procedures discussed are illustrated by the following case.

RWR: The Nation's Most Famous Patient

A 70-year-old man was brought to the emergency room at approximately 3 P.M., having sustained a gunshot wound to the left chest. Although alert, he felt weak and his blood pressure was slightly low. Examination of the chest showed evidence of bleeding in the thoracic cavity. For this reason a chest tube was inserted, through which was removed over a liter of blood. Because the bleeding did not rapidly stop, he was taken to the operating room where he was intubated and a thoracotomy was performed. This consisted of a six-inch incision between the ribs on the left side near the breast muscles. After much searching the bullet was located and the lung was repaired, stopping the bleeding. Two chest tubes were left in place to drain air and fluid and the chest incision was closed. The patient was removed to the recovery room with the endotracheal tube still in place, and was attached to an *artificial ventilator.* He complained of some shortness of breath and required morphine for pain. Arterial blood gases showed a low O_2 tension and a chest X-ray showed a large amount of haziness on the left side. To help clear secretions fiberoptic bronchoscopy was attempted by passing the bronchoscope through the endotracheal tube already in place. An unexpected kink or narrowing in the endotracheal tube prevented complete passage of the bronchoscope and the procedure was abandoned. At this time nurses began aggressive suctioning of secretions from his airway, and he rapidly improved over the next several hours. By 3:30 A.M. the next morning his blood gases and chest X-ray improved to the point that the endotracheal tube was able to come out.

He continued to receive chest physical therapy, suctioning, and pain medication as needed. Arterial blood gases showed steady improvement in the oxygen tension. The chest tubes were removed on the third post-operative day. On the fourth post-operative day he developed a fever; because of possible plugging of his airways fiberoptic bronchoscopy was again attempted. This time the flexible scope was successfully passed through his mouth without the endotracheal tube in place. Recovery progressed and he was discharged the 11th hospital day.

This patient experienced many of the procedures commonly performed in patients with medical and surgical chest problems: thoracotomy, bronchoscopy, arterial blood gases, chest X-rays, etc. Most of these procedures were either not available or primitive when this patient started out his career as a movie actor four decades earlier.

CHAPTER NINE

Patterns of Lung Disease

WHAT ARE THE PATTERNS OF RESPIRATORY DISEASE?

Doctors often speak of many lung diseases as representing one of two patterns of breathing: restrictive or obstructive. These terms refer only to how a respiratory problem affects a patient's breathing pattern; they say nothing about cause, treatment, X-ray appearance, or prognosis of his condition. Furthermore, the two breathing patterns frequently are seen together in one disease. At best they are merely descriptive of many respiratory problems. Despite their limitations, use of the terms "restrictive" and "obstructive" is so pervasive that they will be defined here and used throughout this book.

WHAT IS RESTRICTIVE RESPIRATORY DISEASE?

This is any respiratory condition where the patient is unable to take in a full, deep breath. It can be due to lung, chest cage, or nervous system disease. By analogy imagine a steel hoop placed around your chest so that you can breathe in a little, but not take a full, deep breath. Your breathing is then restricted. The closer the steel hoop comes to your resting breathing level at the end of a normal breath, the less you can inspire and the more severe is the restriction.

Any respiratory condition resulting in inability to expand fully the lungs is a restrictive problem. Once air is inhaled, however, patients with restrictive disorders can exhale without any impediment or obstruction. Hence, the major distinction between restrictive and obstructive lung disease is between difficulty getting all the air *in* (restrictive) and getting all the air *out* (obstructive). This difference can be appreciated by measuring the forced vital capacity (Figure 9-1).

Respiratory diseases and conditions commonly associated with a restrictive breathing pattern are listed in Table 9-1. Although many of the lung diseases listed here may also be associated with airway obstruction, restriction is usually predominant.

WHAT IS OBSTRUCTIVE LUNG DISEASE?

Asthma, chronic bronchitis, and emphysema are examples of obstructive lung disease. Characteristic of this group is difficulty getting all the air out. As a group obstructive lung diseases are the greatest cause of respiratory morbidity in the United States. Obstructive lung disease is best diagnosed by a simple pulmonary function test of the forced vital capacity (see Chapter 8). As shown in Figure 9-1, the obstructed patient can take a deep breath but the rate of exhalation is slowed. This is contrasted with a restricted patient, who cannot inhale as much air but can exhale it readily. For comparison the normal FVC curve is also shown.

Table 9-2 lists the most common diseases or conditions that may lead to airway obstruction.

WHAT IS THE DIFFERENCE BETWEEN UPPER AND LOWER AIRWAY OBSTRUCTION?

Asthma, chronic bronchitis, and emphysema are all diseases of the lower airways (bronchial tubes). The trachea, larynx (voice box), and pharynx (area behind the tongue) comprise the upper airway and are not involved in these conditions. Croup,

FIGURE 9-1 Patterns of respiratory disease as shown by measurement of forced vital capacity. See also Figure 8-4.

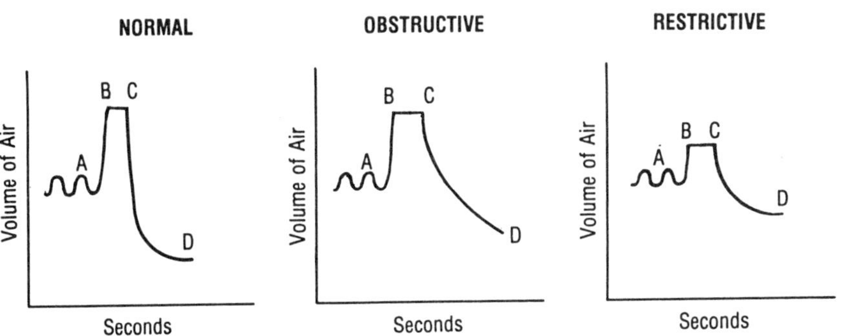

A = Quiet breathing
B = Point of maximal breathing
C = Beginning of exhalation
D = End of exhalation

TABLE 9-1 Respiratory diseases and conditions commonly associated with a restrictive breathing pattern

CENTRAL NERVOUS SYSTEM AND CHEST BELLOWS	LUNGS
Polio	Pneumonia
Obesity	Sarcoidosis
Myasthenia gravis	Lung fibrosis
Guillain Barré syndrome	Acute respiratory failure associated with pulmonary edema
Flail chest (multiple broken ribs)	Hyaline membrane disease
Diaphragm paralysis	Advanced lung cancer
Spinal cord disease	Congestive heart failure
Pickwickian syndrome	
Pleural effusion and pleural disease	

laryngitis, tracheitis, and epiglottitis are infections or inflammations of the upper airway; they may lead to upper airway obstruction. They are more common in children than in adults; also, children are more prone to upper airway obstruction because of the child's smaller airway.

A tumor or foreign body can also obstruct the upper airway. Any patient with upper airway obstruction can present with expiratory wheezing just like asthma, so the distinction is important. Accurate diagnosis of upper airway obstruction can usually be made by a combination of history and physical examination, X-rays of the neck, and spirometry. Stridor (a high-pitched, inspiratory wheeze) is common in upper airway obstruction and is not usually heard with asthma and other forms of lower airway obstruction. (Complete airway obstruction is a medical emergency. See Chapter 5.)

TABLE 9-2 Diseases or conditions that may be associated with obstruction to airflow

Lower Airway Obstruction:	Asthma
	Chronic bronchitis
	Emphysema
	Cystic fibrosis
	Sarcoidosis
Upper Airway Obstruction:	Croup
	Laryngotracheobronchitis
	Epiglottitis
	Various tumors and foreign bodies that may involve the upper airway

Note that central nervous system and chest wall conditions do not ordinarily lead to an obstructive breathing pattern, whereas they are a common cause of a restrictive pattern. This is because the process of expiration is passive and requires only normal airways once the air has been inhaled. By contrast, the process of inspiration is active, requiring an intact brain control center, chest wall, and lungs. Finally, some diseases, such as sarcoidosis (Chapter 16), can manifest both an obstructive and restrictive pattern.

CHAPTER TEN

Asthma: "Hypersensitive Airways"

WHAT IS ASTHMA?

Asthma is a condition of hypersensitive airways. Normally the airways of our lungs stay open continuously so that the air we breathe can enter without difficulty. The airways of asthmatics have a tendency to narrow or close down when excited by many types of stimuli. For this reason they are said to be hypersensitive or hyperreactive. (Also descriptive of the asthma condition is the term "twitchy airways," as though the asthmatic's airways are primed to narrow when the right stimulus comes along.)

The basic reason for this hyperreactivity, and hence for asthma, is unknown. Regardless of the stimulant, the end result is the same for the patient; the bronchi (another name for the airways) tend to narrow or constrict (hence called bronchoconstriction) and there is trouble breathing.

When the airways constrict the patient usually wheezes. A wheeze is a high-pitched sound produced as air is forced through the narrowed air passages. Also characteristic of asthma is its reversibility—the airways can (almost always) be opened up. Often they open up on their own or perhaps after the stimulus has been removed. Frequently, however, medication has to be given to aid in opening up the airways.

The lungs consist of multiple branching airways that become narrower and narrower as the number of branches increases (Figure 10-1). During normal breathing these airways stay open. During an asthma attack the walls of the airways are thickened. In addition, the smaller airways may become partially or completely

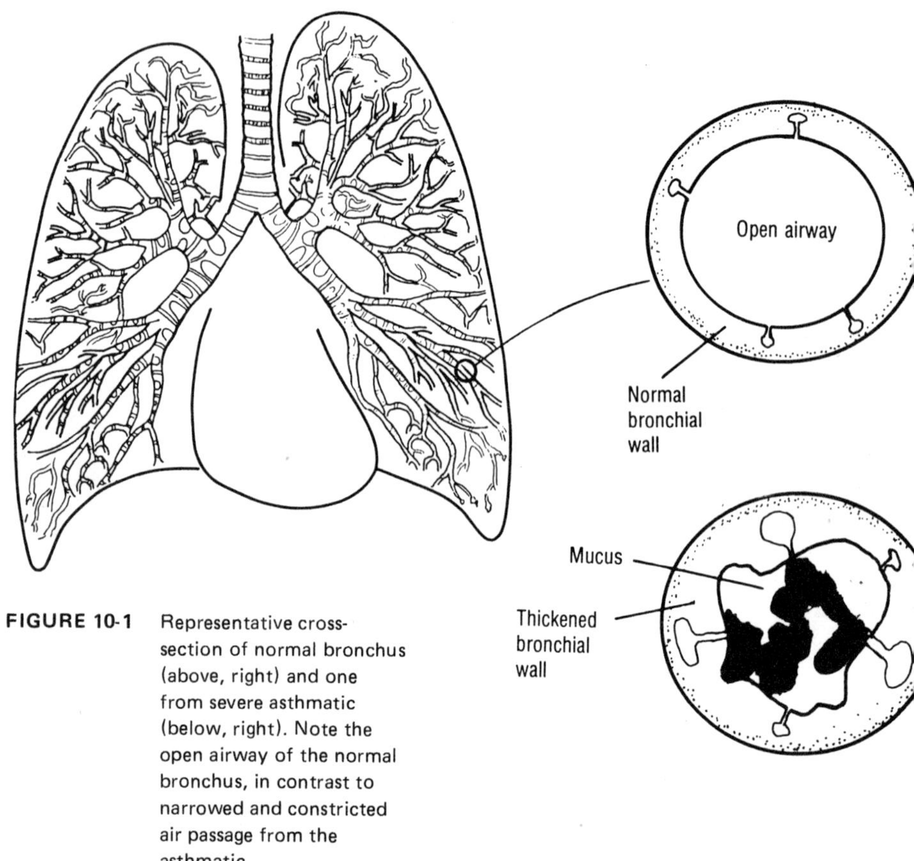

FIGURE 10-1 Representative cross-section of normal bronchus (above, right) and one from severe asthmatic (below, right). Note the open airway of the normal bronchus, in contrast to narrowed and constricted air passage from the asthmatic.

filled with tenacious mucus. Thickened walls and increased mucus result in narrowing of the airways and obstruction to the flow of air (Figure 10-1). To the extent these airway problems can be relieved patients will also be relieved of their asthma symptoms.

WHAT CAN TRIGGER AN ASTHMA ATTACK?

We only know some of the stimulants that make asthmatic patients wheeze. Fortunately, however, treatment is usually effective regardless of the cause. Airways of all asthmatics react in a common way no matter what the stimulus and thus respond to medications similarly. Table 10-1 lists common stimuli that may precipitate or exacerbate wheezing and shortness of breath, a condition described as an asthma attack.

Our current understanding of asthma can be diagrammed in simple fashion, as is shown in Figure 10-2. Asthma is a condition of unknown cause that can flare up (asthma attack) on exposure to certain stimuli. In a way not yet understood, these stimuli can make the airways of an asthmatic narrow and produce excessive mucus.

TABLE 10-1 **Stimuli that may bring on an asthma attack in a patient with hyperreactive airways**

Irritants	Various air pollutants, tobacco smoke, perfumes, petroleum solvents, etc.
Allergens	Pollens, ragweed, certain foods, molds, etc.
Infections	Virus and bacteria-like organisms
Temperature and Climate	Particularly cold air
Exercise	May exacerbate asthma under any weather conditions, but usually worse in cold, dry air
Emotional Factors	May exacerbate some asthmatic conditions
Aspirin & Other Analgesic Drugs	May affect some asthmatics through a non-allergic mechanism

Exposure to the same stimuli, in a non-asthmatic, does not lead to this reaction. Treatment, which can completely reverse an asthma attack, does not cure the underlying asthma condition, and the asthmatic remains at some risk for further attacks.

Not all asthmatics react to the same stimuli, but a single attack can usually be traced to one or more of the stimuli shown in Table 10-1. The number, frequency, and severity of asthma attacks can vary tremendously from patient to patient.

HOW COMMON IS ASTHMA IN THE UNITED STATES?

It is estimated that asthma alone afflicts approximately nine million people in the United States, including those who have hay fever symptoms along with their asthma. However, the number of Americans who have ever had asthma, even though they may no longer be symptomatic, is approximately seven percent of the entire population or about 16 million people.

The vast majority of asthmatics have a mild or moderate condition easily controlled by either avoiding known stimuli of bronchoconstriction or by taking simple medication when wheezing or other asthma symptoms occur. Approximately five percent of the asthma population suffers from severe, recurring attacks,

FIGURE 10-2 Simple model for asthma.

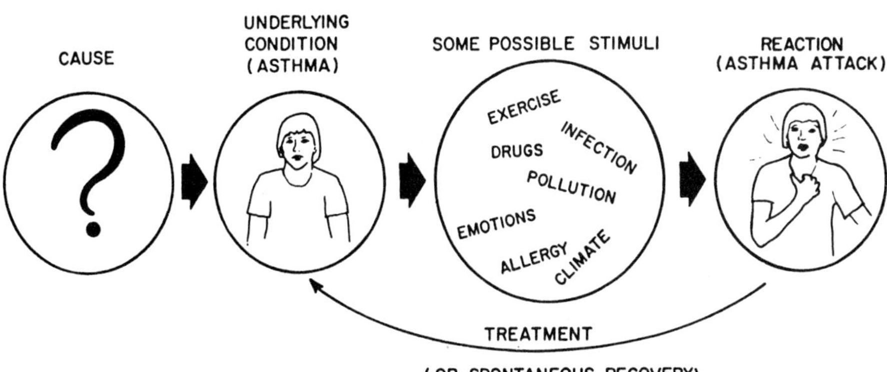

often requiring hospitalization. For this group of patients daily medication is the rule.

DO PEOPLE DIE FROM ASTHMA?

Unfortunately, yes. Although the exact number of deaths is not known, an estimated 2,000-4,000 Americans die annually from asthma alone. This does not include the much larger group of patients whose basic problem is chronic obstructive pulmonary disease combined with an asthmatic component (see Chapter 12).

Based against the approximately nine million who have asthma in this country, or the estimated four to five hundred thousand who suffer from severe asthma, two to four thousand is a small percentage. Although asthma is a treatable condition, and ideally no deaths should occur, there are still patients who, for unclear reasons, do not respond. When death occurs, it is usually from intractable respiratory failure (see Chapter 25).

IS ALL ASTHMA DUE TO ALLERGY?

No. Although all asthmatics have hypersensitive airways, most adult asthma is not related to allergy. In only a minority of adult asthma patients can an allergic mechanism be found. Allergy is only one of many possible stimuli of an asthma attack (see Table 10-1).

Generally speaking there are two broad categories of asthma. One type is caused by allergy, and is triggered by things inhaled, ingested, or touched that the patient has previously been sensitized to. This means antibodies have formed to something in these substances, and when the latter enter the body an allergic reaction occurs. This allergic reaction is a more common form of asthma in children than in adults. When specific allergens can be identified as provoking symptoms the asthma is called extrinsic, since the cause is outside the body. Extrinsic asthma is synonymous with allergic asthma. In extrinsic asthma the stimulant (such as pollen) enters the body and combines wth the patient's antibodies to produce the bronchoconstriction. In such patients allergy skin tests to the stimulating substance will often be positive and the amount of allergy antibody measured in the bood will be elevated.

WHAT TYPE OF ASTHMA DO ADULTS HAVE?

A non-allergic form of asthma is usually present in adults. In most adult asthma the cause is not allergy and there are no specific substances that can be identified as provoking the asthma. This is true even though many adult asthmatics have a history of atopy—or hypersensitivity—preceding the onset of asthma. There may be a history in childhood of hay fever, various food allergies, or even mild asthma that remitted before or during adolescence, only to flare up as an adult. For an adult asthmatic, an atopic or allergic childhood history does not prove an allergic mechanism for the asthma.

The term intrinsic asthma is used to describe most cases of adult asthma, implying the cause is from within the body. Intrinsic asthma is synonymous with non-allergic asthma.

Actually the term intrinsic is something of a misnomer. Originally intending to mean from within the body, we now know many of the non-allergic causes are from the environment. A good example is the inhalation of cold air, particularly on exercise, that exacerbates many asthmatics. Perhaps the most common stimulus for intrinsic asthma attacks is a viral respiratory infection, a cause that certainly comes from outside the patient.

DOES IT MATTER IF ASTHMA IS INTRINSIC OR EXTRINSIC?

Yes, in two important ways. First, if the asthma is truly extrinsic (allergic), it may be possible to completely avoid the precipitating stimulus. For example, pollen or cat fur can and should be avoided if they cause wheezing.

The second reason is that for the small percentage of patients who have allergic asthma, desensitization shots may be effective. The shots work by building up an immunity to the stimulus of the asthma attack, and they are occasionally helpful. However, most adult patients do not have allergic asthma. Experience indicates also that most adults will know if they are allergic to a specific agent since their symptoms (shortness of breath or wheezing) get worse on exposure and better when the stimulus is avoided. This is illustrated by the following case.

Eric S.—A Case of Extrinsic Asthma

Eric S. is a 25-year-old patient with a history of a runny nose and watery eyes every spring; he has never wheezed or experienced shortness of breath. He brought a cat home one day and three days later began having chest tightness and wheezing. He thought he might be allergic to the cat and left it with a friend, after which he improved. A week later, when he picked up the cat, his wheezing recurred. He gave up the cat and has felt well since.

Such a patient likely has extrinsic or allergic asthma to cat fur. In obvious situations such as this the precipitating agent should just be avoided.

DOES THIS MEAN ALLERGY SHOTS ARE OF NO VALUE?

Not necessarily. The value of allergy shots depends on the individual patient and the type of asthma. In some children allergy shots may be very beneficial. Also allergies can manifest in ways other than asthma, such as hay fever with a runny nose and watery eyes. If hay fever symptoms are a seasonal problem allergy shots may help a great deal. However, for most adults who suffer from asthma, allergy shots are simply not helpful. If given, they certainly should not take the place of asthma medications when there is wheezing or shortness of breath. At best allergy shots work over the long range and are not helpful immediately.

DOES CIGARETTE SMOKING CAUSE ASTHMA?

No, not directly. Smoking can, however, cause bronchitis that can then lead to wheezing and shortness of breath and for all practical purposes behave just like asthma. We use the term asthmatic bronchitis to describe such patients.

Asthmatic bronchitis when due to cigarette smoking differs from asthma in that there is underlying lung damage from prolonged smoke exposure. In such patients lung function is often impaired. By contrast lungs of true asthmatics (nonsmokers) usually show normal function between asthma attacks. Also, patients with asthmatic bronchitis (when due to cigarette smoking) can go on to develop emphysema; as far as is known this does not occur in true asthmatics. (Emphysema is a diagnosis that is best made by special breathing tests; see Chapter 12).

WHAT IS OCCUPATIONAL ASTHMA?

This is an asthma condition arising from inhaling dusts or other noxious material at the workplace; it is discussed in more detail in Chapter 4.

IS WHEEZING ALWAYS PRESENT IN AN ASTHMA ATTACK?

Wheezing is both a sign and a symptom. Patients frequently know when they are wheezing. Usually, however, it is something the doctor is more aware of than the patient, since wheezing is easily heard with the aid of a stethoscope. The absence of wheezing does not rule out asthma. (In fact, patients can suffer from asthma without ever wheezing).

Some patients have asthma whose only symptom is cough or shortness of breath on exertion. Although the asthma may remain undiagnosed because there is no wheezing, these patients would respond to asthma medication just as well as those who wheeze. To be sure of the diagnosis, lung testing is carried out (see pulmonary function testing, Chapter 8). If such testing cannot be done, asthma medication may be tried anyway. Because there are many causes other than asthma for cough and shortness of breath, treatment should only be under medical supervision.

DOES WHEEZING ALWAYS MEAN ASTHMA?

Just as asthma may be present without wheezing, the presence of wheezing does not always indicate asthma. It does indicate airway narrowing or obstruction, of which there are several other causes. Chronic obstructive pulmonary disease (Chapter 12) commonly is accompanied by wheezing and may even have a true asthma component (have some reversibility of the airway obstruction).

So-called cardiac asthma is a heart condition that may be accompanied by wheezing (Chapter 17). Another cause of diffuse wheezing that may masquerade as asthma is upper airway obstruction (Chapter 9). Causes of localized wheezing (confined to one side of the chest) include lung cancer (Chapter 21) and pulmonary embolism (Chapter 22).

Most patients with diffuse wheezing have asthma or an asthma component to their illness. However, "not all that wheezes is asthma."

WHAT ROLE DO EMOTIONS PLAY IN ASTHMA?

A common misconception is that asthma is of psychological origin or is a psychosomatic disease. There is simply no basis in fact that asthma is caused by psychological factors. Most physicians accept that asthma attacks can be triggered by emotional factors, but emotions are simply one of the many stimuli to which the hypersensitive airways of asthmatics may respond (see Table 10-1 and Figure 10-2). Not being able to breathe comfortably is emotionally distressing, so it is difficult to even know if emotional upset is a stimulus or a result of the asthma attack.

Psychoanalytic thought has in the past emphasized a faulty mother-child relationship involving asthmatic children. This is a myth not substantiated by scientific evidence; in fact many asthmatic children have a normal, healthy mother-child relationship. Certainly the relationship between a mother and her asthmatic child can be unhealthy from a psychological point of view and make the affliction worse. However, this is also true with many chronic diseases, and does not in any way imply a cause and effect relationship.

WHAT DRUGS SHOULD ASTHMATICS AVOID?

Probably the most important group of drugs for anyone with asthma to avoid is the beta-blockers. These work directly opposite to the beta-adrenergic drugs used to treat asthma. The generic name of all beta-blockers ends in "-olol." Beta-blockers are used to treat some forms of heart disease, high blood pressure, and many other conditions such as glaucoma and migraine headache. Examples of commonly used beta-blockers are listed in Table 10-2.

All of these drugs, except the eye drops, are used in treating high blood pressure and some forms of heart disease. Unfortunately, all of them can also exacerbate asthma.

Even Timoptic eye drops (used for glaucoma) can exacerbate an underlying asthma condition. Several patients using the eye drops are reported to have died

TABLE 10-2 Beta-blockers

Generic Name	Brand Name
Propranolol	Inderal
Nadolol	Corgard
Atenolol	Tenormin
Metoprolol	Lopressor
Timolol	Blocardren
Timolol	Timoptic (eye drops)

from asthma and many others suffered adverse reactions. All patients with a tendency for asthma and wheezing should avoid beta-blocking drugs in any form.

Other drugs can have adverse effects in some asthmatics. These include aspirin and other arthritis medications, discussed in the next section. Also, some drugs used for colds and flu may dry up secretions and have an adverse effect on asthma. Any person who suffers wheezing or shortness of breath along with a cold or flu syndrome should consult a physician before using non-prescription remedies.

Sedatives and anti-anxiety medications may depress breathing and should not be used during any asthma attack, although at regular doses these drugs should cause no breathing problem in symptom-free asthma.

Many drugs can interact with each other and cause problems. Patients taking drugs for any non-respiratory problem (hypertension, seizures, headache, anxiety) should consult with their physician to find out about potential interference with asthma medication.

WHAT ROLE DOES ASPIRIN PLAY IN ASTHMA?

For years it has been recognized that some people get asthma attacks when they take aspirin. Various studies have estimated that up to 20 percent of adult asthmatics may wheeze after aspirin ingestion. This reaction does not appear to be allergic in nature and so the term aspirin-intolerance is preferred to aspirin-allergy.

Aspirin is actually one of a group of drugs that can inhibit body compounds called prostaglandins or PGs. PG's are one of a large group of long-chain fatty acids that normally serve diverse functions. One type of prostaglandin–PGE–appears to function as a bronchodilator and open up the airways; another type–PGF–opposes this action and tends to narrow the airways.

Normally, along with other compounds in the body, the opposing prostaglandins balance each other and so keep the airways from narrowing. Aspirin (and other drugs) appear to work by blocking the formation of prostaglandins. It is postulated that people who wheeze from aspirin probably have more PGE (bronchodilating) than PGF (bronchoconstricting) effects and when all the PGs are inhibited bronchoconstriction predominates.

Aspirin-induced wheezing is also associated with nasal polyps (abnormal swellings inside the nose) and sinusitis in some asthmatics; the true incidence is unknown. When all these conditions are present the patient is said to have the asthma triad (sinusitis, nasal polyps, and aspirin-intolerance).

The treatment of asthmatics who have aspirin intolerance or the asthma triad is no different from any other asthma patient. However special emphasis is placed on avoidance of aspirin and aspirin-containing products. Aspirin, also known as A.S.A. for acetyl salicylic acid, is a ubiquitous drug; it is present in many over-the-counter (O.T.C.) and prescription (Rx) analgesics. Some of the more common aspirin and aspirin-containing compounds are listed in Table 10-3.

For patients requiring mild analgesia who may be intolerant of aspirin the analgesic acetominophen is widely recommended. However, like any drug acetominophen can be toxic in large amounts (liver damage can result).

Other analgesic drugs that may cause wheezing by inhibiting prostaglandin formation include (brand names(s) in parentheses): indomethacin (Indocin),

TABLE 10-3 **Commonly used aspirin and aspirin-containing compounds**

Available O.T.C.	Available by Rx
BC Tablets & Powder	Empirin with Codeine
Bufferin	Fiorinal with Codeine
Anacin	Percodan Tablets
Alka Seltzer	
Ascriptin	
Excedrin	
Fiorinal	
Coricidin	
Vanquish	

In addition, numerous compounds with the following initials in their name contain aspirin:

A.S.A.
APC
P-A-C

mefanamic acid (Ponstel), ibuprofen (Motrin; Rufen), fenoprofen (Nalfon), phenylbutazone (Azolid; Butazolidin), and zomepirac sodium (Zomax).

These drugs are available only by prescription, for pain and other symptoms of arthritis. A history of aspirin intolerance does *not* predict the same intolerance to these prescription drugs. Asthmatic patients should check with their physician for any questions regarding use of these drugs.

HOW DOES EXERCISE EXACERBATE ASTHMA?

Much research has been done in recent years on exercise-induced asthma (EIA). Many asthmatics experience wheezing and shortness of breath during or after strenuous exercise. Physicians in Boston and elsewhere have shown that inhaling large volumes of cold, cool, or dry air during exercise is associated with airways obstruction in asthmatics.

Apparently the exercise, by itself, is not the culprit. When patients perform the same amount of exercise breathing heated, humidified air, wheezing does not occur. This may also explain why many asthmatics prefer swimming over other exercises; the air inhaled during swimming is usually warm and wet.

Many episodes of EIA can be prevented or ameliorated by prior treatment with inhaled bronchodilators; Cromolyn sodium (see Chapter 11) is also recommended by some physicians for prevention of EIA.

HOW IS ASTHMA TREATED?

The answer to this is as variable as the number of patients who have the condition. Asthma can present in varying degrees, from very mild to life-threatening. Treatment depends on the clinical condition of the patient when seen, as well as on the past history available to the physician. Chapter 11 will be devoted to the treatment of asthma and reversible airways disease. An example of severe asthma is shown by the following case.

Cheryl L.—A Case of Severe Asthma

Mrs. L., 35, has suffered from mild hay fever since childhood. Every year, in late summer, she develops a runny nose and itchy eyes, and finds relief with antihistamines and decongestants. She has never wheezed or suffered shortness of breath and has never received treatment for asthma. One sister has mild asthma. Her mother had asthma as a child but has since outgrown it and is now doing well. Her father developed emphysema after many years of smoking and died at age 68 of a heart attack. Mrs. L. does not smoke.

She experienced her usual hay fever symptoms in August and by Labor Day they were gone. She developed a cold in October and noticed some shortness of breath shortly afterwards. Her doctor heard some wheezing in her chest and prescribed oral theophylline. This seemed to help for a few days, but then it made her sick to her stomach and she quit the medication. Respiratory symptoms continued and she was prescribed an inhaler; this helped some but never gave complete relief.

About 10 days after her cold began she became very short of breath and was rushed to the emergency room. There she was found to be in some respiratory distress; after a brief history and examination she was given a shot of epinephrine, without noticeable relief. A peak flow test (one determination of asthma severity) was 26 percent of predicted, a very low value. She was next begun on intravenous aminophylline and given another shot of epinephrine. An hour later she felt a little better, but her peak flow was only 28 percent of predicted. Her chest X-ray was normal. Blood gas revealed some lowering of her oxygen tension and only slight lowering of her CO_2 tension. Because there was no improvement after three hours in the ER and she was becoming very tired, Mrs. L. was admitted to the hospital. Diagnosis: severe asthma attack.

Intensive treatment was begun after she arrived at her hospital bed. She was given four different drugs. She received aminophylline and corticosteroids by vein (see Chapter 11), a beta-adrenegic drug by inhalation (Chapter 11), and oxygen by a nasal cannula. Although she complained of being very tired and not being able to sleep, her doctor expressly forbid any sleeping medication or sedatives, for fear they would depress her breathing.

Mrs. L. made slow but steady progress. On the third day after admission her peak flow was 65 percent of predicted and she felt much better. Her doctor still noted wheezing, but explained to her this was often the last thing to clear after an asthma attack. On the fourth hospital day her intravenous medication and oxygen were stopped and she was given only oral drugs plus the inhalation treatments. On the seventh day her peak flow was 80 percent of predicted and she was discharged, with prescriptions to continue the oral medication.

This case exemplifies a common pattern in severe adult asthma. There is often a personal or family history of asthma or allergies, but the severe attack is not usually allergic in origin. As with Mrs. L. it usually follows an upper respiratory viral infection. Almost everyone gets these infections, but asthmatics, with their hypersensitive airways, are prone to wheezing and bronchospasm as a result. Finally, once a full-blown attack sets in, treatment may have to be given intravenously and over several days.

CAN SEVERE ASTHMA ATTACKS BE PREVENTED?

A severe asthma attack is one requiring immediate medical attention and treatment with intravenous medication, usually in the emergency room or hospital. The fact that such attacks can usually be prevented may come as a surprise to those who have suffered the ravages of severe attacks, bouts with intravenous medication, trips to the emergency room, or hospitalization.

But remember that the airway obstruction in asthma is a reversible process. The problem is that, like Mrs. L., the prologue to the severe attack may go either unrecognized or under-treated. Both the patient and physician may be culpable.

The patient is often to blame by not seeking medical help until the attack is well under way, perhaps several days after symptoms have begun; by not taking the medication as prescribed; by continuing to smoke despite symptoms; or by not following up after an initial medical visit.

The physician may be culpable in failing to diagnose the condition as asthma; by not treating with enough medication; by not using steroids when indicated; or by not following up the patient closely enough.

Even with the best treatment and the most compliant patient, severe attacks may still occur. However, the vast majority are preventable.

WHERE CAN I GO FOR HELP IF I HAVE ASTHMA?

Any patient with asthma that is debilitating, limiting, or causing disruption in life-style should seek medical attention. Asthma is a treatable disease and one should not suffer needlessly. The best source for help is your personal or family physician. Most cases of asthma are treatable by most primary care physicians; all that is required is an interested and knowledgeable physician and a compliant patient. The number of available medications is huge and varied, and patients should not rely on over-the-counter medications unless the symptoms are very mild and easily reversible (see Chapter 11). By all means, if you don't feel adequately treated or your physician is unable to devote sufficient time to your problem, you should seek referral. There are many physicians who deal specifically with difficult asthmatic problems, and there should be one or more in your community.

This is not to say that all asthmatics need treatment by a specialist; most do not. Severe asthma, refractory to regular therapy, is relatively uncommon. Other reasons for lack of improvement are physician failure to treat adequately and patient non-compliance. Frequently, patients who don't respond with one physician will be referred on the initiative of that physician. However, if your personal physician is unable (for whatever reason) to manage adequately your case, you should do one of two things: Ask for referral to an allergist or pulmonary physician who specializes in the management of asthma; or if this is not possible, contact your local medical society for a referral in your area.

Several lung organizations (listed in Appendix A) may also be contacted for help in securing more information and referral to a specialist.

For no other lung disease is proper treatment so critical; asthma is a reversible and eminently treatable condition. It may require above average effort to achieve a proper balance of medical care and patient compliance, but for patients who can't breathe the effort is warranted. Until both the patient and physician are assured everything feasible has been tried there is no reason for anyone to suffer from asthma.

CHAPTER ELEVEN

Treatment of Asthma and Other Reversible Airway Problems

HOW IS ASTHMA TREATED?

Although there is usually no cure for asthma, the disease responds remarkably well to treatment. The specifics of treating asthma are highly variable and depend on its severity, prior patient response to medications, and so forth. Below are listed types of therapy commonly used in treating asthma.

Therapies 1 and 2 are usually used to prevent asthma symptoms or an asthma attack. Drugs are also used for this purpose, as will be discussed below. Therapies 3 through 6 are used in the active treatment of symptoms: shortness of breath, coughing, and wheezing. For practical purposes the treatment of asthma symptoms *is* drug therapy, the main subject of this chapter. Other therapies will be mentioned insofar as they interact with drug therapy. Although asthma symptoms will abate

TABLE 11-1 Therapy used in treating asthma

P	1. Avoidance of exciting stimuli
P	2. Allergy shots
Rx	3. Chest physiotherapy
Rx	4. Reassurance
Rx	5. Increased fluid intake
P,Rx	6. Drugs

P = prevention of asthma symptoms
Rx = treatment of symptoms

when a known stimulus is removed, the foundation for treating an asthma attack is drug therapy.

HOW ARE DRUGS USED TO TREAT ASTHMA?

There are hundreds of different medications used to treat asthma, but they can be divided into a few basic groups. The large number of drugs is in part due to manufacturers' combining several key ingredients in various ways to create a different *brand* of drug. In some cases a basic drug molecule will be altered slightly and then introduced as a "new" drug, although it is not really much different from the old one. For a list of oral and inhaled asthma formulations and combinations, see Appendix C.

A simple classification is useful; Table 11-2 groups all asthma drugs according to how they are administered. More than anything else, a patient will always remember how a drug is taken.

WHAT TYPES OF DRUGS ARE USED IN TREATING ASTHMA?

There are three fundamentally different types of medical compounds widely used in asthma. They are usually given to treat asthma symptoms, but may also be used to prevent an asthma flare-up. Virtually all patients who receive any asthma treatment will be taking one or more of these three basic drug types:

1. *Beta-Adrenergic Drugs.* Adrenergic drugs are related to adrenalin, a compound made by the adrenal gland. There are two broad types of adrenergic drugs, alpha and beta. Beta-adrenergic drugs are powerful bronchodilators. Alpha-adrenergic drugs may constrict the airway; hence, pure alpha drugs are not used in treating asthma.

   During an asthma attack the body's own adrenal output increases, but not nearly enough to open the airways. Amounts of beta-adrenergic drugs given for asthma are far in excess of what the body produces. These drugs act by stimulating nervous system endings in the airway muscles. This causes the muscles to relax, helping to open up the airways.

TABLE 11-2 Classification of drugs used in treating asthma by route of administration

Inhalation	Inhalation is usually of a powder or fine mist delivered from hand-held device; medicine may also be inhaled from a machine device.
Oral Ingestion	This includes all tablets, capsules, and liquids that are swallowed.
Rectal	This route is used for suppositories and enemas that contain medication.
Subcutaneous/Intramuscular	Some medications are administered by injection either under the skin or into the muscle.
Intravenous	Intravenous medications are given through a fine tube placed safely in a vein; this route is reserved for hospitalized patients.

2. *Theophylline.* Theophylline and derivatives of theophylline are a separate class of drugs from the adrenergic group. Theophylline is chemically related to caffeine, the stimulant in coffee and tea; like caffeine, theophylline is a mild stimulant. Theophylline drugs are potent bronchodilators.
3. *Corticosteroids.* This group of drugs is also found naturally in the body's adrenal gland, but in a different part than the adrenergic agents. Like the adrenergics, the body simply cannot produce enough corticosteroids during an asthma attack to keep the airways open.

Table 11-3 shows examples of the three major drug groups along with their routes of administration. A dash (–) means this class of drug is seldom or never used via that route. The drug examples given are generic–the common chemical name. Appendix C lists generic and brand names of most inhaled/oral asthma preparations used in the United States.

HOW DO THE ASTHMA DRUGS WORK?

Beta-adrenergic and theophylline drugs work by increasing an important body chemical called cyclic AMP. Normally present in small amounts, cyclic AMP is one of the major chemicals responsible for keeping the airways open. Any drug that tends to increase cyclic AMP has a bronchodilating (airway-opening) effect.

Fortunately, these drugs tend to increase cyclic AMP by different pathways. Beta-adrenergics increase the production of cyclic AMP. Theophylline helps prevent its natural breakdown in the body. The net result for either action is a buildup of cyclic AMP. (An analogy: your bank account can be increased by putting more money in–increased production–or by not taking any out; in the latter case, interest accumulates and your account is not broken down.) Because they operate by two different pathways, the two drug types are often used together for added benefit.

TABLE 11-3 Three major drug groups used in treating asthma

Route	Beta-Adrenergic	Theophylline*	Corticosteroids
Inhaled	Epinephrine Isoproterenol Isoetharine Metaproterenol Albuterol	-	Beclomethasone
Oral	Ephedrine Terbutaline Metaproterenol	Theophylline Aminophylline Dyphlline	Prednisone Methylprednisone
Suppositories	-	Aminophylline	-
Subcutaneous/ Intramuscular	Epinephrine Terbutaline	-	-
Intravenous	-	Aminophylline	Hydrocortisone Methylprednisone

*Including derivatives of theophylline.

The action of corticosteroids (usually abbreviated "steroids") is unknown. They don't act by increasing cyclic AMP. Steroids probably work by decreasing the inflammation and edema (swelling) present in the airways during an asthma attack. How they do so is unclear, but this doesn't deter from their use. They are the most powerful asthma drugs available and the sicker a patient the more likely steroids will be used. Also, since their action is different from adrenergic and theophylline drugs, steroids can and should be used in conjunction with them.

WHAT ARE THE DRUG REGIMENS USEFUL IN TREATING ASTHMA?

Ideally, asthmatics should never require treatment. By avoiding whatever excites the hypersensitive airways, an asthmatic should be able to breathe comfortably without medication. Unfortunately, this ideal is seldom realized for many, which is why drugs are so commonly used. The need for drugs may arise infrequently (once a year) or may be continuous, even life-long.

The variability of asthma is such that it's difficult to generalize about the type and frequency of drugs. Table 11-3 lists the types of drugs available and routes they can be given. For a particular patient in an individual situation, intelligent selection from the list is necessary. Possible drug combinations are shown in Table 11-4.

For *treating a patient* with asthma symptoms, the more severe the attack the more likely all three types of drugs will be used. Beta-adrenergic agents and theophylline may be used alone and can be effective in mild cases. Both together, plus steroids, will provide maximum pharmacologic treatment in most conditions, including those requiring hospitalization.

For *preventing an asthma attack* in someone free of symptoms the situation is a little different. Often just *one* drug on a continuous basis will suffice, usually oral theophylline or an inhaled steroid. Thus, oral theophylline can be used continuously to prevent exacerbations *or* to treat an exacerbation of asthma once begun. By contrast inhaled steroids are not effective once an attack has begun, since the dose is too small to be effective. (Cromolyn sodium is also used to prevent asthma symptoms; it is discussed in a later section).

The seven basic combinations allow for *thousands* of different therapeutic regimens when other factors are considered (for example: route of administration; dose of drug; brand name of drug; other compounds added to one of the basic three asthma drugs).

TABLE 11-4 Possible drug combinations for treating asthma

1. Beta-adrenergic drug alone
2. Theophylline drug alone
3. Corticosteroid alone
4. Beta-adrenergic + theophylline
5. Beta-adrenergic + corticosteroid
6. Theophylline + corticosteroid
7. Beta-adrenergic + theophylline + corticosteroid

Thus it is possible, indeed likely, that *patients with similar or identical symptoms can be treated equally well with different regimens.*

WHAT ARE THE SIDE EFFECTS OF ASTHMA MEDICATION?

Side effects are unwanted effects. All medication has the potential for producing side effects and asthma drugs are no exception. Fortunately, most side effects from asthma drugs are dose-related; by adjusting the dose the side effects will usually subside or disappear. Occasionally side effects are so severe that the drug must be stopped completely. Despite being generally dose-related, both the occurrence of side effects and tolerance to them vary greatly among individuals.

Principal unwanted effects from the three main drug types are discussed below.

Beta-Adrenergic Drugs

Most side effects from beta-adrenergic agents are due to stimulation of the nervous system and include nervousness, tremor, headache, palpitations, tachycardia (increased heart rate), sweating, and occasional muscle cramps. In addition some of these medications may cause drowsiness, nausea, and vomiting. The most common problem seems to be flushing and rapid heart rate soon after ingestion or injection of an adrenergic drug. Severe side effects are uncommon except in patients with underlying heart disease; such patients should use these drugs cautiously.

Theophylline and Theophylline Derivatives

The most frequent side effect of theophylline is gastrointestinal (GI) upset: nausea, vomiting, abdominal pain, or diarrhea. For unclear reasons, equivalent doses of theophylline are tolerated much better by some patients than others; this does not appear solely related to the blood level of the drug. Stopping the drug for a short period, or lowering the dose, will help relieve most GI symptoms.

Another potential problem is heart effects, similar to what can occur with adrenergic agents. Palpitations, tachycardia (fast heartbeat), and flushing may all occur with theophylline, as may low blood pressure. Taken to excess, or in the presence of underlying heart disease, severe heart arrhythmias (irregular heartbeats) may occur.

With very high doses seizures may occur; however, this is not a problem if recommended blood levels are maintained. Any patient with headaches, irritability, restlessness, insomnia, or muscle twitching should have a blood level test if the drug is to be continued.

Very severe side effects can often be prevented by checking the amount of theophylline in the blood and adjusting the dose accordingly. We now know that many factors can interfere with theophylline metabolism, including cigarette smoking, certain antibiotics, some anxiety medications, some antacids, and the presence of liver or heart disease. Also, theophylline is metabolized faster in younger patients than in older ones.

Corticosteroids

These drugs rarely cause immediate side effects like the above two groups, but are much more likely to cause long-term problems, particularly when maintained at high doses. The two most bothersome side effects are stimulation of appetite leading to weight gain and increased puffiness of the face, referred to as "moon face." Much more serious over the long term are development of diabetes and weakened bones; these don't happen to everyone on long-term steroids, and usually only occur if the dose has been maintained at a high level.

Another major and potentially serious side effect is permanent adrenal suppression. The body's adrenal glands (which sit on top of the kidneys) normally produce several types of steroids necessary for life. When steroids are given as a drug for treating asthma, the adrenal glands sense the high blood levels and shut off their own production. If the steroids are given for less than two weeks, the adrenal glands will start making the hormones again without difficulty. However for longer periods, especially after several months, the adrenal glands may not respond when the asthma drug is removed. Abrupt removal of steroid medication in the face of such adrenal suppression has proved fatal in a number of patients. One way to counteract this is to taper the steroids very slowly over several months, giving the adrenal glands a chance to respond.

Serious effects of corticosteroids are usually avoided if patients take only a short course of steroids—two weeks or less. Fortunately this duration is sufficient to treat most asthma flare-ups. Patients should not be maintained on long term oral steroids without a clear and compelling reason.

Despite the best intentions of physicians, many asthmatics do have to take steroids for months or years. Although the drugs are crucial for such steroid-dependent patients, every attempt should be made to minimize the risks. Physicians often try several stategies to help minimize side effects from prolonged use of steroids, including:

1. Substituting an inhaled steroid, called beclomethasone (brand name: Beclovent or Vanceril), for oral steroids. Beclomethasone is much safer to use long-term than steroid tablets. This is because when inhaled in recommended doses, it is not absorbed enough to give serious side effects. Substituting inhaled beclomethasone is most feasible in patients needing 10 milligrams or less of daily oral prednisone. Inhaled beclomethasone should only be used during stable asthma, when the patient feels comfortable and the dose of all asthma drugs is constant from day to day. During asthma attacks, the drug can be irritating and should not be used. Another potential problem is the confusion that sometimes arises between inhaled beclomethasone and inhaled beta-adrenergic medication. Both come in identically-shaped canisters, but only the beta-adrenergic will provide relief during an asthma attack. Unfortunately, some patients who have both drugs mistakenly rely on the beclomethasone during attacks, to no avail. Despite these limitations, inhaled beclomethasone is an excellent drug, and should be tried in all steroid-dependent asthmatics.
2. Using the lowest oral dose compatible with patient comfort and ability to function. Steroids should not be maintained solely to normalize breathing tests, but to allow the patient to be relatively symptom free and comfortable. Regardless of the dose used, frequent and continuing attempts should be made to wean off steroids completely.

3. Using an alternate day schedule, where the dose of oral steroid is taken every other day. This minimizes some of the adrenal suppression and other side effects, although it may also lead to flare-up of symptoms on the day steroids are not taken.
4. Using antacids. Steroids can cause an upset stomach, and may aggravate peptic ulcer in patients susceptible to this condition, particularly when high doses are used. This effect can be minimized if antacids are taken along with the steroids. Antacids are not routinely needed for most asthmatics taking steroids.
5. Monitoring the blood periodically for its acid content. Steroids tend to cause an imbalance in blood acidity that can be corrected with potassium chloride or other medication.

WHAT IS THE PROPER DOSE OF ASTHMA MEDICATION?

There is no simple answer to this question. Appendix C lists well over a hundred different tablets, capsules, sprays, and elixirs marketed for asthma. Within each group (such as theophylline preparations, Table C-2) there are enough different compounds (and strengths of each compound) to make any generalization meaningless. However, the problem of proper dose of asthma medication far transcends the cornucopia of drugs provided by the pharmaceutical industry. The answer to this question must take into account both the *extreme variability of asthma as a disease* and the equally marked *variability of patient response to asthma drugs.* For these reasons equivalent asthma drugs, taken as prescribed, may help one patient and not another, or help one patient through an attack the first time, but not the second.

The variability of asthma has been discussed. Once an attack has set in, its course may be slow or fast, mild or severe. Any experience with previous attacks is probably the best guide to current management. Drugs that worked before (number, dose, duration of therapy) are likely to work again.

Beta-Adrenergic Drugs

The bulk of beta-adrenergic medication in this country is taken via simple, hand-held nebulizers. These should always be used as prescribed, or as directed in the specific product circular (drug-insert); generally one puff or two puffs a minute apart are enough to provide relief from mild asthma symptoms.

The tablet and liquid forms of beta-adrenergic drugs provide longer-lasting effects. The actual milligram (mg) dose depends on the type of drug. For ephedrine the recommended dose is 25 mg, three to four times a day. This is a popular component of combination bronchodilators, each tablet of which usually contains 25 mg ephedrine.

Terbutaline and metaproterenol are designed to provide longer bronchodilating action with less of the jittery side effects of ephedrine. The dose of terbutaline is between 2.5 and 5 mg, three to four times a day. The recommended adult dose of metaproterenol is 20 mg three to four times a day. The recommended dose of albuterol is 2 to 4 mg, four times a day.

In practice, all of the oral beta-adrenergic drugs may give side effects; their continuous or prolonged use should be under physician supervision. Also, as will be discussed below, *any recommended dose of asthma medication may have to be modified depending on the patient's course and response to therapy.*

Theophylline Preparations

When inhaled or oral adrenergic drugs are not sufficient to relieve symptoms, a theophylline preparation is usually added. Depending on severity, *both* an adrenergic and theophylline drug may be started together. Also, many physicians prefer to start with theophylline, adding an adrenergic drug if needed.

Specific dosage guidelines for beginning therapy with oral theophylline are shown in Table 11-5. Note that the recommended dose varies according to age and the presence of an underlying disease that might interfere with the drug. These are guidelines only; *in actual practice the subsequent maintenance dose may have to be modified often.*

Corticosteroids

Corticosteroids are usually employed for severe asthma; this includes asthma symptoms unresponsive or poorly responsive to beta-adrenergic and theophylline drugs. Since steroids have the potential for severe side effects when used at high doses for prolonged periods, the goal is always to stop steroids in less than two weeks if possible. Sometimes this is not feasible because of the severity of the asthma; in such cases the lowest possible maintenance dose that will help the patient is employed.

TABLE 11-5 Recommended dosage of theophylline for treating patients suffering asthma symptoms*

Age of Patient	Initial (Loading) Dose	Maintenance Dose
6 months-9 years	6 mg/kilogram (kg)+	4 mg/kg every 6 hours
9 yrs-16 yrs & young adult smokers	6 mg/kg	3 mg/kg every 6 hours
Otherwise healthy adults (non-smokers)	6 mg/kg	3 mg/kg every 8 hours
Older patients and patients with chronic lung disease	6 mg/kg	2 mg/kg every 8 hours
Patients with heart failure or liver disease	6 mg/kg	1-2 mg/kg every 12 hours

* These guidelines are for patients not currently receiving any theophylline preparation. The dose given here is based on pure theophylline. For theophylline derivatives the equivalent amount of pure theophylline is given in Appendix C, Table 2.

\+ Kilogram is a metric unit of weight. 1 kg = 2.2 pounds. The maintenance dose is a general recommendation and in practice is modified often depending on patient response, tolerance, and measurement of theophylline in the blood. The maintenance dose is based on ideal or lean body weight, whereas the loading dose is based on actual or total body weight.

The steroid dose most frequently prescribed for outpatients is about six to ten times the body's own daily output of this hormone. Since we normally make the equivalent of about 5 mg of prednisone a day, the asthma dose is roughly 30-50 mg a day, *to start.* A tapering method is commonly used to get the patient off the drug in less than two weeks. The following case illustrates the use of drugs in asthma.

Howard G. is a 33-year-old mechanic referred for continued shortness of breath interfering with his work and sleep. He has suffered intermittent asthma symptoms for many years, usually controlled with puffs of inhaled bronchodilator. Since a viral infection two months ago he's had continued problems with cough and wheezing, and hardly a night goes by that he doesn't wake up to use his inhaler. He has also been taking an over-the-counter drug containing theophylline and ephedrine, which has helped a little.

He is wheezing at rest and gets short of breath walking across the room. His breathing test shows definite airway obstruction. Clearly the combination pill is not sufficient; it is stopped and he is prescribed the following regimen (Table 11-6):

TABLE 11-6 Regimen for patient Howard G.

	Beta-Adrenergic Drug	Theophylline Drug	Corticosteroid
Day 1	Two puffs of albuterol inhaler 4 times a day, plus as needed (not more frequently than every 3 hours)	Sustained-release theophylline tablets, 300 mg each; take 2 initially, then one every 12 hours	Prednisone, 5 mg tablets Take 8 the first day (total 40 mg) all in the morning
Day 2	Same as day 1 (this is maintenance regimen and is continued daily)	1 every 12 hours (this is maintenance regimen and is continued daily)	7 Prednisone tablets (total 35 mg) as above
Day 3	As above	As above	6 Prednisone tablets (30 mg)
Day 4	As above	As above	5 Prednisone tablets (25 mg)
Day 5	As above	As above	4 Prednisone tablets (20 mg)
Day 6	As above	As above	3 Prednisone tablets (15 mg)
Day 7	As above	As above	2 Prednisone tablets (10 mg)
Day 8	As above	As above	1 Prednisone tablet (5 mg)
Day 9	As above	As above	No Prednisone tablets

Several points can be made about this case.

1. Mr. G. is suffering from severe asthma but does not, in my opinion, require hospitalization. He *does require* treatment with all three drug types used for symptomatic asthma.
2. Although the above regimen is *prescribed* for Mr. G., I will be in frequent telephone contact and may well make changes, depending on side effects, change in symptoms, and so forth (See next section). Mr. G. understands that the steroids are to be tapered, but that the beta-adrenergic and theophylline drugs may be continued at a level amount.
3. The specific drug used within each group (beta-adrenergic, theophylline, and corticosteroid) is not critically important (see Appendix C for many possibilities). What is important is a definite regimen for beginning therapy, and close patient follow-up.

There is marked improvement in Mr. G's symptoms by the third day. Two weeks later breathing tests confirm definite improvement in airflow; by this time the steroids have been discontinued. The dose of inhaled albuterol is lowered to an "as needed" basis and theophylline is maintained for a few more weeks until it too is discontinued.

WHY IS THERE A VARIABLE RESPONSE TO ASTHMA THERAPY?

It has long been known that asthmatics with similar symptoms may vary markedly in response to identical asthma therapy. There are several possible reasons for this.

1. *Different causes* of asthma attack. As defined earlier the asthma syndrome is one of hypersensitive airways and can respond to a variety of stimuli. Although attacks may appear similar in severity, the underlying stimulus may affect drug response. For example, a patient who is allergic to cats and who remains around them may not respond as well as another patient whose asthma is exacerbated by a common cold that soon runs its course. Similarly, long-term cigarette smokers may develop asthma that doesn't respond as well as asthma in nonsmokers, though examination and breathing tests may be similar before initiating treatment.
2. *Type of obstruction.* Asthmatics whose airway obstruction is mainly from bronchospasm respond better than those whose airways are filled with thick, tenacious mucus (mucus plugs). On initial examination there is no way to know for sure the relative components of each. Generally, the more mucus plugs, the more severe the asthma. The lungs of patients who die from asthma are invariably filled with mucus plugs.
3. *Variability of drug metabolism.* Different patients may metabolize, or break down, the drug theophylline at different rates. For this reason, four tablets of theophylline/day may be toxic for one patient and have no effect on another. When blood levels of the drug are measured, we find the former patient has too much, the latter too little of the drug. Why?

   We know that theophylline metabolism (breakdown to inactive compound) can be influenced by many factors, some tending to *decrease* metabolism (and hence *raise* the amount of effective medication in the blood), others tending to have the opposite effect. These factors are all relative, so that physicians need only be aware of them and adjust the manufacturer's recommended dose (which tends to be an average) for each patient.

4. *Taking drugs incorrectly.* Whenever multiple drugs are prescribed there are many chances for patient error. Lack of expected response can often be traced to improper use of prescribed drugs. The common mistakes are:
   a. Quitting medication prematurely. After the patient feels a little better he stops the drugs, only to have symptoms flare again in a day or so. Many asthma attacks are not over when a patient begins to feel better; proper treatment may require prolonged medication. This is best gauged by breathing tests or by the experience of the physician managing the problem.
   b. Misunderstanding the difference between medication prescribed to *prevent* symptoms and medication prescribed to *treat* symptoms once they occur. This most commonly occurs with inhaled beclomethasone and inhaled cromolyn; both are prescribed only to prevent asthma flare-ups, not treat them. Patients may incorrectly stop these drugs when they feel better or first use them when they have trouble breathing.
   c. Improperly using beta-adrenergic inhalers. This is a common error. Some coordination is required to inhale the spray that comes from these devices; careful observation of some patients shows they don't inhale the medication properly and hence do not receive the intended dose. Proper technique is discussed in a later question.

To a great extent you—or any patient—can prevent these problems by learning about these drugs. This means asking questions, reading package inserts, and going over a new drug with your doctor whenever it is first used.

WHAT ELSE CAN AFFECT PATIENT RESPONSE TO ASTHMA DRUGS?

There are many other possible reasons for variability of patient response. Emotional reaction to illness, disruption of work or lifestyle, patient-physician interaction—all are factors that may affect the outcome of asthma therapy. It is only on follow-up, over days, weeks, or longer that the pattern and degree or response will become evident.

For outpatients the best course is to take the medication recommended, then have it adjusted either at follow-up visits or over the phone. Proper adjustment will depend on side effects, response of the asthma, and, when necessary, measurement of drug levels of theophylline. This method makes drug therapy for asthma a dynamic process and necessitates frequent interaction between the patient and his or her doctor. For mild attacks or chronic asthma, once the patient has been evaluated or is already well known to the doctor, much of this drug manipulation may be handled over the phone. For patients unresponsive to oral therapy, hospitalization and intravenous therapy are usually required.

ARE GENERIC DRUGS USED IN ASTHMA?

Generic drugs are those marketed under their chemical name only, without a brand name. For example, a drug sold simply as "theophylline" would be a generic; it is also available under several brand names and marketed as such (Appendix C). In theory the chemical and biologic nature of any generic drug should be equivalent to its brand name counterpart. Since generics are not advertised heavily, many people think prescribing generically is a way of getting the same drug at a lower price.

In fact this is not always the case. Generic prescribing is a complex issue about which few generalizations hold. For some drugs, such as the widely used heart pill digoxin, the generics have been found to be not as good as the same drug sold under its brand name, Lanoxin®. For other drugs there is no generic available, the medication being so new that the original pharmaceutical developers are the only ones currently marketing the drug. This is the case for the adrenergic drug terbutaline (Appendix C), marketed under only two brands, Brethine® and Bricanyl®.

For other drugs, generics are available but not generally stocked by individual pharmacies. A patient who has been prescribed theophylline without a specified brand name will still likely receive a brand name product. There are so many theophylline brands on the market and physicians are so used to writing for a specific company's product that many pharmacies do not bother stocking a generic product and will fill a generic prescription with one of the available brands.

For corticosteroids the situation is reversed. Pharmaceutical manufacturers do not advertise or push particular brands of steroids for asthma therapy and physicians usually prescribe this group generically.

In summary, generic drugs are rarely used in outpatient asthma when an adrenergic or theophylline drug is prescribed and almost invariably used when a corticosteroid is given. This is a result more of advertising patterns and physician prescribing habits than of any inherent advantage in terms of cost and efficacy.

WHAT OTHER DRUGS ARE USED IN ASTHMA?

Adrenergics, theophylline, and corticosteroids are universally used in treating symptomatic asthma. However they are frequently given along with other medications. These are listed in Table 11-7 and discussed in questions that follow.

None of these drugs is specific for treating asthma symptoms or an asthma attack. For the symptoms of asthma–cough, shortness of breath, chest tightness, wheezing–one or more of the three basic drug types (adrenergics, theophylline, corticosteroids) will invariably be used.

WHAT IS CROMOLYN SODIUM?

Cromolyn sodium is a relatively new type of asthma medication altogether different from the basic drugs discussed earlier. Cromolyn is used only by inhalation and

TABLE 11-7 Other medications commonly received by asthmatics

Cromolyn sodium
Cough medications, including expectorants
Mucolytics
Antihistamines
Antibiotics
Sedatives

only to prevent asthma symptoms, not to treat them. (Research is under way on using the drug in tablet form.) The brand name is Intal and it is available only by prescription.

Cromolyn can be inhaled either as a drug powder or in a nebulized solution; the drug powder comes in a capsule that is placed in a device called a spinhaler; the spinhaler punctures the capsule and allows the powder to be inhaled. The spinhaler is the same size as other hand-held inhalers and so is easily portable.

The nebulized solution of cromolyn comes in a capsule and requires a power-driven nebulizer and face mask. Although this can be set up at home, the requirement for a piece of special apparatus confines its use mainly to hospitals.

Cromolyn is used more in children than in adults, although it should not be used in children under age five. Many physicians feel cromolyn is the best drug to prevent asthma attacks caused by animal dander and other allergens; such attacks seem to be more prevalent in children than in adults. Cromolyn is also useful in all ages for preventing attacks of exercise-induced asthma. As an asthma preventative cromolyn can be taken alone or with other drugs.

WHAT ARE EXPECTORANTS?

As a group expectorants are probably one of the least understood of the commonly used drugs. The word expectorate means to cough or spit out material from the lungs. An expectorant is a drug that is supposed to aid the patient in coughing up mucus. Because expectorants are widely prescribed for cough many patients mistakenly think they are for suppressing the cough. In fact, expectorants are not cough suppressants; if anything they are given to encourage more effective coughing.

Expectorants are frequently combined with bronchodilators* and marketed for asthma since thick, tenacious sputum is often part of the asthma condition. Expectorants used in conjunction with bronchodilators are:

- Guaifenesin (also known as glycerylguaiacolate or GG)
- Potassium Iodide (KI since K is the chemical symbol for potassium)
- Iodinated glycerol

Appendix C lists asthma preparations containing these compounds. Another expectorant widely employed for cold remedies is terpin hydrate, not apparently used in asthma drugs.

Expectorants are also available as separate drugs and, in the case of guaifenesin, advertised widely and sold over-the-counter. Unfortunately, unlike bronchodilators, the efficacy of expectorant drugs has never been proved. Although some studies have purportedly found them effective in mobilizing sputum, the doses employed were invariably much greater than commonly prescribed and certainly greater than available in combination drugs. Despite the lack of scientific

*A pill or liquid preparation containing an expectorant and bronchodilator is technically termed a "combination." However, these drugs should be carefully distinguished from combination asthma drugs that contain two bronchodilators. Each drug in the latter group is footnoted in Appendix C.

proof of efficacy, expectorants enjoy wide popularity as can be seen from reviewing Appendix C, Table 2.

Perhaps the safest and cheapest expectorant is *water.* Asthma patients are routinely advised to drink plenty of water, in the belief that it will help thin the bronchial secretions. Dehydration can certainly make an asthma condition worse, so there is a ring of common sense to this advice. However, there is no evidence that extra water (in excess of what would normally be ingested) is all that beneficial. At the very least asthma patients should avoid becoming dehydrated.

Water is also frequently given by inhalation in the form of a hot or cold mist; different patients prefer different temperatures. Some patients are irritated by inhaling water in this form so it cannot be universally recommended. (If tap water is used in any inhalation equipment it should first be boiled to remove impurities.) Inhaled salt water (saline) is also commonly used and is a definite expectorant in concentrated solution. However, in any strength saline may worsen bronchospasm; when used in asthma therapy it should be given along with an inhaled bronchodilator.

WHAT ARE MUCOLYTICS?

These are drugs designed to lyse or break up the mucus, hence the term mucolytic. Currently the only mucolytic recommended is a chemical known as acetylcysteine. A problem with acetylcysteine, and one reason it is not more widely used, is its potential to cause bronchospasm in asthmatics. Acetylcysteine is used mainly in hospitals and then only in conjunction with a bronchodilator drug to help prevent bronchospasm.

At least one manufacturer now markets a liquid combination of acetylcysteine and isoproterenol (a quick-acting bronchodilator) that may be nebulized and inhaled by patients at home. It is available only by prescription and should be used cautiously.

IS THERE ANY ROLE FOR ANTIHISTAMINES IN ASTHMA?

Histamine is a chemical responsible for many abnormal body reactions: the nasal swelling and stuffiness we get with the common cold; the red, itchy blotches on our skin from some allergic reactions; and, in part, the wheezing seen in asthma. For reasons that are unclear however, antihistamines are *not* effective in treating asthma symptoms or in preventing them. In fact antihistamines tend to cause drying of mucous membranes; this may be good for the nose but can make mucus in the bronchial tube harder to cough up.

For these reasons antihistamines should not be used during asthma attacks except under a physician's recommendation.

WHEN SHOULD ANTIBIOTICS BE USED IN ASTHMA?

This question is harder to answer than it may seem. Respiratory infections are the most common trigger of asthma attacks. But they are invariably *viral* infections, not bacterial. And viral infections do not respond to antibiotics.

Despite this fact many physicians commonly prescribe antibiotics during an asthma attack. This is not necessarily wrong since it is possible some bacteria-like organisms (not full-fledged bacteria) may precipitate an asthma attack, and these are sensitive to antibiotics. Yet the exact cause of infection is almost never documented during an asthma attack. Proof of viral infections, the most common infectious cause, comes long after the attack has subsided, usually by examining blood collected over a period of time.

In practice, antibiotics are not routinely recommended for asthma symptoms unless other findings are present, including:

- Underlying chronic bronchitis, which may be exacerbated by bacterial or bacterial-like infection
- Fever and/or sputum examination that suggest a bacterial or bacterial-like infection

In such conditions it seems wisest to use either tetracycline or erythromycin, since these are effective against both bacteria and bacteria-like organisms. In any case antibiotics are only adjunctive therapy in symptomatic asthma and should not be used without concomitant bronchodilators.

ARE SEDATIVES USEFUL?

Sedatives are included in many combination asthma medications (see Appendix C). Their purpose is to counteract the jitteriness from the bronchodilators and not to treat the asthma per se. Anxiety and nervousness are of course also part of the asthma syndrome. Do sedatives have a role in treating these asthma symtpoms?

Definitely not! Sedatives should *never* be used in the setting of an acute asthma attack. First, they may depress breathing, and have been thought responsible for some sudden deaths in asthma. Second, they are a poor attempt to treat a manifestation of trouble breathing; the problem is shortness of breath, not the anxiety that results. Third, sedatives may blunt this anxiety (as they are intended to do) and give a false sense of security to both patient and physician. By lowering the level of anxiety and apprehension, without at the same time improving airflow, the severity of the asthma may be underestimated. This could prove fatal.

The mild, stable, chronic asthmatic patient may safely take anti-anxiety medication, Valium® and Librium® being among the safest. But note the important distinction. Unstable, actutely ill patients–those whose asthma is clearly changing for the worse or not improving–should NEVER take sedatives as part of their asthma treatment.

HOW SHOULD INHALERS BE USED IN TREATING ASTHMAS?

An inhaler is a hand-held device that contains asthma medication under pressure. A push on the inhaler delivers a predetermined dose of drug into the airways. If the patient synchronizes the push with the proper inspiratory effort, the medication will enter the airways; if this synchrony does not occur, the medication will not be effectively delivered. Figures 11-1a-e outline proper steps in using an inhaler.

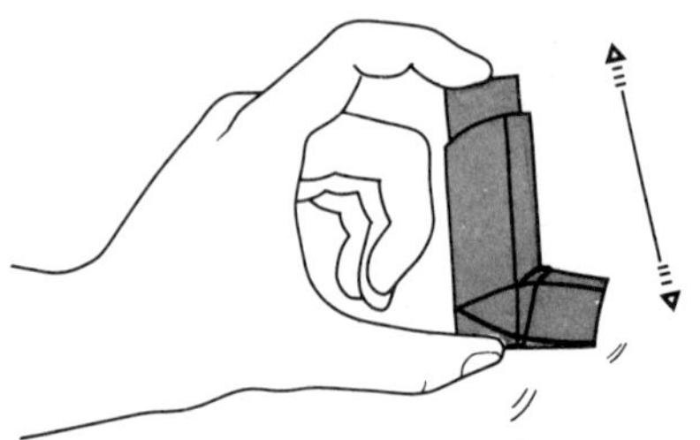

FIGURE 11-1a After removing cap from mouthpiece, shake the inhaler for a few seconds.

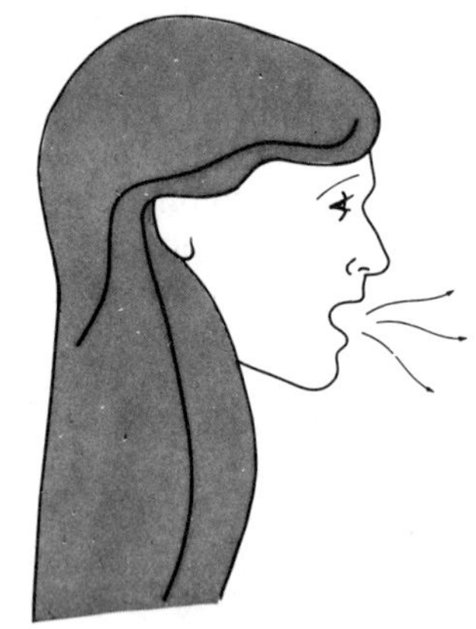

FIGURE 11-1b Breathe out fully, blowing out as much air as possible from your lungs.

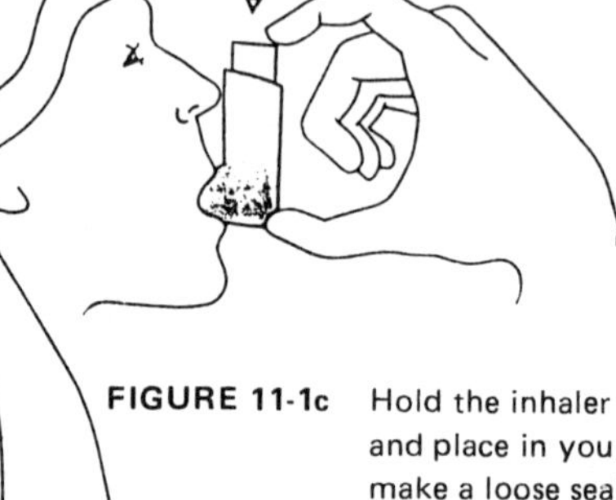

FIGURE 11-1c Hold the inhaler upright and place in your mouth; make a loose seal with your lips around the inhaler.

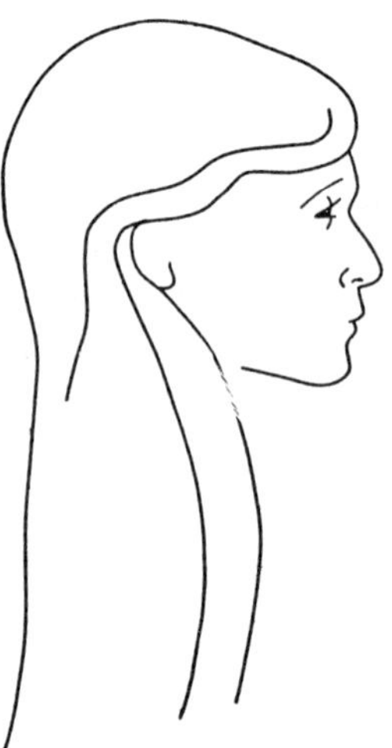

FIGURE 11-1e Remove the inhaler and hold your breath for a few seconds; then resume normal breathing. Wait at least one minute before repeating steps outlined in Figures 11-1, a-d. (Most inhaler medication calls for taking two puffs at a time; these puffs should be at least one minute apart.)

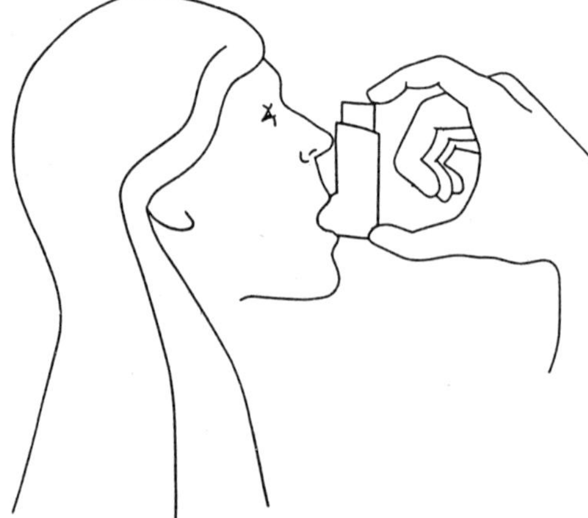

FIGURE 11-1d Breathe in deeply and *at the same time* press the inhaler between your forefinger and thumb. This will expel the medication from the inhaler into your throat and lungs.

Treatment errors frequently occur with the use of inhalers, the most common being improper use of the device. For example, if the canister is pressed only *after* taking in a deep breath, medication will not enter the lungs.

Another common error is using the wrong inhaler (the wrong medication) for a particular problem. There are three basic types of asthma medication that can be delivered via hand-held inhalers: beta-adrenergic agents, corticosteroids, and cromolyn sodium*. Note that theophylline is not available as an inhalant. The list of currently available inhalers, and their uses, is shown in Table 11-8.

Cromolyn is only used to prevent asthma flare-ups, not to treat them once begun. Of the corticosteroids, only beclomethasone is in common use today and it is designed only for prevention of symptoms. (Another corticosteroid, dexamethasone, is also available for inhalation to treat asthma symptoms, but is rarely used.) Thus, only the beta-adrenergic agents are routinely used as inhalants for treating asthma symptoms.

Several different types of beta-adrenergic drugs can be inhaled (Table 11-8). They all can provide quick relief when used properly for mild symptoms. Many asthma patients carry an inhaler with them wherever they go, to use on an as needed basis.

Cromolyn sodium and beclomethasone, on the other hand, should only be used for prevention. To be effective these drugs must be inhaled regularly, usually three to four times a day, while the asthmatic patient is *well.*

WHAT ARE COMBINATION DRUGS?

Combination drugs contain more than one active bronchodilator compound. A drug that contains both an adrenergic and a theophylline compound in the same tablet or capsule is a combination drug. Combination drugs never include a corticosteroid.

Many patients can be treated effectively with combination drugs. Besides theophylline and an adrenergic agent, the combination often includes a mild sedative to counteract side effects of the bronchodilator, or an expectorant to help raise phlegm. A commonly used combination drug is Tedral**, each tablet of which contains:

24 milligrams ephedrine
130 milligrams theophylline
8 milligrams phenobarbital

TABLE 11-8 Inhalers for asthma (brand names in parentheses)

To Prevent Attacks	To Treat or Prevent Attacks
Cromolyn (Intal)	Metaproterenol (Alupent; Metaprel)
Beclomethasone (Beclovent; Vanceril)	Epinephrine (Primatene)
	Isoetharine (Bronkosol)
	Albuterol (Proventil; Ventolin)
	Isoproterenol (Isuprel)

*A fourth type, called "anti-cholinergic," is under active investigation.

**A list of most oral and inhalation drugs used in the treatment of asthma, including combination preparations by brand name, is in Appendix C.

The phenobarbital is a barbiturate, given in a very low dose (100 milligrams is the usual dose when used as a sleeping pill); it helps counteract the side effects of ephedrine, which are mostly a mild jitteriness and fast heartbeat.

Other ingredients that have been added to the major asthma compounds (adrenergics, theophylline, and steroids) include:

- guaifenesin, an expectorant
- potassium iodide, an expectorant
- hydroxyzine, a mild sedative
- butabarbital, another barbiturate

You can begin to appreciate the large number of combination drugs possible by varying the ingredients, dosages, and form of the drug (most can be taken as either tablet or liquid).

ARE COMBINATION DRUGS BETTER THAN SINGLE DRUGS TAKEN SEPARATELY?

Combination drugs have been used for many years and are certainly more convenient to take than several single drugs. Also, they are often cheaper than comparable products taken separately. Combination drugs are used widely in mild cases of asthma, particularly when over-the-counter products are purchased in lieu of prescription drugs.

For more severe or protracted cases of asthma combination drugs have several disadvantages:

1. *Inability to control the dose of each ingredient.* If the asthma condition worsens there may be less need for some of the ingredients and more for others. As we discussed earlier, asthma treatment often requires medications specifically tailored to individual circumstances. This cannot be done as well with combination preparations, since to increase or decrease a combination drug is to change all the components at the same time. For example, to increase Tedral because the patient needs more theophylline is to increase both ephedrine (that may make one jittery) and phenobarbital (that may make one drowsy).

2. *Inability to attribute side effects.* All asthma medications have potential unwanted effects. If they occur from a combination drug it is often difficult (if not impossible) to tell which ingredient is the culprit. Separate drugs could be stopped one at a time without removing all asthma-relieving medication at once. This is not possible with combination drugs.

3. *Inclusion of drugs with marginal or no benefit.* Although subject to some controversy, the best medical evidence has not shown any direct benefit in asthma from the extra, added ingredients in combination drugs. This includes all the expectorants, sedatives, and other agents added to the three basic asthma drugs. Some of these added compounds may help counteract side effects of the active drugs, but even this is of doubtful benefit.

4. *Toxicity from ignorance of what is being taken.* When a patient has seen more than one physician and has multiple prescriptions, or is taking over-the-

counter medications plus prescription drugs, toxicity may result. For example, a patient may be taking Marax by prescription, but later obtains Tedral (over-the-counter) for extra relief. Since both contain theophylline there is risk of resulting theophylline toxicity. If the patient knew he was already taking this active compound, there would be less likelihood of taking another drug containing theophylline.

WITH THESE PROBLEMS WHY ARE COMBINATIONS USED AT ALL?

People will always prefer a single pill to two or three. Also combinations *do work* for many asthmatics–although this no doubt because of the active compounds and not the extra ingredients. There is a shift away from combinations and toward individual drug use; the last several years have seen introduction of more single drug brands than of combination brands.

Combination drugs will probably remain popular over-the-counter medications. These are bought and used by many asthmatics and are fine for uncomplicated, responsive, mild asthma. Beyond that–and this distinction is up to the patient–medical care is necessary and the patient is more apt to be prescribed non-combination drugs.

Regardless of what is used, it remains most important that the patient know *what it contains* and that *it helps.* If you take asthma medication look up your drug(s) in Appendix C to be sure you are not taking different drugs that contain the same or similar ingredients.

ARE NON-PRESCRIPTION DRUGS EFFECTIVE FOR ASTHMA?

Several non-prescription drugs for asthma are identical in potency to those available only with a doctor's Rx (Appendix C). Tedral, a popular combination asthma drug, is available without an Rx in those states where low dose phenobarbital doesn't require a prescription. Primatene tablets, another popular non-Rx asthma medication, comes in two formulations so it can be sold without a prescription everywhere:

PRIMATENE P	PRIMATENE M
Theophylline 130 mg	Theophylline 130 mg
Ephedrine 24 mg	Ephedrine 24 mg
Phenobarbital 8 mg	Pyrilamine 16.6 mg

Note the similarity of Primatene tablets to Marax, which is available only by a doctor's prescription:

MARAX

Theophylline 130 mg
Ephedrine 25 mg
Hydroxyzine 10 mg

In each of the combination drugs the active ingredients are theophylline and ephedrine, both effective for mild asthma symptoms. The added compound (phenobarbital, pyrilamine or hydroxyzine) is to counteract the side effects (jitteriness) of ephedrine and is not a bronchodilator. It is also the non-bronchodilator compound that determines the drug's prescription status; pyrilamine or phenobarbital are allowed in some states, hydroxyzine is allowed in none (requirement of the Federal Food and Drug Administration).

Because of vagaries in both diagnosis and treatment of asthma, one should not self-medicate without a prior established diagnosis of asthma. Nor should these non-prescription drugs be taken for long periods without physician guidance. They also should not be used whenever symptoms truly limit you in daily activity.

CAN PREGNANT PATIENTS TAKE ASTHMA MEDICATION?

Asthma is an unpredictable condition. Thus, it is no great surprise that during pregnancy–a time the mother experiences normal physiologic stress and profound hormonal changes–underlying asthma can stay the same, get worse, or improve. In fact a review of the reported cases in the medical literature reveals that about one-third of pregnant asthmatics fall into each category.

As a general rule, useful asthma medication should not be withheld during pregnancy. Although no drug can ever be certified completely safe during gestation, experience and animal studies show each of the three major drug types useful in asthma can be taken by pregnant patients. No pregnant patient should ever suffer an asthma attack for fear of harming the fetus with drugs that may help the mother. Indeed the most significant risk to the fetus is hypoxia, so every attempt should be made to relieve pregnant patients of respiratory distress.

Thus, the treatment of pregnant asthmatics differs little in principle from treating other patients: use the number and amount of drugs that give the most benefit with the fewest side effects. In addition of course, avoidance of any potential asthma triggers is mandatory, such as cigarette smoke, known allergens, and drugs a particular patient may react to (such as aspirin). Other drugs commonly used in treating asthma, that should be avoided by all pregnant patients, are the antibiotic tetracycline (may stain teeth of fetus), preparations containing iodine (may interfere with fetal thyroid function), and sedatives (may cause fetal deformities).

HOW ARE ASTHMA MEDICATIONS USED IN CHRONIC BRONCHITIS AND EMPHYSEMA?

Chronic bronchitis and emphysema are discussed in the next chapter. For now it is important to point out that they may overlap with asthma and thus be treated with the same medications outlined in this chapter. Whenever a physician diagnoses reversible airways obstruction, regardless of whether the underlying disease is pure asthma, bronchitis, emphysema, sarcoidosis, or cystic fibrosis, the treatment modalities and principles outlined in this chapter apply.

WHAT IS THE FUTURE FOR ASTHMA THERAPY?

Drug therapy should become far more effective, although real breakthroughs uncovering the basic cause of asthma are still in the future. In the near future a new type of bronchodilator that works on a mechanism different from both the beta-adrenergic and theophylline drugs should enter the drug market. Called anti-cholinergic, this type of medication has already been used for several years in Europe. Although a different type of medication, it does not promise to add significantly to the regimens already in use.

There are many other potential drugs, of a more experimental nature, that will probably enter the market for asthma therapy in the next decade. An example is some type of prostaglandin, a compound normally in our body (see question on Asthma and Aspirin).

One exciting breakthrough has been uncovering the structure of some of the chemical mediators of asthma, such as SRS or slow reacting substance. This is one of a number of compounds released when a stimulus triggers an asthma attack. Perhaps this will lead to an anti-SRS medication.

Based on past experience, none of the conceivable new drugs will be a wonder drug. Several new asthma medications have recently been introduced, each heralded widely and advocated strongly by some physicians and patients. But the fact remains that all asthma drugs have major limitations or side effects and none has proved a dramatic breakthrough for the majority of patients. No medication on the horizon is likely to be curative (as penicillin is for some pneumonias) or fully preventative (such as polio vaccine). The cause of asthma is unknown and any possible cure remains elusive.

CHAPTER TWELVE

Chronic Bronchitis and Emphysema: "COPD"

WHY ARE BRONCHITIS AND EMPHYSEMA CONSIDERED TOGETHER?

Chronic bronchitis and pulmonary emphysema are the main causes of chronic respiratory disability in the United States today. They account for over 50,000 deaths each year; between five and ten million Americans are partially or totally disabled from these conditions. Because the diseases share many common characteristics, they are often referred to as chronic obstructive pulmonary disease or COPD for short. (Some physicians use the term chronic obstructive lung disease or COLD; since this can be confused with the common cold, COPD is a preferred abbreviation).

Chronic bronchitis and emphysema are due mainly to long-term cigarette smoking. Both conditions lead to damaged airways and shortness of breath. (Figure 12-1 illustrates how most physicians view the two conditions). Although there are specific differences, and patients may manifest predominantly chronic bronchitis or emphysema, many patients suffering from COPD have elements of both.

To put these diseases in perspective, questions on bronchitis will be answered first, followed by questions on emphysema. Keep in mind the common cause and clinical overlap in most cases.

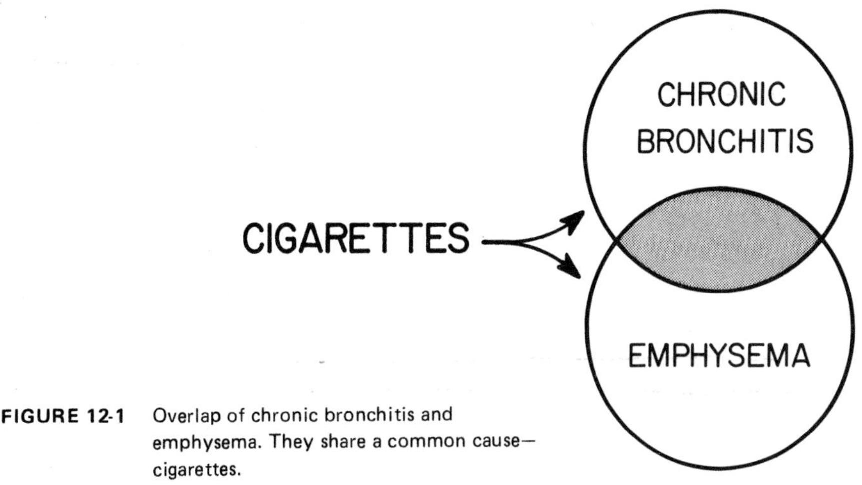

FIGURE 12-1 Overlap of chronic bronchitis and emphysema. They share a common cause—cigarettes.

WHAT IS BRONCHITIS?

Bronchitis is inflammation of the airways of the lungs that leads to increased mucus production, making people cough. It can occur in various forms but is usually divided into "acute" and "chronic." In acute bronchitis you feel very sick and have a hacking cough; this is usually accompanied by fever and flu-like symptoms. In the chronic form you cough up mucus daily for at least several months each year but don't feel acutely ill. People with chronic bronchitis are usually able to work unless the disease is far advanced. Because everyone coughs sometimes, the medical definition for chronic bronchitis requires daily cough and mucus production for at least 3 months of the year for 2 consecutive years.

Acute bronchitis is usually due to a virus or bacterial infection; the infecting organism settles in the airways and leads to inflammation and increased amounts of mucus production. Acute bronchitis may occur in nonsmokers as well as in patients with COPD. Treatment with antibiotics leads to recovery within a few days unless there is a complication.

Chronic bronchitis is most commonly due to cigarette smoking, although there are other causes (see below).

IS CHRONIC BRONCHITIS JUST A "REACTION" TO IRRITANTS, OR IS IT A SPECIFIC DISEASE?

Chronic bronchitis is really a type of reaction of the airways to many irritants. It can also be called a disease but one with many possible causes. Regardless of the cause the symptoms are usually the same: chronic cough and expectoration of mucus. Cigarettes, the principal cause of chronic bronchitis, probably act via the "tar" in the smoke; this irritates the airways and damages the ciliary clearing mechanism, impairing the lungs' ability to handle mucus. Some patients who have never smoked develop chronic bronchitis. Some of the conditions that can lead to chronic bronchitis in nonsmokers include:

Exposure to industrial pollutants
Severe asthma
Cystic fibrosis
Chronic lung infections

Cystic fibrosis (CF) is an inherited disorder that manifests itself in childhood and affects the lungs, pancreas, and other organs. CF patients almost always have chronic coughs and mucus production. (See Chapter 23).

Chronic bronchitis patients also have an increased risk of developing acute bronchitis. Thus, acute bronchitis can occur *on top of* chronic bronchitis. (People without chronic bronchitis infrequently get attacks of acute bronchitis; when they do it's of short duration. By contrast, patients with chronic bronchitis may suffer frequent attacks of acute bronchitis.) The condition may progress even further to pneumonia, which is infection of the small air spaces at the end of the airways.

WHAT IS THE NATURAL HISTORY OF CHRONIC BRONCHITIS?

Natural history refers to the usual or expected course of a disease. For chronic bronchitis, as with so many lung diseases except perhaps lung cancer, the natural history is highly variable. One can have mild, moderate, or severe disease. Generally, the longer the symptoms have been present and the longer the exposure to cigarettes (or whatever cause), the more severe will be the disease. However, there is great individual variation in susceptibility. For this reason physicians perform breathing tests (pulmonary function tests) on patients with suspected COPD. These are tests of lung function and require the patient to exhale quickly and forcefully through a tube attached to a measuring device (spirometer; see Chapter 8). Another test, an arterial blood gas, is performed on a sample of arterial blood and determines whether or not the patient's lungs are bringing in enough oxygen or getting rid of enough carbon dioxide. These tests (pulmonary function and arterial blood gas; see Chapter 8) give the best idea of disease severity and what the long-term outlook may be.

HOW DOES CIGARETTE SMOKE CAUSE CHRONIC BRONCHITIS?

Healthy lungs produce mucus constantly. It comes from the millions of cells that make up the lining of the airways, and forms a "blanket" over the tops of these cells. Underneath this blanket are cilia, tiny hairs that extend from the tops of the cells. Acting in unison, these cilia move the mucus blanket up the airways to the throat, where much of it is normally swallowed. This is possible since the trachea (the large air tube in the neck) and the esophagus (which leads to the stomach and lies behind the trachea in the neck) have a common opening in the back of the throat.

This mucus blanket effectively gets rid of the everyday air pollutants and dusts we inhale. If the dust is not excessive our lungs won't be damaged and the normal defense mechanisms won't be overcome. However, when cigarette smoke or another pollutant is inhaled, the ciliary action is impaired. Inhalation of cigarette smoke over a period can destroy the ciliary blanket. The cilia don't beat normally, and in some cases the cells lining the airways are also destroyed and the lining is denuded. Without a normal ciliary mechanism the inhaled pollutants won't be swept out. Also, the increased mucus secreted in response to these pollutants won't be cleared. When this occurs the result is usually a cough.

In the mildest cases this mucus may be coughed up in the morning and either swallowed or expectorated by the patient; this is known as morning cough or in some cases smokers' cough. If the condition persists throughout the day, the result is a chronic smokers' cough. In the most severe cases the airways themselves are permanently damaged, beyond any natural healing process, and the patient then has one type of chronic obstructive pulmonary disease (see Figure 12-2).

WHAT IS ASTHMATIC BRONCHITIS?

In many case chronic bronchitis blends in with asthma (see Chapter 10). Patients with chronic bronchitis may later develop an asthma picture; conversely, patients with long-standing asthma may develop chronic mucus production and chronic bronchitis. In either case the resulting condition is referred to as asthmatic bronchitis. (Interestingly, chronic asthma does not lead to emphysema–unless the patient smokes.) Although most cases of COPD are due to cigarette smoking, the cause of asthma is unknown.

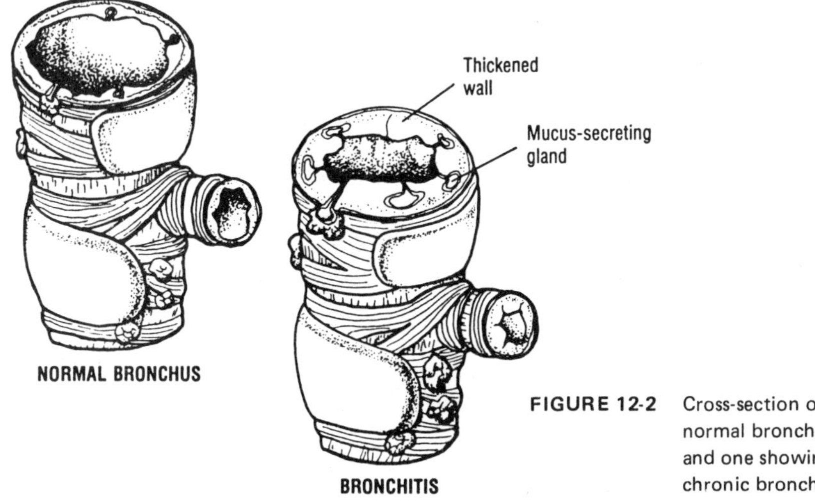

FIGURE 12-2 Cross-section of normal bronchus and one showing chronic bronchitis.

Patients with predominant emphysema may also develop an asthma picture. Since asthma is a reversible condition, many of the asthma drugs are also commonly used to treat COPD patients, with the goal of reversing whatever airway narrowing is amenable to bronchodilators.

With this concept we can expand our two-circle diagram to three circles, as shown in Figure 12-3.

HOW IS CHRONIC BRONCHITIS TREATED?

There are several therapeutic modalities; not all are used simultaneously in every patient. The only one that should be universally applied to every patient is *stop smoking or never start.*

Treatment Modalities for Patients with Chronic Bronchitis

Stop Smoking Almost all patients with chronic bronchitis are or have been cigarette smokers.

Bronchodilators These are drugs designed to open up the airways. See Chapter 11.

Steroids These drugs are very helpful in some severe cases of chronic bronchitis, especially when there is an asthmatic component. See Chapter 11.

Antibiotics These are widely used for exacerbations of chronic bronchitis.

Oxygen This is reserved for the sickest, usually hospitalized, patient. See Chapter 13.

Chest Physical Therapy This is a form of treatment that attempts to mobilize secretions by mechanical and gravitational methods. It is used mainly in hospitalized patients. Although its efficacy is not proven, many physicans and patients feel it is beneficial.

FIGURE 12-3 Overlap of asthma, chronic bronchitis, and emphysema.

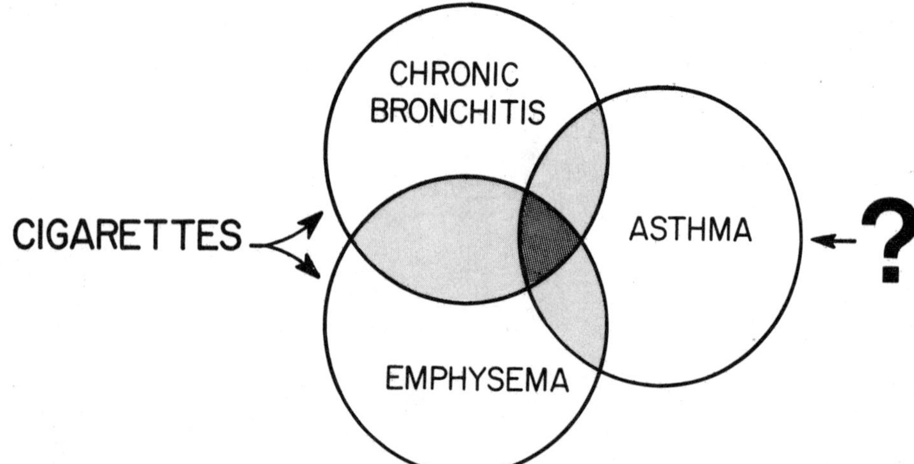

Patient John T.—Severe Chronic Bronchitis

Mr. T. is a 57-year-old car salesman who has had a hacking cough and a low grade fever for several days. Except for several colds a year he has enjoyed good health. He has a long history of cigarette smoking, at least a pack a day since age 17. He also admits to having a daily morning cough that brings up small amounts of whitish sputum; this has been going on for several years and has never bothered him–in fact he considers it normal. His current cough is much different in its intensity and in the color of the sputum produced–now it is greenish-yellow.

Examination of his chest with a stethoscope reveals a few wheezes. A chest X-ray is negative–no abnormal shadows are seen. The negative X-ray helps to rule out pneumonia or lung cancer as the cause of his current problem. The sputum is examined under the microscope and shows many bacteria. The diagnosis of acute bronchitis is made, and Mr. T. is given a prescription for ampicillin, an antibiotic. He is also told in no uncertain terms to quit smoking.

Four days later he is better and able to return to work. He notices, however, some shortness of breath after exertion, such as climbing stairs; the shortness of breath was not present before his actute illness. Although he does not resume smoking, his dyspnea on exertion persists, and pulmonary function tests are ordered.

In the pulmonary function laboratory Mr. T. undergoes both a blood test and spirometry. First, an arterial blood sample is drawn and analyzed for carbon dioxide, oxygen tension, and blood acid levels. Next, he is asked to breathe in deeply and blow all his air out into a hose connected to a spirometer. This test is repeated after he has inhaled some medication designed to open up the airways.

The test results are abnormal. The blood test shows that, while he is ventilating adequately (at rest he is moving enough air in and out of his lungs) and has normal blood acidity, he is not transferring oxygen into his blood properly; his blood oxygen tension is lower than it should be. The spirometry test shows he has airway obstruction–he cannot blow the air out as fast as normal men his age. In addition, the medication has no effect in opening up his airways.

These tests, plus the history, confirm the diagnosis of chronic obstructive pulmonary disease and chronic bronchitis. The chronic bronchitis is due to cigarette smoking and at this point is not reversible. The airways, were they examined under a microscope, would show abnormal thickening and swelling due to repeated insults from cigarette smoke.

Although he claimed no symptoms before his acute bronchitis, it is suggested from his history that Mr. T. had chronic bronchitis for many years. Had breathing tests been done a year earlier they would have shown airway obstruction also, though perhaps less severe. When he developed acute bronchitis he was at the threshold of symptoms; the acute infection "tipped" him over and now he notices his pulmonary impairment (see Figure 12-4). Normal function will not return and continued smoking will only hasten lung destruction, perhaps causing emphysema as well (not yet evident). Hence, complete cessation of smoking is a critical part of his medical management. In addition, Mr. T. will receive antibiotics at the first sign of another acute lung infection. Fortunately, his blood oxygen tension is not low enough to warrant home oxygen therapy and his lung disease is not end-stage. He has a moderate case of COPD and with good medical management may continue to work until retirement.

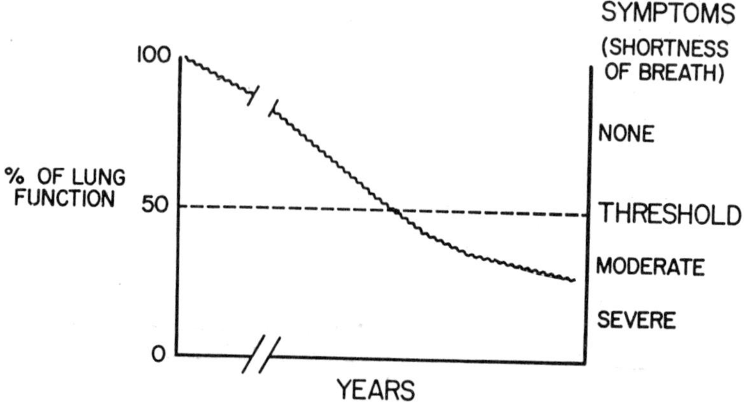

FIGURE 12-4 Decline of lung function in patients with chronic obstructive pulmonary disease (COPD). Patients don't suddenly develop COPD. As shown here, lung function declines over many years. When the threshold for symptoms is reached (shown at 50% of lung function in this figure—the exact point will vary among individuals), the patient notices shortness of breath. Lung function may continue to decline, leading to progressive worsening of symptoms.

WHAT IS THE VALUE OF BREATHING TESTS IN COPD?

The previous case illustrates how a patient can smoke for years and "suddenly" develop symptoms. In fact, COPD develops over many years, yet shortness of breath occurs late in the course. Figure 12-4 illustrates what happens. Breathing tests may fall way below normal, but the patient has no symptoms. Then with a little further decline in function, the patient has noticeable shortness of breath. Often the symptom "shortness of breath on exertion" appears to have come on suddenly; in fact the underlying airway damage builds over years and continues until the threshold is finally reached.

Although not everyone's threshold for developing symptoms is the same, most COPD patients will have years of gradually decreasing lung function before they finally become short of breath. Thus breathing tests can help detect and quantify this impairment before it is too late.

WHAT IS THE DIFFERENCE BETWEEN CHRONIC BRONCHITIS AND EMPHYSEMA?

Although both diseases are caused by cigarette smoke, the damage in the two cases is different. Chronic bronchitis starts with ciliary damage; in the most severe cases the airways themselves are irreversibly damaged, yet the basic architecture of the lungs remains intact. In emphysema not only are the airways damaged, but many of the alveoli and their accompanying blood vessels are destroyed. They are evaporated by the effects of the cigarette smoke, leaving only empty air spaces that cannot effectively transfer oxygen and carbon dioxide. For gas exchange to occur the patient has to literally work harder to bring more air into the remaining normal air spaces. For this reason emphysema is generally a more severe clinical condition than chronic bronchitis and not usually amenable to any specific treatment. (Figure 12-5 diagrams the basic differences in airway structure between the two conditions.)

WHY DO SOME CIGARETTE SMOKERS GET CHRONIC BRONCHITIS AND OTHERS EMPHYSEMA?

As stated earlier, most patients who contract chronic obstructive lung disease have elements of both chronic bronchitis and emphysema, although one or the other may be predominant in a given individual; physicians can usually determine which process predominates.

Chronic bronchitis is found most commonly in patients who have inhaled tremendous amounts of cigarette smoke so that the "tar" has had a direct, toxic effect on their bronchi. It's possible that anyone inhaling comparable amounts of smoke would have similar changes. This doesn't rule out a genetic or constitutional factor, but the end result (chronic bronchitis) does seem related to the dose of toxic material ("tar") inhaled.

Patients who develop predominant emphysema, where the lung tissue is destroyed, may have a genetic or constitutional basis. Emphysema patients are probably more susceptible to cigarette smoke than the general population. Evidence for this comes from the small percentage of emphysema patients who lack a certain enzyme called alpha-l-antitrypsin. This enzyme, normally present, functions to break down another enzyme (trypsin) that tends to destroy lung tissue. If trypsin accumulates, as it might with alpha-l-antitrypsin deficiency, the result can be lung destruction (emphysema).

FIGURE 12-5 Two alveoli from a normal lung, and from lungs involved with chronic bronchitis and emphysema. Blood vessels are not shown in this figure. In chronic bronchitis the airways are narrowed but intact. In emphysema the damage is more extensive, involving actual destruction of alveoli and blood vessels; note the coalescence of two alveoli into one larger, ineffectual "space" that no longer functions as a normal alveolus. The end result in chronic bronchitis is thickened air tubes and loss of the ciliary blanket. The end result in emphysema is literally "holes" in the lung.

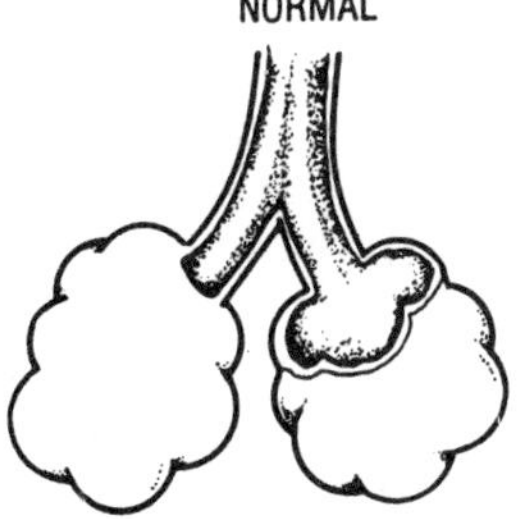

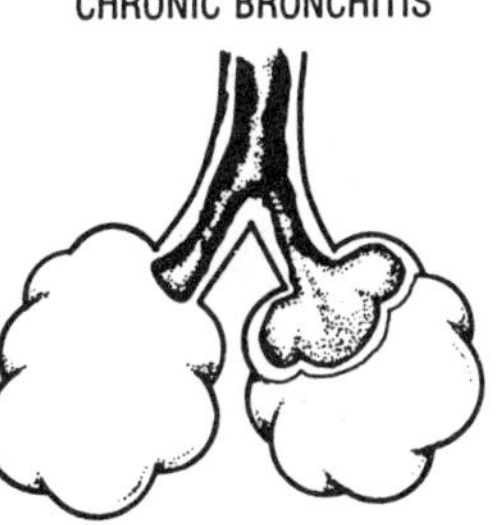

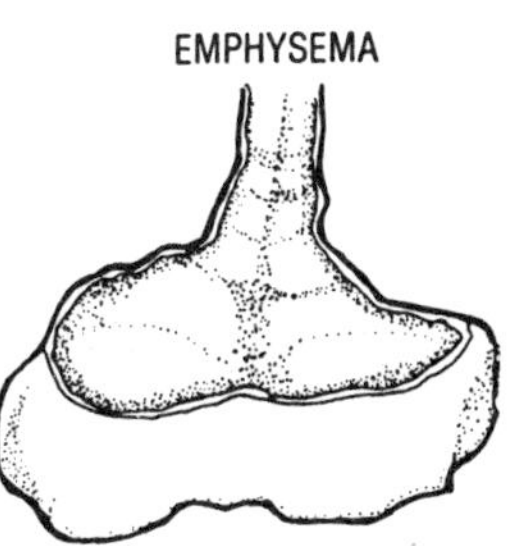

Deficiency of alpha-l-antitrypsin is an inherited disorder present in less than 2 percent of the population. Fortunately, this deficiency itself rarely causes severe lung disease unless the patient smokes. There is a synergistic effect between this inherited deficiency and cigarette smoke, presumably leading to destruction of the lung tissue by the body's enzyme system. Although this helps to explain why some people get emphysema, it does not explain all or even most cases. The vast majority of emphysema patients do not lack alpha-l-antitrypsin.

It is likely that other, yet to be discovered genetic or constitutional factors will explain why some cigarette smokers develop emphysema, other smokers chronic bronchitis, and still other smokers no major impairment. (Similar information may help explain why some smokers get lung cancer.) If such highly susceptible people could be identified early in their smoking career (or before they begin), this information could be a definite incentive to stop smoking.

WHAT ARE THE SEVERE EFFECTS OF CHRONIC BRONCHITIS OR EMPHYSEMA?

The major symptom of either chronic bronchitis or emphysema is difficulty breathing, or shortness of breath. If this occurs only on exertion, most people are able to live comfortably with it. However, in some patients shortness of breath occurs with the slightest effort or even at rest! These people, severely limited, may require daily medication and oxygen at home (see Chapter 13).

The end-stage of these conditions is known as respiratory failure, a failure of the lungs to bring in oxygen and get rid of carbon dioxide in an efficient manner. Some patients are still able to live if their respiratory failure is chronic and they have had time to adapt to this very abnormal situation. When respiratory failure occurs acutely, the situation is indeed critical and intensive care is necessary.

R.J.G.—A Case of Respiratory Failure Due to COPD

Mr. G. first developed symptoms of lung disease at age 62, although by history he had a chronic productive cough for over 20 years. His main symptom was shortness of breath on exertion. Breathing tests confirmed emphysema with severe airway obstruction, and he was strongly advised to quit smoking. He tried, but the stress of business plus the heavy smoking by associates at sales meetings made it difficult; he continued to smoke at least a pack a day.

At age 64 he developed pneumonia and severe respiratory distress and was hospitalized. On admission to the hospital he was "blue" and confused; an arterial blood gas showed severe oxygen deficiency and a high CO_2 tension in the blood. Because of this and his mental confusion he had to be artificially ventilated. Mr. G. was put in the intensive care unit, and a tube was placed in his throat (intubation) and connected to a ventilator. He had a stormy course, but after five days he was able to be disconnected from the ventilator. In another 10 days he was well enough to go home.

During his hospital convalescence he also resumed smoking, at first hiding the fact, but then smoking openly, despite repeated protestations by his family and his doctor. Pulmonary function studies done just prior to his discharge showed worse lung function than two years earlier; in addition his oxygen tension was low, but better than on his admission and not yet severe enough to warrant home oxygen therapy.

Mr. G. cut down his smoking to about half a pack a day. He was now severely limited and could walk no more than a block without disabling shortness of breath. He retired from his job. Two months after his 65th birthday he noted swelling of his feet and increased shortness of breath. His doctor diagnosed heart failure due to lung disease, prescribed water pills, and told him to quit smoking. Three months later he became somnolent, turned blue, and was quickly admitted to the hospital. His blood oxygen tension was again very low, with high carbon dioxide tension and increased blood activity. Initially treatment was attempted with judicious amounts of oxygen and bronchodilators. However, Mr. G. continued to deteriorate; six hours after admission he had to be intubated and artificially ventilated. During this time he developed severe pneumonia, and despite antibiotics, oxygen, and various other medications, he died two days later.

An autopsy was performed. It revealed severe emphysema and bronchitis, the former predominating. In addition, his heart was enlarged from the stress of working against such damaged lungs. He had pneumonia in both lungs—the immediate cause of death.

This case represents the most severe stage of COPD—low oxygen levels, heart failure, and death. Had he stopped smoking at age 62 his downhill course might not have been so precipitous; however, even at that age he already had severe, far-advanced disease. It takes years for this advanced state to develop, yet during all that time he was asymptomatic except for his daily cough. Had breathing tests been done, say at age 50, they would have revealed some impairment in lung function. Unfortunately, by the time his case was diagnosed it was end-stage.

CAN ONE DEVELOP 'ACUTE' EMPHYSEMA?

Emphysema, destruction of lung tissue, usually occurs over a period of years before symptoms develop; there is no counterpart to acute bronchitis, which can occur in otherwise healthy people. Some cigarette smokers (particularly those with alpha-l-antitrypsin deficiency) can develop rapidly progressive emphysema leading from symptoms to death in less than a year, but this is unusual.

Patients with emphysema may have such poor lung function that any *added* insult may make them acutely ill. This could be acute bronchitis on top of emphysema or any infection that involves the lungs.

HOW IS EMPHYSEMA TREATED?

For pure emphysema there are no drugs available. The problem in emphysema is destruction of normal lung tissue; the lung tissue remaining does not work any better in the presence of drugs. However, because most patients with emphysema also have some element of chronic bronchitis, the same modalities used to treat bronchitis are often employed in emphysema patients.

Also, as previously mentioned, asthma may develop on top of pre-existing emphysema. The asthma component is potentially reversible and warrants aggressive treatment. As you can well imagine, drugs and other therapy for the emphysema patient are more likely to be beneficial when there is a component of bronchitis or asthma.

WHAT ABOUT FLU SHOTS AND THE PNEUMONIA VACCINE?

There are currently two recommended preventive vaccines for patients with COPD (as well as other groups of patients). Flu vaccine prevents infection with certain influenza viruses. Because the viruses change yearly, the vaccine is updated annually to prevent infection with the current viral strain. The official Public Health Service recommendation is that any patient with chronic lung disease should receive the current flu shot. The basis for this recommendation is that the flu (a viral infection) affects the lungs and in compromised patients could be severely debilitating or even fatal.

In 1978 the Federal Drug Administration approved a pneumococcal vaccine for prevention of one common form of pneumonia caused by the bacteria pneumococcus (also known as *streptococcus pneumoniae*). There are approximately 70 strains of this bacteria that can cause pneumonia; the vaccine is designed to prevent infection with the 14 that are most virulent and potentially fatal. Pneumococcal organisms are also extremely sensitive to penicillin, but elderly people and patients either debilitated or suffering from chronic lung disease have lower host defenses against these organisms. For such patients (and some other groups) the vaccine is recommended once. At this writing repeat vaccination is not recommended.

Both the pneumococcal vaccine and the flu vaccine may be given at the same time.

WHAT KIND OF LIFESTYLE CAN COPD PATIENTS LEAD?

The symptom that bothers most COPD patients is shortness of breath, or dyspnea. It is dyspnea that COPD patients find most limiting, sometimes debilitating, and occasionally frightening. The "chronic" in COPD means the lungs won't rejuvenate—the disease will remain with the patient. Yet even for patients with severe disease much can be done to maintain or improve the quality of life. For the vast majority of COPD patients the answer to this question is "normal and rewarding."

Pulmonary physicians are familiar with the following paradox. One patient with severe COPD is incapacitated, housebound, bitter, and angry. Nothing helps and life does not seem worth living. Another patient—*with identical lung impairment*—lives a full and rich life, stays involved in activities, and enjoys being alive. Both patients have respiratory limitation, but only one has learned to cope. Why the difference?

Some of the reasons may be beyond the capacity for patient or physician to change: differing degrees of family support, basic personality differences, unequal incomes, job status, and so forth. Even so, there are many things that can be altered and, as a result, markedly improve a COPD patient's quality of life.

To a large extent quality of life can be improved just by receiving good medical care, including any necessary medications and correction of whatever reversible disease is present.

Beyond this, the most obvious measure is to stop smoking. This alone may add enough oxygen to the blood to make the difference between breathing easily and still feeling short of breath (see Chapter 2). There is simply no excuse for any patient limited by lung disease to smoke. Period.

Also helpful is weight control. Although a discussion of weight loss methods is beyond the scope of this chapter, diet books (if these are needed) can be found in virtually every bookstore. Weight loss is obviously not easy (or there wouldn't be so many books); nonetheless, it can't be minimized–overweight patients will feel better and breathe easier if they lose the extra pounds.

The combination of taking medications, stopping smoking, and losing weight can make a dramatic difference for many COPD patients. Of course, not all patients fit this picture. What about the patient who takes medication, has quit smoking and is not overweight, but is still limited by breathlessness? Such patients may benefit from oxygen therapy, a determination best made after a blood gas examination (see Chapter 13).

Beyond these few points, there are other measures that can improve the quality of an individual's life. The next few questions–dealing with exercise, postural drainage, climate, sex, and travel–provide specific information that may be helpful for the COPD patient.

ARE BREATHING EXERCISES HELPFUL?

To a certain extent breathing exercises are helpful in COPD. Unfortunately they help the patient only to breathe slightly more efficiently and perhaps feel more comfortable, but they do nothing to alter the basic disease or improve lung function.

Patients with bronchitis and emphysema have trouble getting air out. In emphysema airways have a tendency to collapse from destruction of surrounding lung tissue. If patients purse their lips on exhalation and create a smaller mouth opening, the airways stay open a little longer and allow air to come out more efficiently. Such an exercise is called "pursed lip breathing" and is often practiced reflexly by patients with severe emphysema.

Another helpful exercise for both bronchitis and emphysema patients is to take deep breaths and breathe out slowly. This is particularly helpful for patients who breathe rapidly and experience anxiety over not being able to exhale fully.

Exercise training, extensively tried in a few medical centers, can definitely improve exercise performance as well as the patient's sense of well being. Like breathing exercises however, exercise training will not reverse the damage to the airways nor significantly improve the breathing capacity of already-diseased lungs. There is still much to recommend in progressive exercise training since it can improve overall cardiovascular fitness and perhaps make an important difference in the individual's lifestyle.

For those who wish to embark on a program of exercise training, reference is made in the bibliography to several paperback books on aerobics by Dr. Kenneth Cooper, in which he explains clearly the benefits to be gained from a systematic aerobics program (running, bicycling, swimming, racquetball, and so forth). It cannot be overemphasized that anyone with heart or lung disease should undertake exercise training only after first checking with his or her physician.

WHAT IS POSTURAL DRAINAGE?

Postural drainage (PD) is a mechanical method of draining secretions from the bronchi. When the patient lies in various positions, with his head lower than his feet, secretions can be mobilized and coughed out.

As practiced in hospitals, postural drainage (PD) involves 3 important steps.

1. The patient inhales an aerosol bronchodilator to help break up secretions and open up the airways (any of the aerosols listed in Appendix C, Table 1 should be adequate).
2. The patient assumes the proper head-down position that will drain the part of the lung desired.
3. While the patient is in position, a therapist "percusses" (taps gently with the fingers) the chest over the part of the lung being drained; this technique is important to help loosen the secretions.

The postural drainage position should be held for three to five minutes and performed once or twice a day (before breakfast and dinner, for example). Postural drainage can easily be performed at home if a family member is available to percuss the chest. Generally, if PD makes the patient feel better, it is worth doing. Not all COPD patients will benefit, but PD may be particularly helpful for patients with copious airway secretions.

DO PATIENTS WITH COPD BREATHE BETTER IN A WARM CLIMATE?

There is no evidence that COPD patients, as a group, breathe easier or live healthier lives in a warm climate as opposed to a cold one. Obviously any patient who becomes sick just because of cold weather should consider living in a warmer place. But a substantial number of people have trouble breathing in hot, humid areas and prefer cooler weather. The decision to move (if that is involved) really has to be a personal one and cannot be based on a disease label. This is true for anyone with allergies and asthma as well as chronic obstructive pulmonary disease.

In addition, many of the sun belt cities are heavily polluted, the worst perhaps being Los Angeles. Altitude is another factor. The higher the city, the less oxygen there is in the air; this makes Denver a miserable place for patients with COPD and hypoxemia. As a general recommendation anyone moving solely for health reasons should research the area carefully and then vacation there at least a week before deciding on the move, preferably during the area's most extreme weather (summer in Florida, for example).

WHAT ABOUT SEX FOR COPD PATIENTS?

During sexual intercourse breathing effort is increased. For this reason patients with severe COPD (or any other chronic respiratory problem) may have difficulty during sex and may even avoid it because of the anxiety of becoming out of breath.

Sexual counseling for the respiratory-impaired patient was, until recently, little talked or written about. There were several reasons for this: patient reluctance to complain to the doctor; doctor reluctance to broach such a sensitive area; and a general lack of information in medical journals. This last deficiency is being remedied because researchers are now recognizing that COPD patients may have sexual problems related to their breathlessness and that counseling can definitely help patients with sexual problems.

The biggest obstacle to helping patients is uncovering the problem. The patient must let his doctor know and not simply wait to be asked (which may never happen).

Once the sexual problem is aired, it is important to know if it is truly from shortness of breath or instead a problem unrelated to breathlessness. Were there sexual difficulties before the onset of lung disease? Are there incompatibilities between the patient and his or her partner that have nothing do do with the lung disease? If so, specific psychological or marriage counseling may be needed.

Ideally, any sexual counseling for the COPD patient (as with anyone else) should include the sexual partner. If the problem is deemed due to shortness of breath, specific measures can be taken to help the patient accomplish–and enjoy–sexual intercourse.

Sexual intercourse is about as stressful as climbing a flight of stairs at a normal pace, so shortness of breath during sex is acceptable if it can be tolerated. Despite the anxiety that some patients have about dying during sex, sudden death is very uncommon during intercourse.

Any steps that can be taken to prolong the sex act or make it more comfortable–unaccustomed positions (woman on top, for example), mutual masturbation, or prolonged foreplay–should be considered, tolerated and encouraged–as long as both partners find them acceptable.

Drugs commonly used to treat COPD (bronchodilators and steroids listed in Appendix C) should have no effect on sexual performance unless side effects (such as fast heartbeat) are present at other times. In fact, use of an inhaler (such as metaproterenol or another beta-adrenergic drug–see Appendix C) just before sex may help relieve subsequent shortness of breath. In addition, use of oxygen during intercourse is worth considering if it helps to relieve any shortness of breath. A nasal catheter (see Chapter 13) can be unobtrusive and not interfere with the act of lovemaking. Drugs to be avoided in this situation are any central nervous system stimulants or depressants, since they may interfere with breathing *and* sexual function. Also, some anti-hypertensive medications may interfere with sexual function.

In summary, sex should not be a casualty of the chronic lung disease. Careful counseling and judicious use of medications may go a long way in improving this important aspect of daily living.

IS FLYING DANGEROUS FOR PATIENTS WITH COPD?

This depends mainly on the patient's blood oxygen tension (or pressure) before flying. If it is very low, flying may not be safe without extra oxygen.

To explain further, consider what happens with altitude. Barometic pressure decreases with an increase of altitude. Although air pressure falls, the percentage of oxygen remains fixed—always 21 percent. Since O_2 is transferred into our blood by virtue of its pressure, it follows that less oxygen enters the blood as we ascend. For this reason mountain climbers often must resort to supplemental oxygen at very high altitudes.

People living in Leadville, Colorado (the highest United States city) breathe 21 percent oxygen, but at a low barometric pressure; hence they have lower O_2 pressure in their blood. Healthy people in Leadville don't need to worry about this, because normal body mechanisms adapt to keep the total oxygen supply adequate.

Problems at altitude may occur in people who have low oxygen tension from lung disease; although not everyone with COPD has low oxygen tension, severe COPD is perhaps the most common cause of low blood oxygen (chronic hypoxemia). If one has a low oxygen pressure and then ascends, the resulting further reduction in oxygen pressure may be harmful.

This problem can easily be overcome by using extra oxygen during flight. For the most part patients requiring oxygen during flight will be those who also need it when not flying. Patients not on oxygen who think they might need it while flying should consult their physicians; this need can only be determined by measurement of the oxygen pressure in arterial blood.

Arrangements for oxygen can be made in advance by informing the airlines reservations personnel of the need. This will also require a physician's prescription for the amount of oxygen required. Airlines provide their own tanks for in-flight use; this is *not* the same oxygen system as the one above every passenger seat, which is only used in the event of sudden decompression.

An excellent guide for patients is *Travel For The Patient With Chronic Obstructive Pulmonary Disease*, published by the George Washington University Medical Center. It is available at nominal cost (see Appendix D).

WHAT IS THE FUTURE FOR CHRONIC OBSTRUCTIVE PULMONARY DISEASE?

Our understanding and treatment of COPD are far more sophisticated than they were 20 years ago, but there have been no dramatic breakthroughs. We understand old drugs much better and have a few new ones. Oxygen is more easily administered and home O_2 is now routinely available for those who will benefit (see Chapter 13). But the basic disease is still chronic, and patients with this condition still suffer. A cure is not on the horizon. Once the damage is done the lung tissues do not fully regenerate even when the insult (cigarette smoke, usually) is removed.

Unfortunately, unlike other vital organs such as the heart and kidneys, lungs have not proved amenable to transplantation. At this writing lung transplants can in no way be considered a viable option for end-stage lung disease.

Experimental work is underway on enzyme replacement for patients with some types of emphysema. The basic idea is that lack of one or more enzymes allows the lung tissue to be destroyed by other body enzymes; replacing the deficient enzymes may prevent this destruction. It is too early to know if this will benefit most patients with COPD.

CHAPTER THIRTEEN

Oxygen: For Some, a Vital Drug

WHAT IS OXYGEN?

Oxygen is a colorless, odorless gas that is vital to life. Without it we would all die within minutes. We normally have more than enough oxygen in our blood. This comes from the air that surrounds us, wherever we are. At all altitudes, air contains 21 percent oxygen (the other 79 percent is mostly nitrogen). A patient who requires oxygen for treatment therefore needs more than the 21 percent normally available. Such patients do not have enough oxygen in their blood from breathing air.

WHEN IS OXYGEN USED?

Giving oxygen is like administering any other drug. There are situations where it is definitely needed and others where it may actually be harmful. Some patients will benefit from this drug, although the vast majority of nonhospitalized patients don't require it.

The best way to show a need for extra oxygen is by a blood test, called an arterial blood gas. A component of this test is the PaO_2, which stands for the pressure (P) of oxygen (O_2) in the arterial blood (a). Its value tells us if the lungs are working properly to bring in enough oxygen. If the PaO_2 is very low the physician must determine if supplemental oxygen will help and how much to give. Since every patient is automatically breathing at least 21 percent O_2 (from the air around us), the decision to administer extra oxygen means choosing an amount between 21 and 100 percent (the maximum). Often the PaO_2 measurement has to be repeated while the patient is receiving supplemental oxygen. In fact, except in brief emergency situations, oxygen should only be used where the dose can be controlled and the level in the blood (PaO_2) easily measured.

Oxygen is most commonly used in hospitalized patients who are acutely ill with respiratory disease. For most patients, once the acute illness is over there is no longer a need for supplemental O_2. Considering the large number of respiratory patients in the United States, only a small percentage will ever receive supplemental O_2.

HOW IS OXYGEN ADMINISTERED?

No matter how oxygen is delivered there must be some method of actually getting the gas to the patient so it can be inhaled.

For most patients, oxygen is simply delivered to the region of the face where it is inhaled. In all systems currently used, a long thin hose leads from the oxygen *source* (either a tank, wall outlet in a hospital, oxygen extractor designed for home use, and so forth) to some facial *appliance* worn by the patient. In adults this appliance takes one of two forms: either a nasal cannula (tube) that fits inside the nostrils, or a face mask that fits loosely over both the mouth and nose.

For most delivery systems, oxygen flowing through the thin hose to the facial appliance is pure, or 100 percent, oxygen. By the time the patient actually inhales the oxygen it has become mixed with surrounding room air (containing 21 percent O_2), so the patient actually receives less than 100 percent oxygen. By varying the flow rate of oxygen through the hose and the specific design of the appliance (there are several types of face masks), physicians can order virtually any concentration of oxygen for the patient, from 24 to 90+ percent.

In infants and small children oxygen tents are sometimes used. These work on the same principle as face masks, but the patient does not actually have anything touching the face. Tents are considered impractical for adults because of their size and requisite need for large amounts of oxygen to be effective.

CAN OXYGEN BE GIVEN ONLY IN THE HOSPITAL?

Oxygen can be administered anywhere. It can be given from special portable oxygen tanks at the scene of an accident or a fire. But oxygen can also be set up for long-term use in a patient's home or in a nursing facility. Special apparatus is available so that patients with a continuous need can be ambulatory while receiving oxygen.

Oxygen is more and more being prescribed for home use in patients with severe chronic lung disease. This is a relatively recent phenomenon but will probably become more common as the ease of delivering oxygen improves and the cost is increasingly borne by third party providers such as Medicare.

HOW CAN A PATIENT KNOW IF SUPPLEMENTAL OXYGEN IS NEEDED?

This question is often asked by patients who are chronically short of breath or have a chronic respiratory illness. However, outside the hospital oxygen is not prescribed lightly. This is for several reasons. Perhaps the most important is that non-hospitalized patients with respiratory disease will usually *not* benefit from oxygen administration.

A patient's symptoms are an unreliable guide to the need for supplemental oxygen. Out of 10 patients with chronic lung disease and identical symptoms (cough, shortness of breath, and so forth), perhaps *one* will actually be low in O_2 and benefit from receiving it. Patients can have severe, even incapacitating lung disease and still *not be deficient in oxygen.* In such patients the incapacitation is usually due to difficulty in moving air in and out of the lungs; they have sufficient oxygen in their blood and giving them more would not help them.

Of course, there is a definite subgroup of patients deficient in oxygen who will benefit from receiving it at home. However, there is no way for the patient to know if he or she will benefit from O_2. In fact, there is no way for a physician to know *without measuring the PaO_2 in the patient's blood.* This is part of the arterial blood gas analysis and is done if the doctor suspects severe respiratory disease and interference with gas exchange.

There are also disadvantages of chronic oxygen therapy, discussed in a subsequent section.

HOW IS OXYGEN GIVEN IN THE HOME?

Hospitals generally have a sophisticated liquid oxygen system that pipes O_2 into all hospital areas. For home use there are three types of systems, all widely used. They are illustrated in Figure 13-1. The oldest in use is oxygen tanks. These large, upright cylinders, always colored green, contain oxygen gas in compressed form. The tank can be delivered and continuously changed by a local oxygen supply company, with delivery frequency determined by how much the patient is using. (For limited portability, smaller tanks can be provided on wheels; one is shown in Figure 13-1). The oxygen is released from the tank by a series of values and travels safely from the tank via a long, thin hose to either a nasal cannula or face mask. The oxygen is odorless, although sometimes one can smell the plastic of the appliance worn by the patient.

A second method is a portable liquid oxygen system, designed for home use. A liquid oxygen container (the two large canisters in Figure 13-1; see also Figure 13-2) is placed in the patient's home and is filled periodically from a truck brought to the residence. Liquid oxygen has the advantage of allowing more oxygen to be stored at one time compared to tanks of compressed oxygen. An additional advantage is that portable walking containers can be filled from the liquid oxygen systems, something not possible with the other two systems (Figure 13-1 and 13-3).

The third method of delivery of home O_2 is via an oxygen extractor, also called an oxygen concentrator, an ingenious device that works from normal house current (in Figure 13-1, it is the large box-like unit next to the tall oxygen tank). This machine extracts oxygen from the air by eliminating the nitrogen, effectively

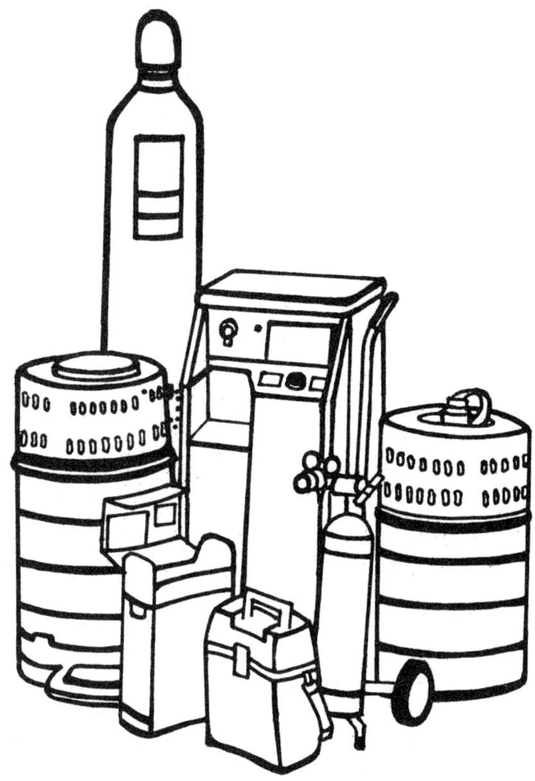

FIGURE 13-1 Equipment used to deliver oxygen in the home. Represents three different systems. (Reproduced by permission, Linde Homecare Medical Systems, Inc.)

concentrating the oxygen and converting it from 21 percent to over 90 percent of the air. As with the other two systems, the actual amount received by the patient will be determined by the liter flow rate ordered by the physician. The therapeutic advantage of all oxygen systems is the delivery to the patient of more than 21 percent oxygen.

WHAT ARE THE DISADVANTAGES OF USING HOME OXYGEN?

Assuming the need for oxygen is established, there are several disadvantages:

1. *Continuous Need.* The need for O_2 is continuous since the body does not store it. Only a few minutes' supply is available in circulating blood; once that supply is exhausted, death ensues. This is in marked contrast to food, which is stored as protein and fat and can keep a fasting person alive for many days. When

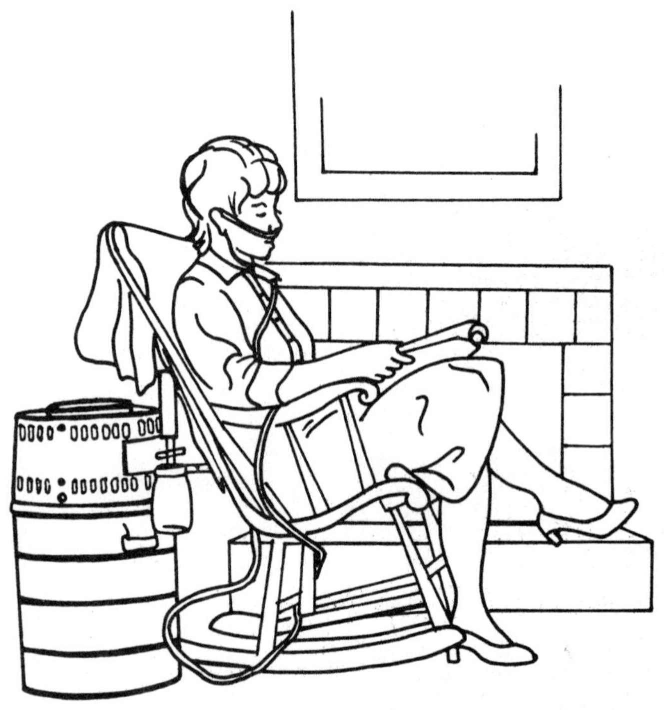

FIGURE 13-2 A woman sitting by the fireplace, using a liquid oxygen system. Note the oxygen tubing leading from the canister to her nose. (Reproduced, by permission, Linde Homecare Medical Systems, Inc.)

patients are low on O_2 they would logically benefit from receiving supplemental O_2 *all the time.* This is impractical because of *inconvenience* and *cost.*

2. *Inconvenience.* The extra O_2 must come from either heavy tanks or a cumbersome electrical apparatus and hence is confining. Practically speaking, patients must be sedentary for continuous oxygen or carry bulky equipment if they are ambulatory (Figure 13-3). In addition, these small canisters do not allow excursions for more than a few hours. Unfortunately, oxygen is available only in gaseous form; there is no pill or elixir one can swallow.

Because of the inconvenience, most patients compromise. They use oxygen mainly at night and during the day when they feel they need it or it is otherwise convenient to use. Many suffer the symptoms of low oxygen rather than be confined, carry bulky equipment, or be seen in public with tubes in their noses. Certainly, both the inconvenience and the stigma some patients feel are an obstacle to continuous O_2 use. Conversely, continuous need is an obstacle to truly effective O_2 therapy.

3. *Cost.* This varies depending on the amount and duration of use. Oxygen at 2 liters per minute for 12 hours a day can range from $100 to more than $300 a month. For some patients a large percentage of the total cost will be subsidized by insurance carriers or Medicare.

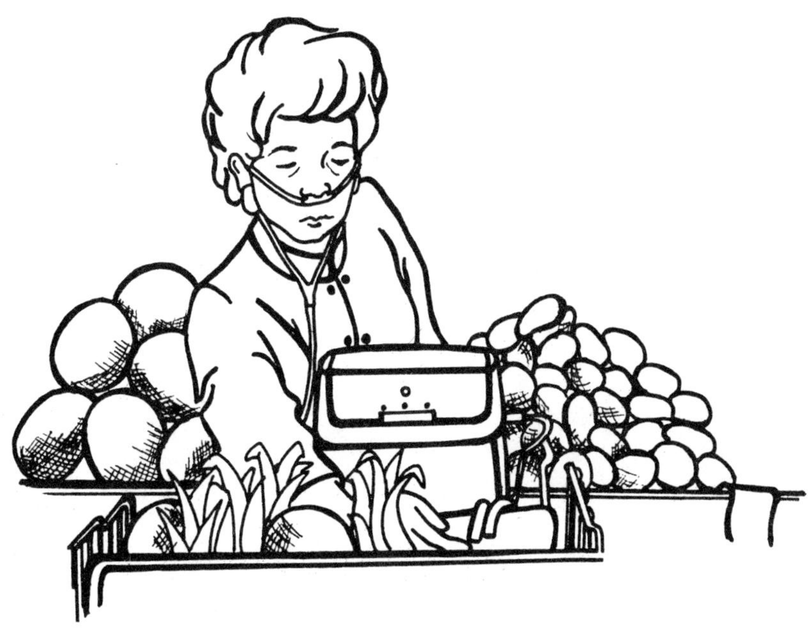

FIGURE 13-3 A woman shopping, while using a portable oxygen system. This system was filled from a canister like the one shown in Figure 13-2; it allows for continuous oxygen use for several hours outside the home. Such portable oxygen systems are continually being made lighter and more convenient to carry. (Reproduced, by permission, Linde Homecare Medical Systems, Inc.)

4. *Discomfort.* Continuous oxygen is given either by nasal cannula or face mask (unless the patient is connected to an artificial ventilator). Prolonged use by either applicance tends to cause irritation and erythema (redness) in the areas of facial contact. Some patients receiving nasal oxygen also complain of a headache, particularly after several hours of high flow oxygen, and find no relief unless they remove the cannula.

5. *Toxicity.* Improperly used, oxygen can be toxic. As with any medication, too much can be harmful to health and can even cause lung disease worse than the underlying condition. This is why O_2 should only be prescribed after blood gas analysis and full evaluation of the patient's respiratory problem.

In summary, determining who will benefit from oxygen requires a thorough evaluation including arterial blood gas analysis. Except in emergency situations, continuous O_2 therapy should never be ordered for a patient without such an evluation.

CHAPTER FOURTEEN

Problems of the Chest Bellows

WHAT IS DISEASE OF THE CHEST BELLOWS?

The chest bellows is one of the three major divisions of the respiratory system (the other two are the central nervous system components that control breathing and the lungs themselves). The system and its components were introduced in Chapter 2.

The chest bellows includes all those structures that make up the thoracic cage (muscles, bones, nerves, and connective tissue), plus the diaphragm muscles and the pleural membranes. The variety of different structures accounts for the diversity of diseases that can affect the chest bellows; the more common ones are listed in Table 14-1.

For example, polio may affect the spinal cord and damage the nerves that innervate the chest wall muscles, leading to respiratory problems. Massive obesity can likewise lead to respiratory difficulty as can severe deformity of the thoracic spine. Although three different conditions, polio, obesity and bone deformity can each interfere with normal movement of the chest bellows and impair breathing. In the most severe cases respiratory failure can result (see Chapter 25). Space does not permit thorough discussion of all conditions that may impair the chest bellows, but a few of the more common ones will be discussed in this chapter.

TABLE 14-1 Diseases that can affect the chest bellows and interfere with normal breathing

A. *Diseases affecting nerves, muscles or bones of the thoracic cage*
   1. *Mainly nerves*
      Polio
      Guillain Barré syndrome
      Spinal cord damage
      Amyotrophic lateral sclerosis
   2. *Mainly muscles*
      Myasthenia gravis
      Multiple sclerosis
      Muscular dystrophy
   3. *Mainly bones*
      Kyphoscoliosis
      Flail chest (from trauma)
      Arthritis (ankylosing spondylitis)

B. *Diseases affecting the diaphragms*
   Diaphragm paralysis
   Massive obesity
   Massive ascites (fluid in the abdomen)

C. *Diseases affecting the pleura*
   Pleural thickening and fibrosis (scarring)
   Pleural effusions

WHAT IS GUILLAIN BARRE SYNDROME?

This is a syndrome named after two French neurologists, Georges Guillain and Jean Alexander Barre, that is also known as "ascending paralysis." In GBS, paralysis usually starts in the legs and then ascends up the body to involve the arms and sometimes the respiratory muscles. Generally a rare condition, GBS is thought to be of viral origin and may strike anyone at any time. Several people who received the swine flu vaccine in the mid 1970s developed GBS and paralysis of their respiratory muscles.

Respiratory failure may result from GBS if it involves nerves of the respiratory muscles. Patients with respiratory muscle paralysis may require artificial ventilation until their condition improves (see Chapter 25). Barring complications, such as pneumonia, recovery usually occurs, although it may take weeks or months.

WHAT IS MYASTHENIA GRAVIS?

A disease that causes muscle weakness, myasthenia gravis is due to abnormal chemical transmission at the "neuromuscular junction," the space between the ends of the nerves and the beginning of the muscle cells. The disease appears due to a decrease in the number of chemical receptors in the muscles. Normally, these receptors are stimulated by a chemical, acetylcholine (ACh), that is released from the nerve endings whenever a muscle is moved. With a decreased number of muscle receptors the released ACh cannot stimulate the muscles normally.

Myasthenia gravis can present in a variety of ways, one of the most common being double vision (from eye muscle weakness) and drooping of the eyelids. Myasthenia can affect muscles anywhere in the body, including the respiratory muscles. Some patients can develop respiratory failure (see Chapter 25).

Once polio or Guillain Barré Syndrome have set in there is no specific treatment. By contrast, myasthenia gravis can be treated by drugs, thymectomy (removal of thymus gland) and/or a technique known as plasmapheresis ('washing' the blood to remove antibodies thought to affect the muscle receptors).

If respiratory failure occurs, ventilatory support will be required until reversal by treatment (see Chapter 25). Although patients with myasthenia may suffer complications such as aspiration pneumonia, atelectasis, or pulmonary embolism, the disease itself does not involve the lungs or airways.

WHAT IS KYPHOSCOLIOSIS?

Kyphoscoliosis is a condition of the bones manifested by abnormal curvature of the spine. "Kypho" refers to hunched over and "scoliosis" to curvature of the spine sideways. The kyphoscoliosis patient has a spine that causes him or her to be slightly hunched over and bent to one side. There are many degrees of kyphoscoliosis. The most severe spinal curvatures can lead to lung disease, respiratory failure, and death. Initially, patients with severe kyphosoliosis may only have decreased lung volumes (restrictive lung disease) and decreased exercise tolerance. Compression of the bottom parts of the lungs due to the bent spine (and compressed thoracic cavity) may lead to recurrent lung infections, ultimately leading to a form of chronic bronchitis. Over many years this can eventually cause respiratory failure. Fortunately, most patients with kyphoscoliosis do not end up with chronic lung disease and respiratory failure.

HOW DOES SEVERE OBESITY LEAD TO TROUBLE BREATHING?

Obesity is a common and widespread condition. Distinction should be made between moderate obesity and so-called morbid or massive obesity, the latter being defined as in excess of 50 pounds overweight. When patients with morbid obesity are studied in the pulmonary laboratory, their routine breathing tests and blood gas analysis are usually normal or near normal.* However, some massively obese patients *do* manifest respiratory impairment, for which there are several possible explanations.

Perhaps the simplest explanation is that excess weight of the chest wall caused by the fat makes it difficult to take a deep breath. Also the massive weight

*This is at rest. As a group, morbidly obese patients who are otherwise healthy will always have decreased exercise ability compared to a group of thin, healthy people.

of the abdominal fat makes it difficult to move the diaphragms. However, weight alone cannot be the only explanation for respiratory impairment, since patients equally overweight often have very different breathing test results.

Also contributing to the abnormal test results of some overweight patients is a decreased drive to breathe. This affects obese patients variably. On their own, some obese patients underbreathe, but when coached they can increase their breathing. A decreased drive to breath plus excessive weight make up the Pickwickian Syndrome (see Chapter 24).

Finally, any underlying lung disease (not a disease of the chest bellows), such as bronchitis or emphysema, can certainly be aggravated by excess weight.

In summary, obesity per se may not lead to respiratory impairment at rest. When coupled with problems of decreased central drive to breathe or underlying lung disease, obesity may be a significant and aggravating factor.

WHAT DISEASES AFFECT THE DIAPHRAGMS?

The diaphragms are the major muscles of breathing. They sit at the bottom of the thoracic cavity and divide it from the abdominal cavity. The diaphragms are powered by nerves that arise from high up in the spinal cord in the neck region.

Injury to these nerves (called the phrenic nerves) or to the area of the spinal cord from which they arise can paralyze the diaphragms and lead to respiratory failure. Uncommonly a viral infection can affect these nerves and cause diaphragm paralysis.

Often only one diaphragm may be paralyzed, either from prior surgery (which involved the phrenic nerve), trauma, or tumor. Most patients with unilateral paralysis have no major problem with breathing. Bilateral or complete diaphragm paralysis definitely interferes with normal breathing. If only the diaphragms are paralyzed, patients can still breath using their abdominal muscles. However, this requires sitting up; recumbency makes the abdominal muscles ineffective and results in severe shortness of breath. If bilateral diaphragm paralysis is due to spinal cord damage, then all the muscles of breathing (including abdominal muscles) will be paralyzed. This is incompatible with life and artificial means must be used to support ventilation.

An artificial ventilator is one method of supporting patients with complete diaphragm paralysis who cannot use other muscles of breathing (see Chapter 25). A sophisticated technique called "diaphragm pacing" has also been tried on some patients. This involves attaching a pacing wire to one or both of the phrenic nerves and stimulating them via a battery that is located outside the body. To prevent nerve fatigue, pacing is only done for part of the day. When the pacer is not used, the patient has to go back on the ventilator (if that was required before pacing).

Complete diaphragm paralysis is rare and unilateral diaphragm paralysis does not cause major difficulty. A more common diaphragm problem is compression and immobilization from above (in the thoracic cavity) or below (in the abdomen). The diaphragms may be partly immobilized by many processes, including pleural disease and effusions from above, and obesity, pregnancy, ascites (fluid in the abdomen), and abdominal infection from below. A common problem in patients who have undergone major abdominal surgery is fluid or infection underneath the diaphragms; this can limit diaphragm activity and cause respiratory problems. When coupled with the effects of anesthesia and possible underlying lung disease the abdominal problem may precipitate respiratory failure (see Chapter 25).

WHAT ARE PLEURAL EFFUSIONS AND PLEURAL DISEASE?

The outside covering of the lungs and inside covering of the chest wall are very thin, transparent membranes called pleural membranes. They provide a smooth surface so the lungs can slide up and down within the chest cavity during breathing. When the membranes become inflamed, thickened, or involved with a disease process (such as cancer) we speak of the patient as having pleural disease. Pleural fluid, also known as pleural effusion, may be one manifestation of pleural disease.

Pleural effusion is an abnormal collection of fluid within the pleural space—actually the "potential" space between the membrane lining the lung and the membrane lining the inside of the thoracic cavity. Normally, these two membranes touch each other as the lungs slide up and down during breathing. Pleural fluid may accumulate between these two membranes, spreading them apart and filling the potential space with fluid; this creates an abnormal shadow on the chest X-ray, as shown in Figure 14-1. Pleural disease can also occur without any apparent fluid; in such cases the chest X-ray may only show scarring and thickening of the pleural membranes.

Pleural effusions and pleural disease may occur in a wide variety of disorders. The specific cause of a pleural effusion can often be diagnosed by examination of the fluid, obtained via a thin needle inserted into the chest cavity. This procedure is

FIGURE 14-1a X-ray appearance of normal lungs. Figure on right shows enlargement of area in box. Between the pleura membranes lining the lung and the inside chest wall is a "potential" pleural space. It is called this because, under normal conditions, the two membranes come together. When pleural fluid forms, as shown in Figure 14-1b, the space enlarges and the two membranes move apart.

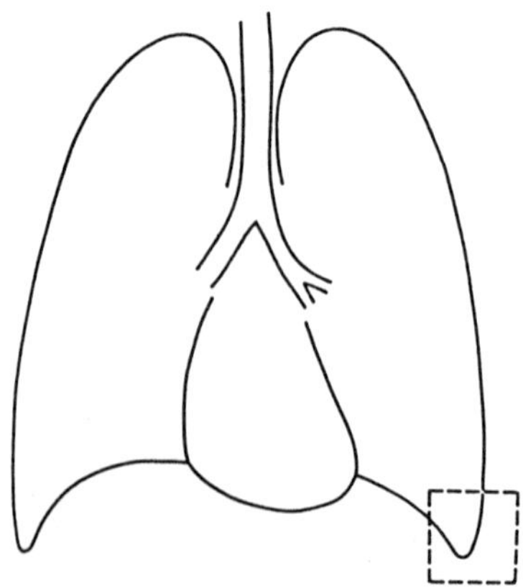

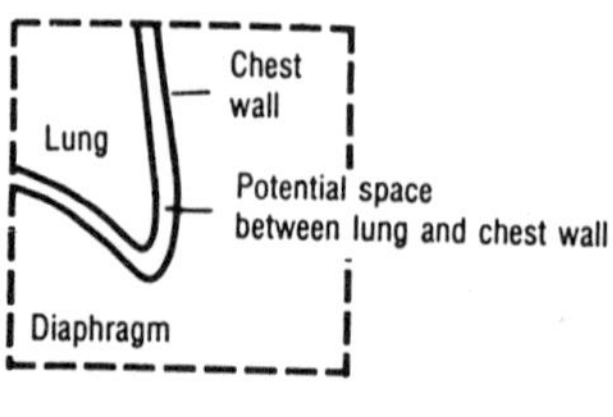

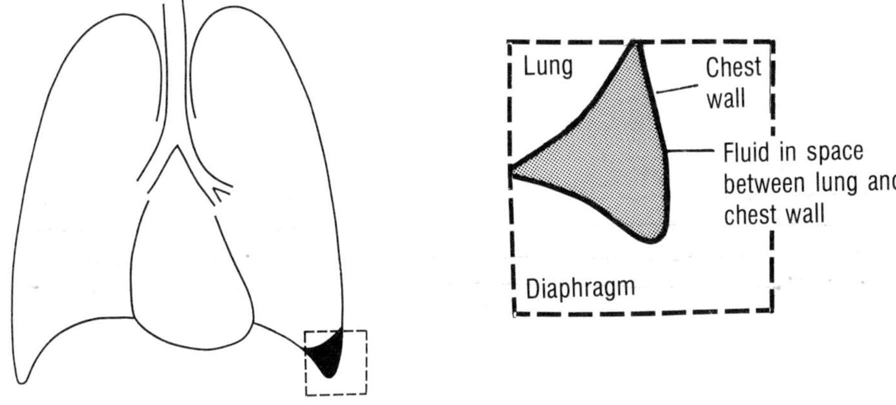

FIGURE 14-1b X-ray appearance of patient with small pleural effusion; figure on right shows enlargement of area in box.

called a thoracentesis. Fluid removed this way is analyzed for several compounds and chemicals, such as protein and glucose.

On occasion, a piece of the pleural membrane itself will have to be removed—this is called a pleural biopsy, and is performed with a larger needle than is used for thoracentesis. Pleural biopsy is generally useful only when the physician suspects either tuberculosis or cancer of the pleura. Cancer and TB in the pleural membranes cause specific changes that can be viewed under the microscope. Pleural biopsy is not helpful for other diagnoses because the pleura only shows non-specific changes under the microscope.

HOW DOES PLEURAL DISEASE INTERFERE WITH BREATHING?

Regardless of the underlying disease, pleural effusions and pleural disease may interfere with breathing. This generally occurs in one of three ways:

1. Inflammation of pleural membranes may cause pain. Pleural or pleuritic-type pain is worse on inspiration and keeps the patient from taking a deep breath. When due to a viral infection this is commonly called pleurodynia. Pleurisy is a more general term for pain due to pleural inflammation of any cause.
2. Pleural disease and pleural effusion may interfere with breathing even without causing pain. If the membranes are very thickened or scarred, the patient may not be able to take a deep breath. Normally these surfaces are smooth and slide easily over each other; when inflamed they may move not at all or only with difficulty.
3. Large effusions may simply occupy so much of the thoracic cavity that the lung behind the fluid is compressed and the patient does not have a normal amount of room in which to expand the lungs.

Any of these mechanisms may led to a breathing problem or a feeling of shortness of breath.

WHAT IS PNEUMOTHORAX?

Pneumothorax is an abnormal collection of air between the pleural surfaces. It is the air counterpart of a pleural effusion; instead of fluid accumulating in the potential space between the pleural membranes, air accumulates. Normally this space is air-free. As with fluid, the air can compress the lung and cause trouble breathing.

How does this are get into the pleural space? The space is normally under negative pressure; if there is any contact between the pleural space and the outside atmosphere, air will rush in. An analogy is the whoosh of air rushing in when a vacuum can is opened. A puncture of either pleural surface (the one lining the lung or the thoracic cavity) may allow air to rush in.

If the pleural membrane covering the inside of the thoracic cavity is violated, as may occur from a stab or bullet wound, air from the outside can enter and create a pneumothorax. If the pleural membrane lining the lung is punctured, as may occur from a ruptured lung bleb or cyst, air from within the lungs will enter the pleural space. A large amount of air from either entry point may compress the lung and require chest tube insertion to suction out the air. The chest tube often has to be left in place several days, until there is a secure seal between the pleural surfaces.

Pneumothorax may occur in many disease conditions, including asthma, severe pneumonia, prolonged artificial ventilation, and trauma. Spontaneous pneumothorax may also occur in otherwise healthy people; it is probably due to spontaneous rupture of a small bleb or cyst in the outermost part of the lung. When the resulting pneumothorax is large, a chest tube has to be inserted to suction out the air.

CHAPTER FIFTEEN

Interstitial Lung Disease: When the Lungs Form Scar Tissue

WHAT IS INTERSTITIAL LUNG DISEASE?

Interstitial lung disease (ILD) refers to a large and heterogenous group of pulmonary disorders characterized by inflammation in and around the interstitium of the lung, the gigantic boundary that separates the air spaces from the blood supply. Figure 15-1 is a schematic cross-section of several alveolar-capillary units showing the interstitium; multiply this by several hundred million such units and you can appreciate the relative size and importance of this anatomic area.

Symptoms of ILD are usually dry cough and shortness of breath, but there may be other complaints related to the underlying cause, such as stiff joints in rheumatoid arthritis. Occasionally patients with ILD have no symptoms, the condition being found on a chest X-ray done for some other reason. The chest X-ray appearance of ILD is characteristic: diffuse "stringy" and/or fine "fluffy" infiltrates throughout both lungs (see Figure 15-2).

On pulmonary function testing ILD invariably gives a restrictive breathing pattern, with a reduced forced vital capacity (see Chapter 9). Unless the large airways are involved, the rate of airflow is normal or increased and airway obstruction is not a problem.

The large number of diagnoses associated with ILD is given in Table 15-1. These are divided into known and unknown causes. Not that many of the known causes of ILD are discussed elsewhere in this book: the pneumoconioses in Chapter 4, infectious diseases in Chapters 18-20, and pulmonary edema in Chapters 17 and 25. The most frequently observed ILD of unknown cause is sarcoidosis, discussed separately in Chapter 16.

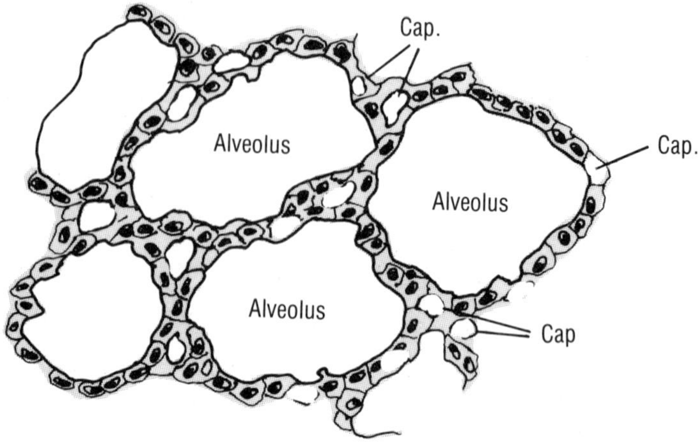

FIGURE 15-1 Area between the alveoli is the interstitium. It contains cells that make up the alveolar walls, plus capillaries (cap.) and connective tissue.

WHAT IS THE RELATIONSHIP OF ILD TO FIBROSIS?

Fibrosis is the medical term for scarring in the body's organs. Scarring (fibrosis) in organs is similar to scarring in the skin: Once-healthy tissue is replaced by tissue (the scar) that no longer functions as it should. For example, a skin scar will not sweat; lung tissue that is scarred (fibrosed) will not transfer oxygen and carbon

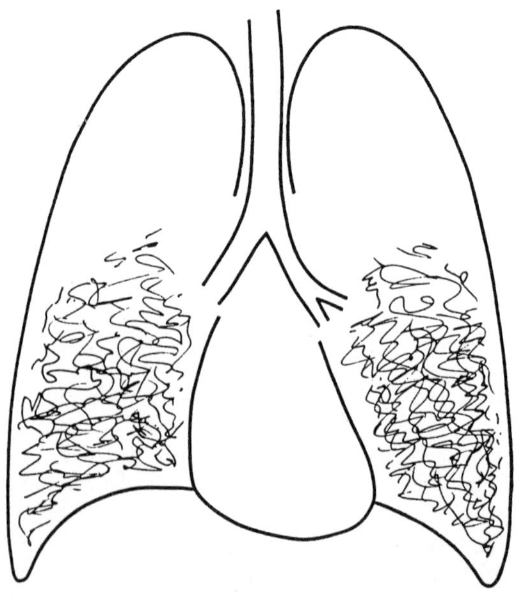

FIGURE 15-2 X-ray appearance of interstitial lung disease (ILD). Given the presence of an interstitial lung pattern as shown here, there is nothing unique on the x-ray for any particular cause, known or unknown.

TABLE 15-1 Causes of interstitial lung disease

KNOWN CAUSES

Drug-Induced

Antimicrobials:	nitrofurantoin (Furandantin), para-aminosalicylic acid (PAS), sulfonamides
Anticancer drugs:	bleomycin, methotrexate, azathioprine, chlorambucil
Epilepsy drug:	diphenylhydantoin (Dilantin)
Arthritis drug:	gold injections
Analgesics:	morphine, heroin, aspirin
Mineral oil	

Paraquat Ingestion—Paraquat is a poisonous herbicide

Radiation Therapy

Inhalation of Inorganic Dusts (Pneumoconiosis)

- Coal cust (coal workers' pneumoconiosis)
- Silica dust (silicosis)
- Asbestos dust (asbestosis)
- Other inorganic dusts

Lymphangitic Metastatic Cancer—Cancer that arises elsewhere and spreads to the interstitium of the lung

Infections

- Miliary tuberculosis (TB that spreads via the blood)
- Legionnaire's disease
- Various viral, fungal, and parasitic diseases that may infect the lungs

Heart Disease (Congestive Heart Failure and Pulmonary Edema)

UNKNOWN CAUSES

Sarcoidosis

Idiopathic pulmonary fibrosis (fibrosing alveolitis)

Collagen-vascular disorders

- Systemic lupus erythematosis
- Rheumatoid arthritis
- Progressive systemic sclerosis (scleroderma)
- Sjogren's syndrome
- Dermatomyositis
- Polymyositis

Eosinophilic granuloma

Goodpasture's syndrome

Idiopathic pulmonary hemosiderosis

Wegener's granulomatosis

Chronic eosinophilic pneumonia

Alveolar proteinosis

dioxide. Perhaps the most important aspect of fibrosis is its irreversibility. Once scar tissue has formed there is no way for it to regenerate into healthy tissue.

Fibrosis is the end result of almost all interstitial lung diseases that progress and do not respond to therapy. Fibrosis may occur over a period of time from days to years, although the latter is more characteristic of most ILDs. Prevention of fibrosis is the ultimate goal of any therapy for ILD.

The difficulty is knowing whether or not a specific ILD is progressive. For most of the ILDs of unknown cause, progression can only be determined by long-term followup of the patient with or without treatment. For diseases of known cause the natural course with and without treatment is usually better appreciated. For example, coal workers' pneumoconiosis is usually not progressive once coal dust exposure has ceased, and no treatment is needed; miliary tuberculosis can be fatal if untreated, but responds readily to appropriate antibiotics; lymphangitic cancer is invariably fatal regardless of treatment.

HOW DO DRUGS CAUSE INTERSTITIAL LUNG DISEASE?

Astonishingly, an estimated 5 percent of all hospital admissions in the United States are because of an adverse drug reaction, and between 10 and 18 percent of hospitalized patients have a drug reaction while in the hospital. Also, as many as 3 percent of all hospital deaths may be drug related (see *Task Force on Epidemiology*, page 59). Many of these drug reactions affect the lungs and cause a pattern of interstitial disease.

The spectrum of drug-induced lung disease is wide ranging, from mild through severe and even fatal reactions. The lung reaction may occur shortly after the drug is taken for the first time or after several months of use, or may not become manifest until after the drug has been stopped. So variable are the reactions that few generalizations can be made about this important cause of interstitial lung disease. Furthermore, while ILD is probably the most common pattern of pulmonary drug reaction, other pulmonary reactions may occur from drugs, including bronchospasm (asthma), pleural effusions, and enlarged lymph nodes.

The mechanism whereby any particular drug causes inflammation in the lungs is unknown. For some agents, such as morphine, heroin, and other analgesics, the lung reaction appears to be dose-related. With other drugs, the reaction appears to be idiosyncratic (a type of allergic reaction peculiar to the patient). It is likely that several mechanisms will ultimately be discovered to explain the diversity of reactions.

Treatment always involves stopping the offending agent. Corticosteroids are also frequently prescribed to reduce the inflammation.

WHAT ARE THE EFFECTS OF RADIATION THERAPY ON THE LUNGS?

Radiation therapy is frequently employed for treatment of pulmonary cancer, including both carcinoma and lymphoma. Unfortunately, 5 to 15 percent of patients receiving such radiation therapy to the chest will also get clinically apparent interstitial lung disease from the therapy (see References, Gross, N.J., page 81) and this may prove fatal before the cancer. Although host factors play an important role (as with drug reactions), the occurrence and severity of radiation-induced lung disease is dose-related. The higher the total X-ray dose the more likely will reactions occur.

To some extent radiation lung disease can be minimized by shielding the good lung tissue from the radiation beam, although for extensive lung cancers this is not always possible.

Treatment is corticosteroids, although the drug may be ineffective in severe or advanced cases.

WHAT IS IDIOPATHIC PULMONARY FIBROSIS?

Idiopathic means of unknown cause. Although all the other unknown causes (see Table 15-1) of ILD are also idiopathic, IPF nonetheless implies a distinct group. A synonym for IPF is "fibrosing alveolitis," since the disease begins with inflammation (alveolitis, or inflammation of the alveolar walls) and ends in fibrosis. What sets IPF apart from all other cases of ILD is the following:

1. The lung biopsy in IPF shows varying degrees of inflammation and fibrosis in a characteristic pattern, without evidence of granulomas to suggest sarcoidosis or tuberculosis, and no evidence of infection or tumor.
2. Other conditions that can lead to ILD, such as collagen-vascular diseases, are not present.
3. Although the clinical course varies widely, IPF is generally progressive, leading to death over an average 4-5 years from the time of diagnosis. Although treatment with corticosteroids may delay progression of ILD, the drugs are not thought to be curative.

After sarcoidosis, IPF is the most common of the unknown causes of ILD and actually accounts for more hospitalizations than does sarcoidosis. There were an estimated 15,000 IPF admissions in 1977 versus 11,000 for sarcoidosis; by contrast asthma accounted for an estimated 18,000 admissions the same year (see *Task Force on Epidemiology*, page 185).

WHAT ARE COLLAGEN-VASCULAR DISORDERS?

Collagen-vascular (C-V) disorders are a group of diseases that share certain clinical and laboratory features that arise from alterations in the connective tissue (which contains the complex chemical collagen) or blood supply of certain issues (hence vascular). As a group C-V disorders are poorly understood. They have also generated some confusion in the medical literature because of their protean manifestations and the difficulty in making a precise diagnosis. There is no known cause for any of the C-V disorders. The two most common are rheumatoid arthritis (RA) and systemic lupus erythematosus (SLE).

Rheumatoid arthritis may appear at any age and in either sex, but it most commonly afflicts middle-aged women. It classically begins with morning stiffness and may lead to deforming arthritis. However, arthritis is only one potential problem in patients with RA. Like all collagen-vascular disorders RA is a *systemic disease*—any part of the body may be involved and the lungs are no exception.

Pleural effusions and interstitial lung disease are the most common lung problems in patients with RA. However, only a minority of RA patients have these lung problems; also, there are many other causes of ILD and pleural effusions. For these reasons, attributing a lung problem to RA requires making a definite diagnosis of RA *and* ruling out other causes of the lung problem. Successful treatment of RA with clearing of the lung condition also helps to establish a relationship.

SLE shares many features with RA but has distinctive diagnostic criteria as well. Although SLE may occur at any age and in either sex, it usually afflicts young women. SLE tends to be a more fulminant process than RA and can be fatal when the kidneys or brain are involved. The lung disease that can occur with SLE is more likely to be pneumonia (due to the lupus itself and not to an infection) and pleural disease; interstitial lung disease may also occur but is less common than in RA. As in RA, attributing any lung problem to SLE requires a definite diagnosis of the collagen-vascular disorder and ruling out other causes of the lung disease.

Although the cause of SLE is unknown, several drugs have been found to cause a syndrome similar to spontaneously-occurring SLE (Table 15-2).

The most common symptom of drug-induced SLE is joint pain. These drugs may also cause pleural inflammation and fluid as seen in SLE unrelated to drugs. The main difference between spontaneously-occurring and drug-induced SLE is that the latter goes away when the drug is stopped.

WHAT OTHER DISEASES CAN LEAD TO INTERSTITIAL LUNG DISEASE?

The diseases discussed below are all rare, of unknown cause and diagnosed with certainty only by lung biopsy.

Eosinophilic granuloma is a systemic disease that may involve the bones as well as the lungs. It is a type of histiocytosis, a tissue reaction that may occur at any age. The childhood form is usually much more serious than the adult variety. Corticosteroids are the preferred treatment, although most adults do not require treatment.

Goodpasture's syndrome refers to a condition that involves both the lungs and the kidneys. It leads to hemoptysis (coughing up of blood) and can be fatal (either from kidney failure or hemoptysis). Treatment is difficult, but corticosteroids and other modalities have been tried with variable success.

Idiopathic pulmonary hemosiderosis is a disease also manifested by hemoptysis. It does not involve the kidneys. Hemosiderosis refers to deposits of heme (from breakdown of red blood cells) in the lung tissue, and the resulting scarring. The disease is usually progressive.

Wegener's granulomatosis is a systemic disease that affects not only the lungs, but also the kidneys and upper airways (nose, throat, sinuses). Until recently there was no effective treatment, but now the drug Cytoxan has produced some remissions. (The generic name for Cytoxan is cyclophosphamide; it is also used as an anti-cancer drug).

Chronic eosinophilic pneumonia is characterized by inflammation of the lungs with eosinophils, a type of white blood cell. Asthma is an accompanying

TABLE 15-2 Some medications implicated in drug-induced SLE

Generic Name of Drug	Type of Drug
Procainamide	anti-arrhythmic (heart medication)
Diphenylhydantoin	anti-epileptic
Hydralazine	anti-hypertensive
Isoniazid	anti-tuberculous
Chlorpromazine	anti-psychotic

feature in many of these patients. Treatment is with corticosteroids and response is usually good.

Alveolar proteinosis is really an "alveolar" disease as opposed to interstitial, but the X-ray may appear similar to any of the ILD's. In marked contrast to any ILD, alvolar proteinosis on biopsy shows deposits of dense, pink-staining material in the alveolar spaces. It is important to make the right diagnosis since there is a specific treatment, different from any other disease discussed in this chapter. Treatment involves washing out the lungs with saline solution, literally removing this dense material clogging up the airways. This is called bronchopulmonary lavage and is done under general anesthesia, one lung at a time. Depending on severity, treatments may have to be repeated. In mild cases of alveolar proteinosis no treatment is needed. Steroids are of no help in this condition.

CHAPTER SIXTEEN

Sarcoidosis: of Unknown Cause after 100 Years

WHAT IS SARCOIDOSIS?

Sarcoidosis is a systemic disease characterized by abnormal tissue swellings throughout the body. These swellings are called granulomas and are most commonly found in the lungs, liver, spleen, and skin. However, they may be found anywhere, including the eyes, ears, bones, and even in the coverings around the brain and spinal cord. Although these granulomas are usually widespread, they are very small and can only be seen with the aid of the microscope.

The cause of sarcoidosis is completely unknown. In the past, organisms such as viruses and bacteria (similar to the tuberculosis bacteria) were suspected. At one time pine pollen was thought to be the cause since many of the cases were found in people who lived near pine forests. The evidence for these and other agents has remained unproved. Sarcoidosis probably results from inhalation of some agent (? virus, ? bacteria), to which certain people react in an abnormal way by developing granulomas.

This disease occurs in all ages and races and in both sexes. It does not favor any socio-economic status, occupation, or level of education, and it is not caused by cigarette smoking, alcohol, or drugs. It is not inherited and does not tend to run in families. In the United States sarcoidosis seems to be most common in black women, but the reason is entirely unknown.

Many patients with sarcoidosis have no symptoms. The granulomas, hidden within the body's organs, are discovered only if carefully looked for. Thus, except for skin lesions, the clinical findings of sarcoidosis are non-specific, and most patients do not have skin involvement. In recent years certain X-ray and blood tests have proven more specific for this condition, so that many patients are now being presumptively diagnosed without resort to tissue examination. However, for the majority of patients a biopsy of some tissue is usually necessary to make the diagnosis.

The lungs are involved in over 90 percent of all sarcoidosis cases. In fact sarcoidosis is usually first suspected by finding an abnormal chest X-ray. It is unusual to see sarcoidosis with no lung involvement or where the chest X-ray is completely normal.

Historically sarcoidosis was not always perceived as a lung condition. For many years after the disease was first described in 1878, it was known as a skin condition only. In fact this is the origin of its name; since the skin lesions so resembled sarcomas (tumors) they were called "sarcoma-like" or "sarcoid." It was only in 1915, 20 years after the discovery of X-rays by Roentgen in 1895, that sarcoidosis was found to involve the lungs.

IS SARCOIDOSIS A SERIOUS ILLNESS?

So variable is sarcoidosis that generalization is difficult. Many people with sarcoidosis have no symptoms. The majority, even with symptoms, tend to suffer no severe impairment. Approximately 20 to 25 percent of patients do have permanent loss of lung function but are still able to live a relatively normal life. In only a small percentage, perhaps less than 5 percent, is the sarcoidosis so severe as to eventually be the cause of death.

Symptoms are often referable to the respiratory system, since the lungs are involved over 90 percent of the time. If lung sarcoidosis is extensive, the patient may have shortness of breath, but this is usually noticeable only on exertion, not at rest. One of the most common reasons to treat sarcoidosis is for difficult breathing. However, any time sarcoidosis causes impairment of a vital organ, such as the eye or heart, treatment is also indicated.

HOW IS THE DIAGNOSIS OF SARCOIDOSIS MADE?

Sometimes this is not easy. To be sure of the diagnosis in most patients, including virtually all cases that require treatment, doctors must obtain a piece of involved organ or tissue and demonstrate sarcoidosis granulomas under the microscope. In most cases a major operation is not needed to obtain the biopsy. Some of the areas that may be involved with sarcoid granulomas, and from which tissue can be readily obtained, are the skin, the eyelid, the lungs, and the liver. Lung tissue may be biopsied by means of the fiberoptic bronchoscope, discussed in Chapter 8. In about 75 percent of pulmonary sarcoidosis cases, a tiny piece of lung tissue taken via the bronchoscope will suffice to make the diagnosis.

In some cases sarcoidosis can be diagnosed without resort to tissue biopsy. Generally this is done only when other likely diseases have been ruled out (such as tuberculosis) and treatment of the sarcoidosis is not being contemplated. One form of sarcoidosis not requiring tissue biopsy is known as Stage 1 (see below), in an asymptomatic patient. Physicians are usually content to follow such patients without treatment. In the event of progression of disease (either on the chest X-ray or by the development of symptoms), a tissue biopsy would be indicated.

At one point a skin test, known as the Kveim test, looked promising for the diagnosis of sarcoidosis. It involves taking a portion of the spleen from a patient with sarcoidosis and processing it in such a way that when injected under the skin of a suspected sarcoidosis patient a sarcoidosis-type reaction occurs. This is proved by a biopsy of the skin reaction area (after six weeks) and examination under the microscope. If this test were widely available and standardized it would be a helpful tool to make the diagnosis. Unfortunately, Kveim antigen (as the spleen extract is known) is available in only a few medical centers in the USA and is not standardized. In addition, the reaction itself is controversial since other diseases have been found to cause the same granuloma reaction. It seems the material injected has to be just the right chemical makeup or it won't be specific for sarcoidosis. Thus, the general unavailability of Kveim antigen and lack of standardization are reasons why it is not widely used to diagnose sarcoidosis.

In recent years two other non-invasive tools have proved helpful. One is the gallium scan, a nuclear medicine scan that may yield a highly specific pattern in patients with sarcoidosis (see Chapter 8).

The other is a blood test called "Angiotensin Converting Enzyme." For unknown reasons the ACE level is elevated in most active sarcoidosis cases. In fact an elevated ACE level and characteristic gallium scan, along with a compatible clinical history and X-ray picture, are virtually diagnostic of sarcoidosis even without a tissue biopsy.

CAN SARCOIDOSIS MIMIC OTHER DISEASES?

Commonly. In fact this is one of the reasons why the diagnosis is sometimes very difficult. Among the diseases that are most often confused with sarcoidosis are lymphoma (tumor of the lymph glands), tuberculosis, and several unusual diseases that may cause the same X-ray picture. Since the treatment of all these is different, it is important to be sure of the diagnosis. That is why, except for the mildest case, a tissue biopsy is usually indicated.

WHAT ARE THE STAGES OF SARCOIDOSIS?

There are three classically described stages of sarcoidosis based on the chest X-ray: Stages I, II, and III.

In Stage I the lymph nodes of the lungs near the center of the chest (the hilar areas) become enlarged, sometimes to the size of potatoes. The lungs themselves don't show any disease on the chest X-ray. Stage I patients are usually asymptomatic and require no treatment (Figure 16-1a).

Stage II shows the enlarged lymph nodes, but there is also an abnormal pattern in the lung fields (Figure 16-1b). Stage II patients usually show some decrease in pulmonary function as well as symptoms (cough or dyspnea), and may require treatment.

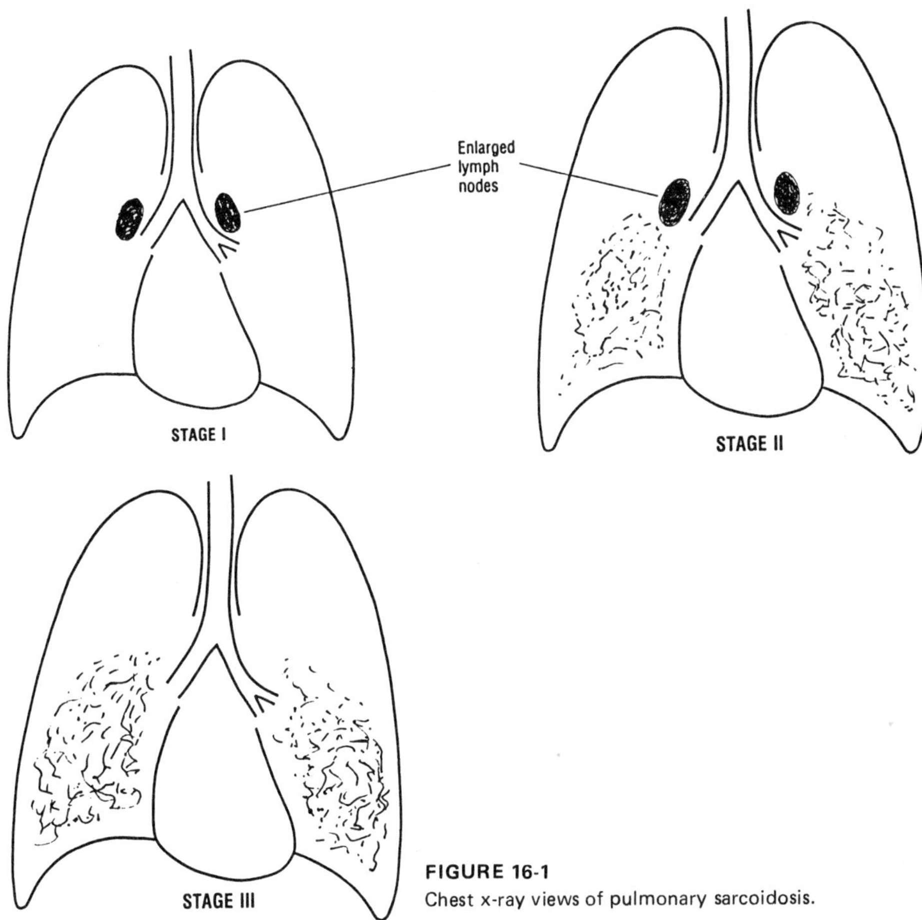

FIGURE 16-1
Chest x-ray views of pulmonary sarcoidosis.

Stage III shows the lung infiltrates without evidence of enlarged lymph nodes in the hilar areas (Figure 16-1c). It is possible these patients once had the hilar "potato nodes," and that progression of their disease had lead to mainly lung involvement and disappearance of the nodes. For most patients who present with Stage III, however, this progression cannot be demonstrated.

Most patients don't actually show progression from Stage I to III or even Stage II to III. Patients may have any one of the three stages, and from that point may stay there, improve (with disappearance of X-ray changes altogether), or worsen (progress in staging). This is another way of saying that the natural history of sarcoidosis is unpredictable.

WHAT IS THE TREATMENT FOR SARCOIDOSIS?

Most patients with sarcoidosis are not treated. Sarcoidosis tends to be a benign disease and its cause is unknown. The available treatment is not a cure, but is only helpful in slowing down (and occasionally stopping) the sarcoidosis process. Since this is non-specific treatment for a disease of unknown cause, physicians only treat sarcoidosis patients if there is a compelling reason.

At present the only effective treatment for sarcoidosis is some form of corticosteroid (steroid) medication. The drug is usually taken by mouth; commonly used are prednisone tablets, one type of steroid. Steroids are the same class of drugs sometimes given for severe arthritis, asthma, and a host of other medical illnesses (see Appendix C). For sarcoidosis, steroids are non-specific treatment. Limited evidence suggests that steroid treatment, once begun, has to be given for at least six months to two years to be effective. The aim of treatment is to improve the patient's function or to at least slow down progression of the sarcoidosis.

Unfortunately, sarcoidosis can never be considered cured, only slowed down or arrested. There are several reasons for this. First, in its early stages the disease sometimes gets better without any treatment whatsoever. Thus, physicians are never sure if a treated patient improves because of the steroids or because of a natural remission. Second, some patients improve after taking the steroid medication, but when they stop, suffer a relapse—the sarcoidosis symptoms and signs flare up. Third, even after prolonged steroid treatment microscopic granulomas can often be found in the body, indicating that some stage of the disease is still present.

Progressive sarcoidosis, unresponsive to steroids, is a medical dilemma. There is currently no other effective treatment for the disease, although experimental drugs are frequently tested. Any patient who has progressive or severe sarcoidosis unresponsive to steroids is likely to have complications, either of the disease or of the treatment, and should come under the care of a physician able to manage the problem. An example is the patient with advanced sarcoidosis who has developed respiratory failure, or the patient who has a metabolic derangement from chronic, high dose steroids. Fortunately, such cases are a small minority of all sarcoidosis patients.

T.R.S.—A Case of Sarcoidosis

Mr. S. is a 27-year-old graduate student who has had a persistent dry cough for the past month. He has also lost 10 pounds. A chest X-ray in the college health clinic shows a diffuse lung infiltrate and enlarged hilar lymph nodes in both lungs (Stage II Pulmonary Sarcoidosis). Because of this he is referred to a chest physician.

On further history we learn he has not been exposed to toxins, chemicals, or tuberculosis (TB). He has no personal history of TB or other lung disease and has never smoked. His last chest X-ray was four years ago and was normal.

He is admitted to the hospital for further tests. Skin tests show no reaction to TB or mumps; since most of the population reacts to a mumps skin test, this suggests a depression in his immune system, a common finding in sarcoidosis. Blood tests are normal, helping to rule out major involvement in his kidneys, liver, and pancreas. Pulmonary function tests reveal some decrease in his vital capacity and other lung volumes, consistent with a restrictive respiratory problem. A gallium scan shows increased activity in both lungs, consistent with an active process such as sarcoidosis. All of these studies are completed within 48 hours and a presumptive diagnosis of sarcoidosis is made. Because he is symptomatic (cough and weight loss) and warrants treatment, an attempt is made to obtain diagnostic tissue. On the third hospital day fiberoptic bronchoscopy and transbronchial lung biopsy are performed. The results show non-caseating granuloma, confirming the diagnosis of sarcoidosis.

He is started on oral prednisone and within three days his cough disappears and he feels better. He is prescribed low dose prednisone for the next 12 months and plans are made to follow his course with serial chest X-rays and breathing studies.

CHAPTER SEVENTEEN

Heart Disease: A Major Cause of Trouble Breathing

HOW CAN HEART DISEASE CAUSE TROUBLE BREATHING?

The right side of the heart pumps venous (de-oxygenated) blood to the lungs where it is oxygenated. This oxygenated blood then returns to the left side of the heart and is pumped out to the rest of the body. In heart failure, a very common condition, the left side of the heart is weakened, resulting in a back-up of blood into the lungs. This is called congestive heart failure (CHF). The pumping action of the heart still works but not as efficiently as normal, and the lungs become congested with extra blood. This congestion of the blood capillaries in the lungs causes shortness of breath (dyspnea); it can be relieved by giving heart pills (such as digoxin) and water pills (diuretics).

Since heart disease is more common than lung disease, the most common organic cause of dyspnea is probably heart trouble. It's important to recognize if the dyspnea is due to primary heart or lung disease, since the treatment is different. This distinction requires a thorough medical evaluation. Often breathing tests and chest X-ray will have to be done to determine the cause. In many patients *both* the lungs and heart are diseased so treatment must be given for both.

WHAT IS THE DIFFERENCE BETWEEN RIGHT AND LEFT HEART FAILURE?

There are two sides of the heart, right and left (see Chapter 1). Each contains two chambers, a right atrium and ventricle and a left atrium and ventricle. Remember that the right side of the heart receives venous blood from the body's tissues and sends it to the lungs to pick up oxygen; the left side of the heart receives oxygenated blood from the lungs and sends it to the body's tissues via the arterial system. Either side of the heart may be stressed to the point of failure. Clinically we speak of patients manifesting either right heart failure, left heart failure, or both. A few generalizations can be made about the two conditions.

Right-sided heart failure is often *due* to lung disease, most commonly chronic obstructive lung disease (see Chapter 12). The right side of the heart suffers increased stress as it pumps blood into a diseased lung. The end result is a large heart (enlargement of the right atrium and ventricle) and fluid backing up in the systemic venous system. This leads to edema (increased fluid) of the legs, bloating, and occasionally abdominal discomfort and ascites (fluid within the abdomen).

Dyspnea in the presence of right heart failure is due to the underlying lung disease, not the heart failure. Treatment is that of the underlying lung condition, since any improvement in lung function will help relieve stress on the right side of the heart. When hypoxemia is present, oxygen is the best single treatment. Diuretics are also frequently used to help mobilize the excess fluid.

R.H.—A Case of Right-Sided Heart Failure

Mr. R.H., 59, was admitted to the hospital because of shortness of breath and leg swelling. He was a heavy smoker for many years, but had no history of heart disease or high blood pressure. In the hospital a chest X-ray showed an enlarged heart and no fluid in the lungs. His blood oxygen level was low.

Mr. R.H. was treated with bed rest, nasal oxygen, and water pills. Within a week he lost 15 pounds and felt much better. His lung function studies showed severe impairment and a need for continuous oxygen at home.

Diagnosis: right-sided heart failure due to severe chronic bronchitis (see Chapter 12). Treatment: For the lung problem, in this case, mainly oxygen and an occasional water pill.

Left-sided heart failure is often due to primary heart disease, usually of the coronary artery blood vessels or of the left heart valves (aortic or mitral valves). Another common cause of left heart failure is severe high blood pressure. In contrast to right heart failure, which results from lung disease, left heart failure may cause lung disease, or at least lead to back-up fluid within the lungs. When this occurs, dyspnea and abnormal gas exchange result. In severe cases of left heart failure the right side of the heart may also fail. However, before the right heart becomes weakened, patients with left-sided failure may experience profound dyspnea without evidence of bloating or edema elsewhere in their body.

L.H.—A Case of Left-Sided Heart Failure

Mr. L.H., 62, was hospitalized because of shortness of breath and leg swelling. He was a nonsmoker, but did have a history of high blood pressure for many years. His chest X-ray showed a large heart, with fluid in and around both lungs. His blood oxygen tension was low.

Mr. L.H. was treated with bedrest, oxygen, heart and water pills, and antihypertensive medication. Within a week he lost 12 pounds. Lung function studies were near normal and his oxygen level was adequate.

Diagnosis: left-sided heart failure due to high blood pressure. Treatment: for the heart problem, in this case heart pills and blood pressure medication to relieve the strain on the heart.

Both conditions may thus lead to congestive heart failure. Right heart failure leads to congestion of the systemic venous system and back-up of fluid in the visible parts of the body (extremities, abdomen). Left heart failure leads to congestion in the pulmonary vessels; this congestion can be seen on a chest X-ray. When left heart failure is severe, the term "cardiac pulmonary edema" is often used. The differences between right and left heart failure are summarized in Table 17-1, along with terms common to both.

Figure 17-1 shows an X-ray picture of normal heart and lungs (17-1a) compared with an X-ray of right heart failure due to chronic obstructive pulmonary disease (17-1b) and an X-ray of left-sided congestive heart failure (17-1c). Lines radiating out from the heart represent exaggerated blood vessels in patient with left heart failure. Figure 17-1d shows X-ray of acute left heart failure: cardiac pulmonary edema. The difference between 17-1c and 17-1d is a matter of degree; in the latter, fluid has leaked out of the capillaries to collect in the alveolar spaces. Such an X-ray appearance, characteristic of pulmonary edema, is often referred to as "batwing."

WHAT IS PULMONARY EDEMA?

Pulmonary edema is water in the lungs. More specifically it is an abnormal accumulation of fluid in the smallest airways and alveoli. This fluid comes from the blood vessels surrounding the millions of alveoli. The most common mechanism for this fluid build-up is increased *pressure* in the pulmonary blood vessels due to failure of the left side of the heart.

Cardiac pulmonary edema is thus one manifestation of congestive heart failure and the terms are sometimes used interchangeably. As commonly used, cardiac pulmonary edema refers to the acute, severe form of left-sided heart failure, not to chronic, insidious cases. The X-ray shown in Figure 17-1c could be inter-

TABLE 17-1 Differences between right and left heart failure

Right-Sided Heart Failure	Left-Sided Heart Failure
Due to lung disease *or* left heart failure	Due to primary heart disease or high blood pressure
Does not cause dyspnea; dyspnea part of underlying lung disease	Causes dyspnea by back-up of fluid within the lungs
Treatment that of underlying lung condition; oxygen often therapeutic and diuretics may also help	Treatment that of underlying heart condition or of high blood pressure
Synonyms often used: Congestive heart failure (right-sided) Cor Pulmonale Right ventricular failure Secondary heart failure	Synonyms often used: Congestive heart failure (left-sided) (Cardiac) pulmonary edema Left ventricular failure Primary heart failure

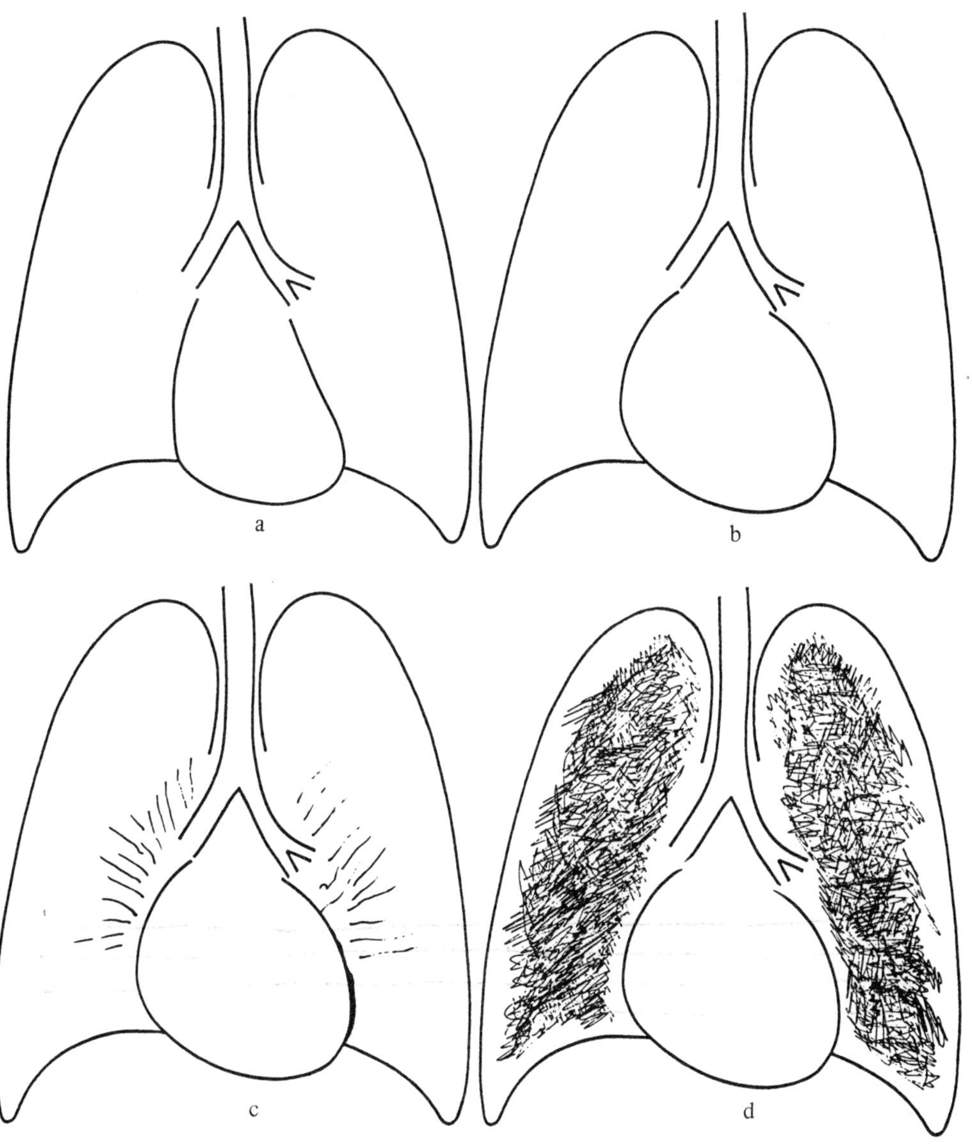

FIGURE 17-1 Chest X-rays of normal heart (a) and of patients with heart disease (b-d). See text for discussion.

preted as indicating CHF or cardiac pulmonary edema, both meaning the same thing. Figure 17-1d shows a more classic example of cardiac pulmonary edema.

Pulmonary edema may also occur unrelated to heart disease or CHF, so-called non-cardiac pulmonary edema. Here, the mechanism is not increased pressure from a failing heart, but pulmonary capillary damage and leakage of blood plasma into the alveoli. The heart may function normally in this condition. In contrast to cardiac pulmonary edema, a variety of diseases may lead to non-cardiac pulmonary edema, a subject covered more fully in Chapter 25 (Respiratory Failure).

HOW IS HEART DISEASE DISTINGUISHED FROM LUNG DISEASE IN A PATIENT WITH DYSPNEA?

There are no reliable physical signs or symptoms that will always distinguish heart from lung causes of dyspnea when either may be present. Difficult diagnostic problems often occur in patients who may have either pulmonary or heart disease as a cause of dyspnea.

Chronic obstructive pulmonary disease (COPD) is a common respiratory cause of dyspnea. Its treatment is different from primary (left-sided) heart failure, yet both can present with nearly identical symptoms and signs.

For example, shortness of breath while lying down, swelling of the legs, and abnormal breathing sounds are all time-honored findings in both left heart failure and COPD.

The most useful test to diagnose left heart failure in such patients is the routine chest X-ray. It shows an enlarged heart and congested pulmonary blood vessels in patients with left-sided CHF. When COPD is accompanied by right heart failure the X-ray will also show a large heart, but not the congested pulmonary blood vessels (unless left heart failure is also present).

Breathing (pulmonary function) tests, along with arterial blood gases, are helpful in diagnosing COPD. These show an obstructive respiratory pattern and (usually) abnormal O_2 and/or CO_2 blood tensions.

Pulmonary function tests and chest X-rays can often distinguish between the two common causes of difficult breathing. When these tests fail, more sophisticated methods such as cardiac catheterization may have to be employed.

WHAT IS CARDIAC ASTHMA?

When left heart failure occurs, fluid backs up into the lungs and leads to dyspnea. The patient may also notice wheezing, or wheezes may be heard by the physician. Wheezing due to the left heart failure is "cardiac asthma." It is not the same asthma as described in Chapter 10, and treatment is for the heart problem and not for a primary pulmonary condition. Although some of the same drugs used in treating regular asthma may be used (particularly aminophylline), heart medication and diuretics are also helpful. Normalizing heart function is usually sufficient to correct the wheezing and dyspnea of cardiac asthma; in regular asthma heart function is normal to begin with (unless the patient has two conditions).

As discussed in Chapter 10 there are several causes of wheezing, only one of which is "pure" asthma. The distinction between cardiac asthma and the more common variety of asthma described in Chapter 10 is best achieved by a chest X-ray and thorough medical evaluation.

CHAPTER EIGHTEEN

From Colds to Influenza: Common Infections of the Respiratory Tract

WHAT IS THE COMMON COLD?

It is impossible to talk about colds without discussing viruses, since these ubiquitous organisms are the cause. Viruses are submicroscopic living particles, smaller than bacteria, that can infect any part of the body and cause symptoms. The lungs and respiratory tract are particularly vulnerable since viruses are easily passed from person to person in the air.

Viruses can cause virtually any type of respiratory infection. The most benign is the common cold. The most serious is a form of pneumonia caused by influenza virus that can spread to involve both lungs and prove fatal (see Chapter 19).

In the United States viral infections of the respiratory tract are responsible for an estimated 250 million lost work days annually. One estimate puts the economic loss at 5 billion dollars each year, of which the common cold accounts for approximately 2 billion dollars.

The common cold, bane of millions, is the most frequent viral infection of the respiratory tract. It occurs with characteristic symptoms: some combinations of runny nose, watery eyes, cough, sneezing, mild sore throat, malaise, and headache. Not all symptoms are present every time. Fever may also occur, but is usually low grade. The symptoms run their course in a week or so, and otherwise healthy people recover without any specific treatment.

Each person has, on the average, two to three colds a year. The virus types responsible for most of them are rhinovirus ("rhino" from the Greek word for nose) and coronavirus ("corona" from the halo formed around the virus's body when seen under the electron microscope). Many other virus types may also cause the common cold.

Rhinovirus is transmitted through the air, often as a result of coughs; it may also be spread by sneezing or even during talking. Rhinovirus and other cold viruses can also be contacted from objects (clothes, phones, books, and so forth) where the virus has settled.

WHAT IS THE BEST TREATMENT FOR THE COMMON COLD?

The old adage about bed rest and plenty of fluids for treating the common cold is as true now as a century ago. Aspirin may help to relieve malaise and discomfort and a nasal spray may ease the congestion, but there is simply no specific treatment for the common cold. Fortunately, recovery usually occurs in a few days no matter what we do.

For the uncomplicated cold antibiotics are not helpful; they will not speed recovery. Antibiotics may help the common cold patient who has underlying chronic lung disease and the possibility of a bacterial infection, or who has a complication of the cold such as sinus or ear infection.

It is a good idea not to take antibiotics for the common cold without consulting a physician. You may be taking an antibiotic inappropriately or the wrong antibiotic. Cold symptoms that should alert you to the possible need for medical evaluation include:

- high fever (above 103°) lasting more than a day
- shortness of breath
- persistent ear pain or drainage from an ear
- coughing up blood or blood-streaked sputum (any sputum during an uncomplicated cold should be whitish in color)
- chest pain
- persistence of debilitating symptoms for more than a few days

IS VITAMIN C HELPFUL?

Vitamin C is ascorbic acid, one of the essential vitamins since it must be supplied in the diet–your body cannot make it. Lack of Vitamin C leads to scurvy, a discovery made in the 1800s when a daily ration of limes was found to prevent the disease in British sailors. True lack of Vitamin C causes malaise, irritability, emotional disturbances, arthralgia (joint pain), nosebleeds, and bleeding under the skin. It is rare for anyone in this country to be truly deficient in Vitamin C, although it can occur in alcoholics, dietary cultists, and some chronically ill patients.

The daily need for Vitamin C at any age is between 35 and 60 milligrams. A glass of orange juice (200 ml) contains 100 mg, so it is not difficult to obtain the daily requirement. Those who recommend Vitamin C for colds and flu advocate megadoses, at least 1,000 mg/day or more. Whether or not this is helpful is problematical. In 1970 Nobel prize-winning scientist Dr. Linus Pauling published a book strongly advocating ascorbic acid for the common cold. Since then there have appeared dozens of scientific articles and statements supporting both sides of the issue. There is no consensus among the medical community about the value of Vitamin C in either preventing or treating colds and flu. This lack of consensus reflects the conflicting nature of the medical findings.

The 1983 edition of AMA DRUG EVALUATIONS makes this statement (page 575):* Since the use of large doses of vitamin C were recommended on theoretical grounds in 1970, claims have been made that large doses prevent or cure the common cold. Numerous experiments have failed to produce any clearcut indication that vitamin C in any dosage protects against or ameliorates the symptoms of the common cold. . . Overall, there is no indication in the current knowledge of biochemistry and physiology or in controlled studies that the use of ascorbic acid (Vitamin C) can prevent or cure acute or chronic respiratory infections.

WHAT IS THE DIFFERENCE BETWEEN THE COMMON COLD AND THE FLU?

The flu refers to a syndrome usually caused by influenza virus, hence the origin of the term "flu." Other viruses can also cause this syndrome, although not usually the same ones as cause the common cold.

Apart from the type of causative virus, the main difference between the flu and the common cold is the degree and type of symptoms. The flu usually appears suddenly and within a day you feel very ill. Profound malaise is characteristic, accompanied by dry cough and fever, often to 103° or higher. By contrast, cold symptoms usually build up over one or more days and, although the symptoms are annoying, you don't feel systemically ill. Runny nose, watery eyes and sneezing–all characteristic of the common cold–are usually absent in the flu.

The flu also tends to last longer than a cold. Once the fever and ill feeling have abated, symptoms of weakness or lethargy may persist for another week or so. The symptoms of a cold are usually completely gone within a week after it began.

Most patients with the flu recover uneventfully. However, complications can occur.

WHAT ARE THE COMPLICATIONS OF THE FLU?

Even without complications most flu sufferers are very ill and feel fortunate to recover in a week or so. Influenza is a systemic disease and for a small number of patients major complications can occur. Most of these are bacterial infections, particularly bacterial pneumonia (see Chapter 19). Bacterial pneumonia was probably responsible for most of the deaths in the great influenza pandemic of 1918.

Other complications are encephalitis (inflammation of the brain), other nervous system disorders, and kidney failure. People most prone to develop com-

*Quoted by permission, The American Medical Association.

plications during flu epidemics are the elderly and debiltated, those with chronic diseases, or those have a compromised immune system. Military recruits and others living in a very close quarters are also at increased risk of flu complications.

ARE SMOKERS MORE LIKELY TO GET THE FLU?

It appears so. And to get it more severely. During a flu outbreak (influenza A) among young Israeli soldiers, doctors were careful to note which patients were smokers and which were not. They found that 68.5 percent of smokers came down with the flu, compared with only 47.2 percent of nonsmokers (see Kark, et al). In other words, smokers were about one and a half times more likely to contract the flu than were nonsmokers. Also, among those recruits who did get the flu, smokers were likely to have a more severe case. This result (more likely to get the flu, and more severely) has been supported by other studies in other countries.

What about other viral syndromes? Another large study (Aronson, et al) found that acute respiratory tract illness (ARTI) was more common and more severe in smokers. Over 1,000 people reporting acute respiratory symptoms (cough, chest congestion, swollen neck glands, sore throat) to an outpatient clinic were asked about their smoking habits. The result? Smokers were much more likely to contract ARTI than nonsmokers, and to get it more severely.

To summarize, not only does cigarette smoking have the severe effects outlined in Chapter 2, it also contributes to thc occurrence and severity of common respiratory infections.

HOW IS THE FLU PREVENTED?

The flu vaccine is designed to prevent influenza. When given before the onset of a flu epidemic, it can prevent an estimated 70 to 90 percent of cases that would otherwise occur. Unfortunately, the viruses responsible for the flu change their characteristics every one to three years, so the vaccine also has to be changed frequently to be effective. Furthermore, these changes in vaccine have to be made in anticipation of the viral strains that will cause the flu. Such predictions are not always accurate. In 1976 many older citizens received the swine flu vaccine in anticipation of an epidemic that fortunately did not occur.

The flu vaccine is made from killed virus, and each year's vaccine includes several strains. For example, the vaccine for 1983-84 contained both A and B influenza virus strains (A/Brazil/78, A/Philippines/82 and B/Singapore/79), in a single 0.5 ml dose for injection.

Vaccination to prevent flu is recommended for patients with chronic or debilitating disease, such as severe emphysema, chronic bronchitis, heart disease that may lead to heart failure, chronic kidney failure, cancer, and so forth. The United States Public Health Service also recommends flu vaccine for individuals over 65. Usage for a pregnant woman should be along the same guidelines as for the general population. There is no evidence that flu vaccine causes harm to mother or fetus (the vaccine does not contain live virus). Even so, if it must be given to a pregnant woman, the PHS recommends waiting until the second or third trimester.

Because it is made from killed virus, the vaccine itself will not cause the flu. However, reactions can occur, though not as often as with the older vaccines used several years ago. Some people will experience a red, tender area where the shot is given. A few may also get a slight fever with chills and headache that abates in one to two days. An allergic reaction can also occur, presumably due to the egg protein since the virus is grown in eggs, but this reaction is very rare.

Perhaps the most dreaded reaction is the Guillain Barré syndrome (GBS). This is ascending paralysis that can lead to respiratory failure and death (see Chapter 14). It is a rare occurence from the vaccine and can also occur from the flu itself. In the 1976 swine flu program GBS occurred in approximately one out of every 100,000 persons vaccinated and was fatal in one in 20 who came down with the syndrome. A GBS surveillance program begun in 1978 has uncovered no excess cases of GBS with influenza vaccine used since then. According to the PHS, "any risk of GBS from influenza vaccine appears to be far lower than the risks associated with influenza among persons for whom the vaccine is indicated" (*MMWR* 31:26, July 9, 1982, 352).

IS THERE ANY TREATMENT FOR THE FLU?

For years the standard treatment for the flu has been bed rest, plenty of fluids, and aspirin to control symptoms. This is still recommended, for in fact the illness is self-limiting and the vast majority of patients get better without complications.

A new anti-viral drug has changed this approach for some influenza victims. Although very few anti-viral drugs are available, one in particular has proved effective against the influenza A strain of virus. The drug is amantadine (trade name Symmetrel). In several studies of patients during small outbreaks of influenza A, amantadine has been shown to:

1. Prevent or greatly ameliorate the flu syndrome when taken before symptoms occur, in essence acting as a prophylactic medication.
2. Attenuate the course of the flu after the illness has begun, when given during the first 48 hours of symptoms.

Most of these studies have been in chronically ill patients who run a high risk of complications from influenza A infections. However, in one study of college students, those receiving amantadine returned to their classes earlier and shed smaller amounts of virus than those receiving a placebo (an inert substance).

Amantadine has relatively minor side effects, mainly lightheadedness; when compared with flu symptoms the side effects appear a reasonable trade-off. At present the drug appears most useful in people who run a definite risk of contracting influenza A infection (as during a defined outbreak). It is not indicated for the individual patient who has the flu syndrome as an isolated case, unless the patient is very ill and the flu can be attributed to the influenza A virus.

WHAT OTHER RESPIRATORY INFECTIONS ARE CAUSED BY VIRUSES?

Besides the common cold and flu syndromes, viruses can cause other types of respiratory infections.

Pneumonia This is an infection of one or both lungs manifested by fluid and inflammation in the alveolar air spaces. Influenza virus can itself cause a pneumonia or can make the patient susceptible to a bacterial pneumonia. Pneumonia is discussed in Chapter 19.

Bronchiolitis This viral infection is limited to the smaller airways, called bronchioles. It is more common in children than in adults.

Laryngo-Tracheo-Bronchitis An infection of the trachea, larynx (voice box), and large bronchi. It occurs most commonly in children where it is also called croup, because of the characteristic "croupy" cough, a high-pitched barking sound.

Pharyngitis An infection of the throat, the area behind and below the tongue.

With any of these infections the patient may feel systemically ill, run a high fever, and require several days for complete recovery.

CHAPTER NINETEEN

Pneumonia and Pleurisy

WHAT IS PNEUMONIA?

Pneumonia* is an inflammation of the lung, usually caused by infection. Pneumonia can also be due to causes other than infection, such as chemical irritants, radiation, aspiration of stomach contents, and so forth. In such cases the pneumonia or pneumonitis is qualified (radiation pneumonitis, chemical pneumonia, aspiration pneumonia, and so on). Unless so qualified in this chapter, "pneumonia" refers to the inflammation caused by infection.

Infection may occur in only a small part of the lung or may involve an entire lung or both lungs (so-called double pneumonia). The infecting organism grows in the lung tissue, causing the body to defend itself by mobilizing infection-fighting cells. In the process the patient develops symptoms such as chills, fever, cough, and general malaise.

These symptoms may range from very mild (often called "walking pneumonia" because the patient can walk around with it) to very severe and even fatal. Pneumonia can be caused by almost any type of organism, although a few specific viruses and bacteria are responsible for most cases, and can occur at any age.

One of the great medical advances has been the development of antibiotics for treating some of the pneumonias. Penicillin, erythromycin, and tetracycline

*Another term often used interchangeably with pneumonia is pneumonitis (from "pneumo" meaning "of the lung" and "itis," "inflammation").

are among the most useful. Despite this miracle group of drugs pneumonia remains a very important problem. In 1936, before the advent of antibiotics, pneumonia was the number one cause of death in the United States. Today pneumonia and influenza (a viral infection frequently complicated by pneumonia) are listed as the fifth leading cause of death.

Most pneumonia fatalities occur in elderly or debilitated patients, or in those who have compromised body defenses as may occur from chronic lung disease, cancer, or after kidney transplantation. However, pneumonia can also be fatal in young adults, particularly when due to organisms such as viruses that do not respond to antibiotics. Fortunately, most viral pneumonias are self-limiting and patients fully recover.

WHAT ARE THE INFECTIOUS CAUSES OF PNEUMONIA?

Pneumonia is caused by microscopic and submicroscopic organisms that infect the lung tissue. There are four main groups of organisms capable of causing this infection:

Bacteria These are the relatively large organisms that can usually be seen under the microscope. They can invariably be killed or retarded with antibiotics; otherwise healthy patients who develop bacterial pneumonia respond favorably when given the appropriate antibiotic. One unusual bacterium has recently been shown to be responsible for Legionnaire's disease (discussed in a later section).

Bacteria-Like Bacteria-like organisms fall somewhere between viruses and bacteria. They share features of both, and microbiologists do not all agree on their classification. One such organism, called mycoplasma, causes a characteristic pneumonia manifested by cough, chest pain, and a patchy infiltrate on the chest X-ray. Such lung infections are called "atypical pneumonia" to distinguish them from "typical" bacterial pneumonia. We now know that pneumonia of any particular cause can have either typical or atypical features, so the terminology is not very helpful.

Fortunately, the biochemical nature of mycoplasma and other bacteria-like organisms allows them to be destroyed or inhibited by antibiotics. Mycoplasma infections usually respond to either erythromycin or tetracycline; penicillin is ineffective.

Viruses These are sub-microscopic organisms very different from the above two groups. They live only in cells and do not respond to antibiotics. However, the body makes a powerful anti-viral substance, interferon, that helps to control most viral infections. Viral infections are difficult to diagnose in the early stages, in part because the organisms cannot be seen with an ordinary microscope. On clinical grounds they cannot be separated from mycoplasma and other bacteria-like infections, and for this reason all patients with presumed viral pneumonia are still treated with antibiotics, usually erythromycin or tetracycline.

Miscellaneous A large group of miscellaneous organisms may infect the lungs, including fungi, molds, parasites, and other unusual organisms that are not classified into one of the three groups above. This miscellaneous group usually infects only patients who are immuno-compromised—whose natural immune system is depressed or compromised enough to allow unusual organisms to gain a foothold. Immune depression may occur either from an underlying disease or from treatment for the disease. Examples include kidney transplant patients who are receiving immunosuppressive agents to help prevent rejection of the kidney, cancer patients receiving drugs that depress the immune system while attacking cancer cells, and patients with blood disorders such as multiple myeloma that directly affect the body's immune system.

HOW IS PNEUMONIA DIAGNOSED?

Doctors generally go through four steps to make the diagnosis. As in any disease, the diagnosis must first be suspected before it can be made. This is not usually difficult. In fact patients will often suspect the diagnosis even before consulting a physician, because of symptoms different from any flu or cold ever experienced. High fever, chills, chest pain, and coughing up dark or foul-smelling sputum are often present in pneumonia and should always make one suspect the diagnosis. By using a stethoscope the physician can hear a "noisy" chest as air goes in and out of the inflamed passages.

In step two the physician confirms the diagnosis by chest X-ray. The chest X-ray is an invaluable test for both diagnosing and following patients with pneumonia, since it shows the extent of the disease as well as any subsequent progression or relapse. Figures 19-1 through 19-4 show some typical X-ray presentations or pneumonia.

In step three the physician attempts to find the cause. This involves ordering certain tests to help determine which organism is responsible for the infection. Such

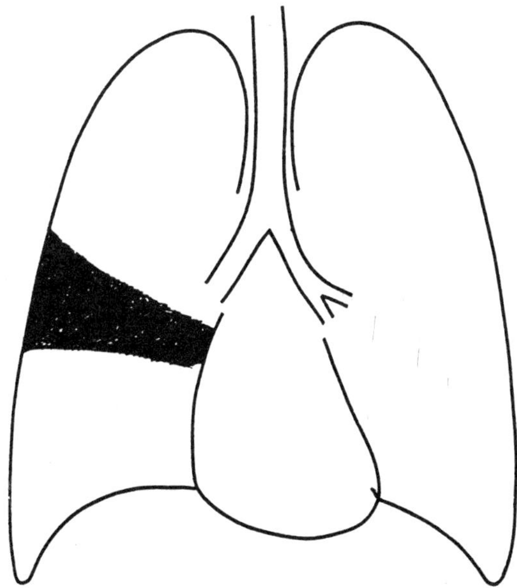

FIGURE 19-1 X-ray appearance of lobar pneumonia involving part of the right lung. The dark area is the pneumonia. Lobar pneumonia results from infection with a bacterial organism, and can involve any part of either lung.

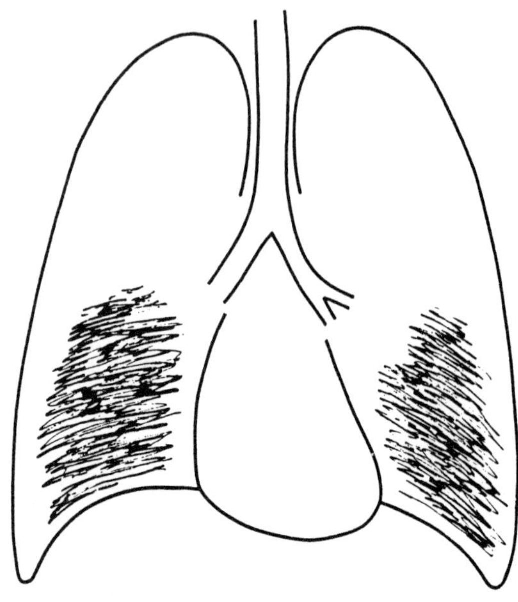

FIGURE 19-2 X-ray appearance of bilateral (double) broncho-pneumonia, also due to bacterial infection.

tests may include a microscopic examination of the sputum, a culture of the sputum, a count of the white blood cells (it goes up in pneumonia), and cultures of the blood to see if the pneumonia organisms have invaded the blood stream. Other tests may be ordered depending on the extent of the pneumonia, degree of symptoms, and past history of the patient.

Finally, step four is to treat with antibiotics. Rapid recovery helps to confirm the diagnosis and type of pneumonia even though the specific organism may not have been identified.

CAN TREATMENT BEGIN BEFORE THE CAUSE IS CONFIRMED?

Yes. In fact this is the rule for most pneumonias. Commonly the presence of pneumonia is confirmed (step one and two) and tests are ordered to diagnose the infecting organism (step three). The white blood cell count, rapidly obtainable, may help distinguish viral from bacterial cause since it tends to be higher when bacteria are the culprit. A sputum exam under the microscope takes only a few minutes and may give a clue as to which specific bacterium, if any, is responsible. More specific information may be obtained from culturing (growing) the organism from the sputum or a blood sample, but this takes one or more days.

Meanwhile, the patient is ill and will likely get worse waiting for culture results. For this reason, an antibiotic is begun soon after the diagnosis (but not the specific cause) is confirmed. The choice of antibiotic is based on the organism most likely responsible, as determined from the patient's history, chest X-ray appearance, sputum examination, white blood cell count, and so forth. For most pneumonias

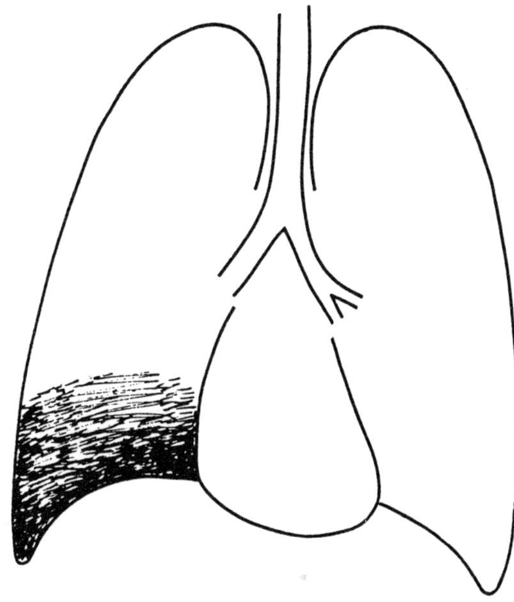

FIGURE 19-3 Extensive broncho-pneumonia with pleural effusion.

the choice of antibiotic is not medically difficult and treatment should not be delayed.

WHAT IS LOBAR PNEUMONIA?

This is pneumonia confined to one specific "lobe," or part of the lung. The lungs are normally divided into five lobes, three for the right and two for the left lung. These are clearly defined by landmarks on the chest X-ray, so lobar pneumonia is easily diagnosed. An example of lobar pneumonia is shown in Figure 19-1.

Lobar pneumonia is probably the most common type of pneumonia seen. It is usually caused by a specific organism, *streptococcus pneumoniae*, also referred to as the "pneumococcus."

Pneumococcal pneumonia is something of a paradox. The responsible organism is exquisitely sensitive to penicillin and patient response is often dramatic. Yet this same bacterium is responsible for thousands of pneumonia deaths each year in this country. The reason appears to be due to inadequate "host defenses" in many patients. For any antibiotic to work, the body must mobilize its own response to the infecting organism. This natural response is in part the increased white blood cells seen in most infections. Without this and other normal host defenses even the best antibiotics are of no use. Although penicillin is very effective in otherwise healthy people, certain patient groups have lowered defenses. They are more susceptible to severe pneumonia and more likely to show decreased antibiotic responsiveness. Such groups include very elderly patients, those with severe and chronic underlying disease (heart, lung or kidney failure), and patients with sickle cell disease, an inherited blood disorder that interferes with the body's natural response to the infecting pneumococcus.

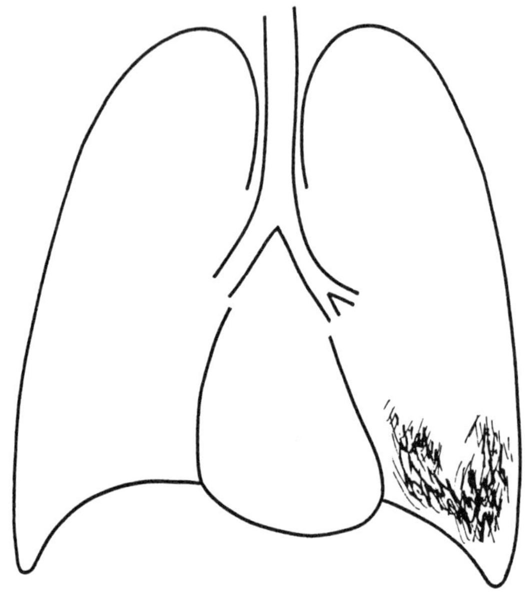

FIGURE 19-4 Patchy viral pneumonia.

IS THE PNEUMONIA VACCINE HELPFUL?

The pneumonia vaccine is pneumococcal vaccine, designed to prevent infection with the most virulent types of pneumococcus. There are over 70 serologic subtypes of this organism, but 14 of them account for most of the fatal cases of pneumococcal pneumonia. The vaccine contains killed strains of these 14 and is given to augment or enhance the body's natural response to infection from these pneumococcal subtypes. It is indicated mainly for the groups of patients mentioned above who are at increased risk and is not necessary for the general population. (See also Chapter 12)

WHAT IS LEGIONNAIRE'S DISEASE?

In July 1976 a "new" disease made the headlines. It began with an outbreak among people attending an American Legion convention in Philadelphia. Many legionnaires staying at one particular hotel came down suddenly with a severe and fatal form of pneumonia. Despite extensive investigation and theorizing, the cause remained elusive throughout 1976. Was it due to water contamination? Air-borne virus? Poison? Would the cause ever be found? Legionnaire's Disease, as the condition is now called, was the medical enigma of 1976.

The answer came in late December, and announced in January 1977. Working at the Center for Disease Control in Atlanta, investigators discovered the culprit: a small bacterium. This unusual organism was officially named *legionella pneumophila* and has now been shown to be sensitive to erythromycin, an antibiotic available for many years. Erythromycin can cure Legionnaire's Disease. Had this been known in 1976, many lives might have been saved.

Even more remarkable is the fact that Legionnaire's Disease is not really new! Investigators have examined stored blood samples from previously undiagnosed outbreaks of pneumonia and found *legionella pneumophila* the cause in hundreds of cases—all occurring before 1976!

We now know that Legionnaire's Disease can be mild or severe. The first few days of illness may be very similar to the flu syndrome and diarrhea may be present. The X-ray appearance is extremely variable and of little help in separating Legionnaire's from other causes of pneumonia. Although it may take some time to confirm the diagnosis (depending on the test used), any patient suspected of having Legionnaire's Disease is immediately treated with erythromycin.

DO PATIENTS HAVE TO BE HOSPITALIZED WITH PNEUMONIA?

Not all pneumonia patients have to be hospitalized. The milder the symptoms and the younger the patient (excluding infants and small children), the less likely is the need for hospitalization. Generally the following groups of patients should be hospitalized:

- Anyone toxic or severely ill from pneumonia or anyone short of breath at rest
- Anyone unable to take oral fluids or unable to receive adequate care at home
- Any patient with a complicating illness, such as heart failure, chronic obstructive lung disease, or chronic renal disease

WHAT IS PLEURISY?

Pleurisy refers to inflammation of the lining of the lung, the pleura (see also Chapter 14). Pleurisy may be due to a variety of causes, most commonly a viral infection. However, any of the organisms that can cause pneumonia can also infect the pleura and lead to pleurisy. Pleurisy (another term is pleuritis) is often painful, in contrast to pneumonia which is not painful (unless the pleura are involved). This is because the lining of the lung is filled with nerve fibers that, when inflamed or stretched, cause pain. Since we normally stretch the pleura with quiet breathing, stretching of the inflamed nerve fibers is often unavoidable. It is common for patients suffering from pleurisy to take only shallow breaths, because deep breaths cause so much pain.

On the chest X-ray pleurisy may be accompanied by fluid around the lung, so-called pleural effusion (see Chapter 14). Occasionally, bacterial infection in the pleural space can cause pus to form. This is called empyema and always has to be drained with a chest tube or by some other technique. Pleural space infected with bacteria may not have the characteristics of "pus," but still require tube drainage. Some physicians refer to any such infected fluid as an empyema or empyema-like.

CHAPTER TWENTY

Tuberculosis and Other Less Common Pulmonary Infections

IS TUBERCULOSIS STILL AN IMPORTANT DISEASE?

Tuberculosis (TB) is certainly nothing like the scourge it was in the nineteenth century, when it was the number one cause of death both in the United States and Europe. In fact, since 1900 there has been a steady decline both in the number of new cases per year (incidence) and in the number of people dying from the disease each year.

For several reasons, however, TB remains an important respiratory illness for the patients who contract it, for society at large, and for the physicians who must always be on the lookout for this treatable condition:

1. TB occurred as a new disease in 27,412 patients during 1981 (as reported to the Communicable Disease Center–*MMWR* 31 (February 12, 1982), 63). For each of these patients the recommended treatment would ordinarily be drugs (called TB chemotherapy) for anywhere from nine months to two years.
2. In addition to those who come down with active disease, the TB organism infects (but does not cause active disease) many thousands more people each year. These people develop a positive skin test to TB but, in contrast to the first group, have no clinically detectable disease or illness. They are usually contacts to patients with active TB disease; contacts always run a greater risk of getting active tuberculosis disease than the general population. Depending on their age and overall health, some of these contacts may be

treated with at least one anti-tuberculosis drug to *prevent* developing active TB disease.

3. TB is a great masquerader and can cause disease in patients debilitated from other conditions such as cancer, kidney failure, and alcoholism. It is a major diagnostic consideration in patients who have a "fever of unknown origin"—fever of at least two weeks' duration for which, despite many tests, a cause cannot be determined.

WHAT ARE THE SYMPTOMS OF TB?

The symptoms of tuberculosis disease are, like many respiratory illnesses, non-specific. Chronic cough, fever, night sweats, and weight loss are the most consistent symptoms of TB, with emphasis on the chronicity. Some patients also have a history of coughing up blood (hemoptysis).

Patients who have a cough, fever, and night sweats for more than a few days should have a chest X-ray; this will pick up most cases of active tuberculosis because the lungs are usually involved. However TB may infect any organ and spare the lungs, although this is not as common as the pulmonary form of tuberculosis.

A typical X-ray pattern is shown in Figure 20-1. Although not diagnostic, an *upper lobe infiltrate* (as shown) is the most common pattern. Not having the infiltrate in the upper lobe also does not rule out TB, since the disease may cause virtually any pattern on the chest X-ray.

Additional tests that can be performed when TB is suspected are the tuberculin skin test and sputum examination. The skin test takes about 48 hours to show

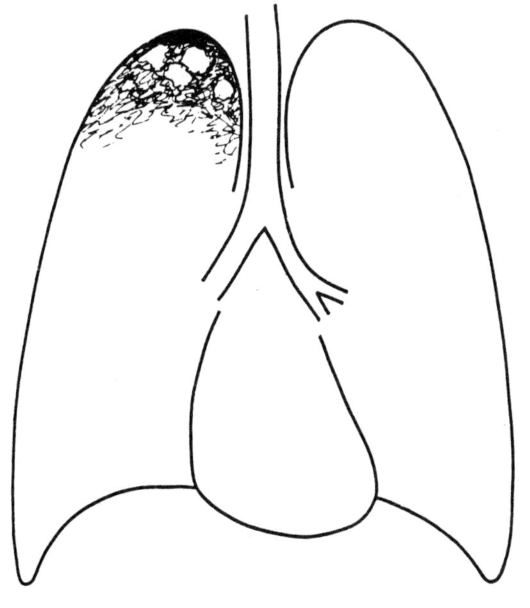

FIGURE 20-1 Chest x-ray appearance of active tuberculosis, involving the patient's right upper lung.

a positive result (redness and hardening of the skin around the injection site); this only means the person has had some contact with the TB organism and does not diagnose TB disease. The sputum exam for TB can be done right away in most hospital microbiology laboratories; if the sputum shows TB organisms under the microscope, this is presumptive evidence of TB disease. Proof of TB disease requires growing the TB organism, which can take one to two months. However, treatment is always begun if the TB organism is tentatively identified under the microscope.

WHAT IS THE DIFFERENCE BETWEEN TUBERCULOUS *INFECTION* AND *DISEASE*?

Tuberculosis is caused by a peculiar organism, called *mycobacterium tuberculosis* (M. TB). M. TB is the size of an ordinary bacterium but behaves very differently from the bacteria usually implicated in respiratory infections. The M. TB is rather tenacious and can live a lifetime (yours) in the body without ever causing any trouble. In some patients, however, the TB bacteria break out of their dormancy and spread to cause "active disease."* People who have had contact with M. TB but have contained it in a dormant state are said to be "infected" with the organism. In contrast, people are said to have TB "disease" if the organisms have multiplied and spread to cause symptoms or if there is evidence the organisms are growing unchecked; the latter is usually diagnosed by careful examination of a patient's sputum, but on occasion other body fluids will show the organism.

Thus, TB *disease* refers to illness that always, when diagnosed, requires treatment. It usually, but not invariably, involves the lungs and causes an abnormal chest X-ray (see figure). TB *infection* means simply contact with the TB organism, but no illness, no disease. This official nomenclature is perhaps confusing, since infection usually implies being sick or having some symptoms; however, that is not the case when referring to TB.

IF PEOPLE WITH TB INFECTION ARE ASYMPTOMATIC, HOW IS IT DIAGNOSED?

TB infection is diagnosed only by finding a positive skin test, called a tuberculin skin test. In this test a small amount of inactivated tuberculin protein (approximately 1/10 cc) is injected under the skin. The area of injection is then "read" at 48 hours; induration (slight hardening of the skin) of the skin at the injection site, of at least 10 mm in width, indicates previous contact with the TB organism.

In practice the test should be performed and read by a trained TB health worker, nurse, or physician. An estimated 7 percent of adults have a positive tuberculin skin test (10 mm or more induration) and are said to be infected. These

*Active disease" is a redundancy in referring to TB; hence "active" will no longer be used as an adjective to "disease."

people have an increased risk of getting TB disease, the amount of risk depending on their age and underlying physical condition.

IS TUBERCULOSIS CURABLE?

Yes. Thanks to modern chemotherapy virtually all patients can be cured *if* they are diagnosed and properly treated before complications occur or another illness proves fatal. Most TB fatalities occur in patients who either delayed seeking help or in whom the disease was completely missed before death.

Treatment is drugs, taken by mouth, for a period of 9 to 24 months. Until recently almost all TB treatment was for 18 to 24 months. Now a relatively new "short course" regimen, consisting of INH and Rifampin, allows for curative treatment in only 9 months, after which drugs are never needed again.

WHAT DRUGS ARE USED TO TREAT TUBERCULOSIS?

Drug therapy for tuberculosis is one of the great milestones in medicine. Before the advent of modern TB chemotherapy the only treatments available were bedrest and surgery, the latter often mutilating and not very effective.

The first drug proven useful in fighting TB was streptomycin, introduced in 1944. Although this drug was helpful in fighting TB, it was not until the introduction of isoniazid in 1952 that really effective therapy became available. Isoniazid (INH) has been the true wonder drug for TB and a "first line drug" for over 30 years.

TB is unlike most bacterial infections. To be eradicated thoroughly, it requires two drugs. INH is almost always one of these, and in the late 1940s and early 1950s it was given along with streptomycin for effective treatment. Because of the tenacious characteristics of the TB organisms effective treatment took two years!

Streptomycin can only be given by injection, so other, oral drugs are preferable to use along with INH. The first to be developed was paraaminosalicylic acid (PAS), introduced in the late 1940s. PAS is no longer used in the United States because of severe side effects. In the last decade ethambutal supplanted PAS as the oral drug to use along with INH. Thus, until recently, a standard oral regimen consisted of daily doses of INH and ethambutal for 18 to 24 months.

Worldwide studies over the past several years have provided another breakthrough. A combination of INH with a relatively new drug called rifampin (introduced into general use in the 1970s) has been found to cure most new cases of TB in about nine months! This so-called "short course" (relative to previous regimens) has greatly simplified TB treatment, particularly for patients who could not comply with the previous 24 month regimen.

Short-course TB chemotherapy is by no means universally accepted or used in the United States. Many patients are still treated with INH and ethambutal or some other combination, depending on the particular situation. But short course chemotherapy is an advance, and it is likely that the next decade will see a greater percentage of TB patients being cured with this regimen.

IF TB IS CURABLE, WHY DO PEOPLE STILL DIE FROM IT?

Many deaths occur in the United States each year from diseases that are potentially curable. Pneumonia is the best example. In pneumonia death may occur because the body's defenses are too weak to help fight the infection, even with the aid of antibiotics. TB is also a curable condition, yet an estimated 2,800 people died from TB during 1980. The reasons for death, despite the availability of currative drugs, are threefold:

1. TB is not diagnosed prior to death. Tuberculosis is a great masquerader. In every hospital patients have been admitted with an unexplained illness and died undiagnosed, only to show TB at autopsy. Many times the clinical diagnosis is not obvious, even in retrospect. In all unexplained illnesses, particularly when fever or weight loss is present, TB must be carefully searched for.
2. TB diagnosis is made too late for drugs to work. This is occasionally the case in some severe alcoholic patients who contract tuberculosis disease but do not seek medical care. They may finally be brought in moribund and die, even if TB is diagnosed and treatment begun, because of the disease's advanced state.
3. TB occurs on top of severe underlying illness. Examples are patients with widespread cancer, patients on maintenance hemodialysis for chronic kidney failure, and patients who have undergone renal transplantation and are immunosuppressed from medication given to prevent rejection of the transplanted kidney. In such patients the body's defenses are compromised and TB disease may be lethal, especially if not diagnosed and treated in its earliest stages.

Fortunately, an otherwise healthy patient who gets tuberculosis and is diagnosed early usually has an uneventful recovery once the proper drugs are given.

DO ALL PATIENTS WITH TUBERCULOSIS HAVE TO BE HOSPITALIZED?

In years past, always. Before the advent of effective chemotherapy in the late 1940s, hundreds of TB sanitaria housed thousands of patients with TB. This was for several reasons. First, TB is communicable and removing diseased patients from society was the only effective way of stopping the spread to other people. Second, there was widespread belief that fresh air and balanced diet were essential for proper treatment. Third, many surgical treatments, such as collapsing part of the lung to help kill the organisms, could be evaluated in specialized hospitals.

With modern chemotherapy TB sanitaria have disappeared from this country. This is one of the most dramatic health revolutions of the century. (Dr. Selman A. Waksman, discoverer of the first effective TB drug, streptomycin, received the Nobel prize in 1952.)

Today, hospitalization is required only for a relatively brief time for a select group of patients, including those with severe underlying disease, such as alcoholism or cancer, those who have an unstable home situation and may not take their medication properly, and those whose TB is either very advanced or who are very ill from the disease.

Even if hospitalization is required, the vast majority of patients are released within two weeks after treatment has begun. By this time they are no longer considered infectious (providing they are taking the medication) and can return to work or school. Patients who are not hospitalized, but who start TB chemotherapy at home, can also return to work or school in about two weeks.

CAN TUBERCULOSIS OCCUR IN OTHER PARTS OF THE BODY BESIDES THE LUNGS?

The tuberculosis organism, *mycobacterium tuberculosis*, can cause disease anywhere in the body. So-called non-pulmonary tuberculosis used to be very common when pulmonary tuberculosis was also a common disease. Although non-pulmonary TB is now seen less often, it simply reflects a diminishing incidence of all tuberculosis.

TB in other parts of the body even has special names. TB of the spine has long been known as Pott's disease after Percival Pott (1714-1788), who first described the spinal deformities that occur from TB. TB of the lymph nodes is also known as scrofula. TB may occur in the bone marrow, where it can cause anemia; in the brain, resulting in confusion and seizures; and anywhere in the abdomen, where it can cause a myriad of gastrointestinal complaints. Tuberculosis can be a great masquerader, and symptoms in any part of the body along with protracted fever have often been found due to tuberculosis. Patients do not have to show tuberculosis in their lungs to have it elsewhere.

Disseminated TB, also known as miliary tuberculosis, occurs when the organisms disseminate via the bloodstream. In the lungs this shows up as scattered, small discrete spots like millet seeds, hence the name "miliary." Patients with miliary TB are usually quite ill but respond within a few days to appropriate anti-TB therapy.

SHOULD HEALTHY PEOPLE WITH A POSITIVE TUBERCULIN SKIN TEST TAKE MEDICATION?

Anyone with a positive tuberculosis skin test (10 mm or greater) has been exposed to the tuberculous bacillus; by the definitions given earlier such a person is said to be "infected" with the TB organism. However, most TB skin test reactors are asymptomatic *and* will never contract TB disease. They have an increased risk (compared to non-reactors) of getting TB disease, however.

Several studies have shown that if positive tuberculin reactors take isoniazid (INH) for a year, their risk of later developing TB disease diminishes. Unfortunately, INH can also cause hepatitis (liver inflammation). A small percentage of adults who in the past took INH for prevention became sick from this side effect; a few of them died. It seems that the older you are the most likely it is that a year of INH medication may also lead to hepatitis. Analyzing all the available data, the

American Thoracic Society in 1974 recommended that skin test reactors under the age of 35 take a year of INH; over the age of 35 the risk of getting hepatitis exceeded the risk of contracting tuberculosis disease and INH prophylaxis was not routinely recommended.

The 1974 recommendation was based on the assumption that one case of hepatitis equals one case of tuberculosis. Since TB is curable and rarely fatal, in contrast to hepatitis which must heal on its own and for which there is no cure, many people might well prefer to risk developing TB disease rather than exposing themselves to the risk of hepatitis. These and other complexities have been analyzed in a 1981 medical article with the interesting title "Should young adults with a positive tuberculin test take isoniazid?" (See references.)

The answer given in the article is "no," not routinely. Each case should be individualized, taking into account not only the skin test reactor's age and known risk factors, but also his or her own wishes. Deciding on a year of medication for a healthy person, with potential adverse consequences either way, should involve the subject as much as the physician.

The controversy thus revolves around young adults who have a positive TB skin test but are asymptomatic and in good health. There are other people for whom it is not controversial to give a year of INH treatment, when the skin test is positive. These include:

1. All children. Tuberculosis disease can be much more severe in children than adults and the risk of contracting hepatitis from INH is almost non-existent.
2. Adults who are at extremely high risk of developing TB disease, including:
   a. people with silicosis (see Chapter 4).
   b. people who have had part or all of their stomach removed (gastrectomy).
   c. people who are being treated with prolonged courses of medication that may suppress the body's immune system (such as cancer chemotherapy).
   d. people whose skin test converted from negative to positive after exposure to someone with active tuberculosis; the risk of contracting TB disease is greatest the first year after skin test conversion (the first year after contact with the TB organism).

WHAT IS "ATYPICAL" MYCOBACTERIAL INFECTION?

The word "atypical" is frequently used when referring to disease caused by organisms that are very similar to mycobacterium tuberculosis but also different in certain ways. These unusual organisms are known as "atypical mycobacteria"; strictly speaking, they do not cause the disease tuberculosis, which is by definition due to M. (mycobacteria) tuberculosis. Atypical mycobacteria go by other names, including M. kansaii, M. scrofulaceum, and M. intracellulare-avium. (This last organism used to be called the "Battey" bacillus after the Battey State Hospital in Rome, Georgia where it was first isolated.)

An important distinction between these atypical mycobacteria and M. tuberculosis is that atypicals are not transmitted from person to person. Rather, they are inhaled from the soil in certain endemic areas. For example, M. intracellulare-avium is common in the South. Like M. tuberculosis, the atypicals can infect an individual without causing any symptoms and can bring about a positive skin test even when regular tuberculin is used. Less commonly, the atypical mycobacteria can cause disease. Although the same drugs used to treat tuberculosis are employed against atypical mycobacterial infection, the latter is usually more resistant to medication and hence more difficult to treat. Proper identification of the mycobacteria and drug sensitivity testing are essential for appropriate treatment.

WHAT IS HISTOPLASMOSIS?

Histoplasmosis is a disease caused by the fungus histoplasma capsulatum. As a fungal infection, it is completely different from infections caused by bacteria, mycobacteria, and viruses, although it may clinically appear like tuberculosis.

The histoplasma fungus is inhaled from the soil and is not spread from patient to patient. This fungus is common in endemic areas, including the Mississippi and Ohio Valley regions of the United States, particularly Kentucky and Tennessee. Many individuals in these areas have a positive skin test to histoplasma fungus, but will never have symptoms or disease from such contact. When histoplasmosis does occur it may cause clinical and X-ray changes similar to tuberculosis but the course of treatment is vastly different. For patients with localized histoplasmosis the best treatment is usually no treatment. Localized, acute histoplasmosis appears as a flu-like illness and the X-ray may show bronchopneumonia; it is usually self-limiting. For disseminated forms of histoplasmosis, which are quite rare, the drug amphotericin is used. This drug can be very toxic, especially to the kidneys, and is one reason why treatment is not given except for life-threatening forms of the disease.

Histoplasmosis is usually in the differential list of difficult-to-diagnose pulmonary infections, especially in areas endemic for the fungus. The diagnosis can be made on special blood tests and by culturing the fungal organisms. Frequently, patients who have had histoplasmosis in the past will retain evidence of this on their X-ray; it may show up as little spots of calcium deposits scattered throughout the chest X-ray.

WHAT IS COCCIDIOIDOMYCOSIS?

Coccidioidomycosis is another fungal infection that occurs in certain areas of the United States. It is particularly endemic in California's San Joaquin Valley and large parts of the Southwest. The fungus responsible, known as *Coccidioides immitis,* can cause problems very similar to histoplasmosis and is treated in a similar fashion. Like histoplasmosis, most infected individuals are asymptomatic. There are certain distinguishing characteristics by chest X-ray and clinical presentation, but like all fungal infections the specific infecting organism must be identified for proper treatment and followup. As in disseminated histoplasmosis, life-threatening coccidioidomycosis requires treatment with amphotericin, a highly toxic drug. Other antifungal drugs have also been tried, with less success.

WHAT OTHER PULMONARY INFECTIONS CAN OCCUR?

The lungs can be "host" to many disease-causing organisms. Dozens of unusual bacteria, mycobacteria, and viruses have been documented as causing disease in humans. Only some of the more common ones have been mentioned in these chapters. Other uncommon pulmonary infections you may hear about include:

North American Blastomycosis (fungus)
Aspergillosis (fungus)
Cryptococcosis (fungus)
Nocardiosis (bacteria)
Actinomycosis (bacteria)
Pneumocystis (protozoa)

These organisms generally cause serious disease only in patients who have a compromised immune system. The interested reader may refer to the bibliography for further information on these and other uncommon infections.

WHAT IS BRONCHIECTASIS?

Bronchiectasis is a lung condition where the air tubes (bronchi) have lost their normal round shape, and are permanently dilated. It is usually due to chronic infection, such as tuberculosis (Chapter 20) or other bacterial disease, but may also occur in cystic fibrosis (Chatper 23) and other uncommon pulmonary conditions. It is usually accompanied by the daily coughing up of infected mucus. Although the symptoms may be similar to chronic bronchitis (Chapter 12), most patients with chronic bronchitis do not have bronchiectasis; the latter term implies a different type of derangement of the air tubes (widening, with flimsy walls) than is present in bronchitis (narrowing, with thickened walls).

Bronchiectasis used to be much more common before the antibiotic era. Often patients had to have part of their lung removed to control the chronic infection. Today, bronchiectasis is diagnosed infrequently. It is difficult to diagnose by a simple chest X-ray; instead, diagnosis requires placement of dye into the airways followed by multiple X-rays, a test known as a bronchogram. Bronchograms, as well as surgery for bronchiectasis, are rarely done today.

With rare exception, patients suffering from bronchiectasis can be treated with antibiotics, and should not need surgery.

CHAPTER TWENTY-ONE

Lung Cancer: A National Epidemic

WHAT IS LUNG CANCER?

Lung cancer is a malignant or unchecked growth in the lung tissues, arising mainly in the tubes (bronchi) that bring air into the lungs. Most lung cancers, over 90 percent, arise from the bronchus and are called "bronchogenic cancer."* (See Figure 21-1.) As with all cancers, cells in the bronchus begin to multiply abnormally until they are either removed, their growth is stopped, or the patient dies. Unfortunately lung cancer is usually not detected until the cells have multiplied in such numbers that the tumor is visible on a chest X-ray. By then it is usually too late for cure.

Infrequently, lung cancer can arise in the air sacs or alveoli. This is called "alveolar cell" cancer and carries the same poor outlook as bronchogenic cancer.**

Cancers can also spread *to* the lung *from* other parts of the body. These are not primary lung cancers (they are not bronchogenic) and their treatment consists of whatever is appropriate for the type of *primary* tumor, such as colon, kidney, bladder, and so forth. When a cancer has spread to a distant site it is said to have "metastasized" and the distant cancer is a "metastasis."

*Another general term for this type of cancer is "bronchogenic carcinoma." Carcinoma is one type of cancer but the terms are often used interchangeably.

**Cancer in the lining of the lungs is called "malignant mesothelioma"; this is discussed in Chapter 4.

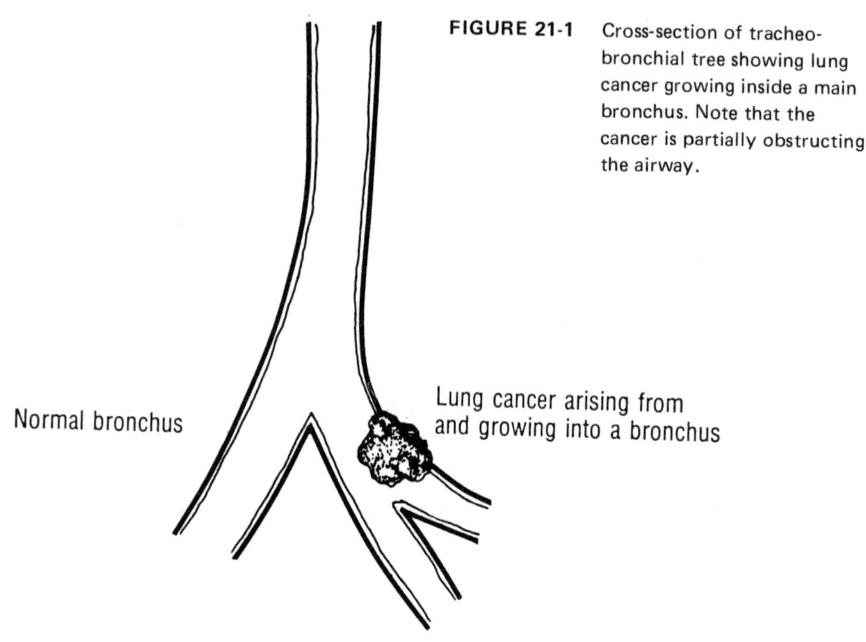

FIGURE 21-1 Cross-section of tracheobronchial tree showing lung cancer growing inside a main bronchus. Note that the cancer is partially obstructing the airway.

WHAT IS THE CAUSE OF LUNG CANCER?

In over 90 percent of lung cancers the cause is cigarette smoking. If there were no cigarette smoking lung cancer would be an uncommon disease. Instead it is near epidemic.

An estimated 120,000 Americans die each year from lung cancer. Treatment for lung cancer is effective only in a small number of patients; for the vast majority, the time from diagnosis to death is less than five years. (Over 90 percent of all patients diagnosed with lung cancer five years ago are not alive today.) The ones who survived may consider themselves fortunate; they are likely cured of the disease. Even so, they remain at increased risk for developing another cancer, particularly if they continue smoking.

Lung cancer occurs in women to the same degree as men, but the absolute number of women afflicted is less because in the past women smoked less than men. Recently however, women have increased their cigarette consumption, so their rate of lung cancer is catching up with that of men.

ARE THERE OTHER CAUSES OF LUNG CANCER BESIDES CIGARETTES?

The other causes are mainly environmental, including such inhaled agents as asbestos, cadmium, and uranium dust. Recently deisel engine fumes have also been implicated as a cause of lung cancer. People who work around these dusts and fumes have a higher incidence of lung cancer than the general population. However, a large percentage of this increased incidence is attributable to cigarette smoking; there is a synergistic effect between cigarette smoking and inhalation of asbestos fibers, cadmium, and uranium dust.

It's true that non-smokers can get lung cancer from long exposure to these compounds, but this is uncommon; even when occupational exposure is heavy, most lung cancers will occur in cigarette smokers.

Not all cases of lung cancer result from inhalation or exposure to cancer-causing cigarettes, dusts, and fumes. A small percentage of patients develop lung cancer without any history of such exposure. Some cancers arise from scars in the lung. These scars are from previous conditions, such as old tuberculosis, silicosis, or old blood clots. For some unknown reason, even without cigarette smoking, these scars have an increased tendency to develop into lung cancer, although this is far less common than when the person also smokes.

There are also a small number of people who develop lung cancer and have never smoked, never worked with cancer-causing material, and have no lung scars. Such "non-exposure" cases usually occur in elderly people. Cancer of the lung in people under age 60 without any history of exposure or lung scars is extremely rare.

WHAT ARE THE SYMPTOMS OF LUNG CANCER?

Lung cancer symptoms are variable and may be obscured by underlying chronic obstructive pulmonary disease (bronchitis or emphysema). The common symptoms of *chronic cough, expectoration of phlegm,* and *shortness of breath* may be found in *both* lung cancer and COPD. A change in the duration, frequency, or severity of these symptoms may occur when lung cancer has developed. In addition, the patient may notice some *blood in the sputum*, a finding that always warrants investigation. The new onset of *wheezing*, particularly if it comes from only one side of the chest, may occasionally be the first lung cancer symptom. *Hoarseness* that occurs without throat infection, or lasts more than a few days, may also be due to lung cancer. Other symptoms such as *weakness, weight loss,* and *bone pain* occur relatively late in the course of lung cancer.

Generally, by the time lung cancer causes symptoms it has grown to the point where it is visible on the chest X-ray. This indicates a size of at least one centimeter in diameter (about half an inch). Hence, smokers experiencing a change in symptoms, or the onset of new symptoms, should have a chest X-ray as a screening test to rule out (or rule in) lung cancer.

Commonly, a small spot or nodule is found on a routine chest X-ray done for other purposes (such as part of an employment physical) and is subsequently found to be early lung cancer. Patients whose cancers are first detected this way are usually without symptoms. For lung cancer there is no substitute for prevention.

WHY NOT DO FREQUENT CHEST X-RAYS TO DETECT LUNG CANCER EARLY?

For many years this in fact was recommended by the American Cancer Society, in the belief that the earlier the cancer was detected, the better the outlook. Theoretically, this makes sense. However, several large studies, involving routine chest X-rays in thousands of male smokers, failed to show any improvement in mortality even though many early lung cancers were detected. It appears that lung cancer is such a virulent disease that even early detection, using currently available X-ray techniques, is too late.

Studies at the Mayo Clinic, Johns Hopkins, and Memorial-Sloan Kettering, tested the use of chest X-rays and sputum cytology to diagnose early lung cancers in high risk individuals. Preliminary data show many more lung cancers are detected early (compared to the group not having chest X-ray and sputum exam), but the overall mortality from lung cancer in the two groups is not different. Hence, chest X-ray and sputum tests do not influence mortality from lung cancer, even though they may detect it earlier. For this reason, and since the tests add to total health cost *and* may cause undue anxiety (as when a spot is seen on the chest X-ray in an asymptomatic person who does not have lung cancer), the ACS issued new guidelines in 1980:

"The society has changed its policy (from yearly chest X-rays in smokers) and does not recommend any tests for the early detection of cancer of the lung, but urges a focus on primary prevention: helping smokers to stop (or to switch to low tar and nicotine cigarettes), and keeping nonsmokers from starting. People with signs or symptoms of lung cancer should consult their physicians."

Not all physicians agree with eliminating routine chest X-rays in high risk patients. Mayo Clinic physicians feel that some early lung cancers can not only be detected but, for the individual patient, such detection may make the difference between successful and nonsuccessful treatment. The Mayo Clinic still recommends frequent chest X-rays and sputum cytology examination for heavy smokers over age 45 because of their higher risk of lung cancer.

The controversy will likely persist, perhaps resolved only when better treatment for lung cancer or easier methods for earlier detection is available. At present there seems to be no proof that routine chest X-rays will benefit an asymptomatic person. Undoubtedly, routine chest X-rays have detected early cancers in some people, but whether the eventual outcome would have been diffeent without the routine chest X-ray is not known.

Asymptomatic people who worry about this should not smoke. That, more than anything else, will decrease their likelihood of dying from lung cancer.

HOW IS LUNG CANCER TREATED?

There are three principal modalities for treating lung cancer: surgery, drugs (chemotherapy), and radiation therapy. Each may be used alone or in combination with the others, depending on the exact type of tumor and its location, plus the current state of knowledge. A dismal fact is that despite several decades of experience with treating lung cancer, the five-year survival rate has not changed! Less than 10 percent of all newly diagnosed patients with lung cancer will live five years, considering all forms of treatment!

However, buried within this grim statistic is hope for *some* lung cancer patients. Not all lung cancers have the same prognosis; the outlook depends both on the tissue type and the stage of growth at the time of diagnosis.

The tissue type is determined by examining a piece of the cancer (removed by a biopsy or at surgery) under the microscope. The size and arrangement of the cancer cells seen under the microscope correlate with the growth pattern of the tumor and, in some cases, determine its treatment. Pathologists now distinguish two broad tissue types of lung cancer: small cell and non-small cell. Another term for small cell is "oat cell," since microscopically the cancer cells are relatively small and look like a bunch of oats. The non-small cell type of lung cancer is further divided into three groups: squamous cell, large cell, and "adenocarcinoma," again depending on its microscopic configuration.

For prognosis and treatment purposes, the distinction between small (oat) cell cancer and non-small cell cancer is crucial. Small cell lung cancer is no longer considered amenable to surgery. By the time of diagnosis, it has already spread to other parts of the body, For this reason, patients with small cell lung cancer always receive some combination of drugs (cancer chemotherapy). As will be discussed below, drug treatment of small cell lung cancer has effected a dramatic turn-around in prognosis for some patients.

Non-small cell cancer is sometimes amenable to surgery. Whether or not surgery is actually offered depends on the stage of the lung cancer.

WHAT IS STAGING OF LUNG CANCER?

Along with determining tissue type (see above), staging of lung cancer helps to determine prognosis and the possibility for surgical treatment (removal). It involves determining, as accurately as possible before treatment, how big the tumor is and how far it has spread. To do this, several diagnostic studies are employed including X-rays, scans, and biopsies. Occasionally accurate staging can only be done after a surgical procedure called "mediastinoscopy"; while the patient is under general anesthesia, the surgeon looks into the region between the two lungs (mediastinum) with a long "mediastinoscope" to take biopsies of lymph nodes. The pathologist can then determine if the area is involved with tumor. The process of staging a lung cancer is principally for non-small cell cancers, since small cell cancer is not considered amenable to surgery.

Basically, the staging procedure asks: How far has the tumor spread both within the chest cavity and beyond, to other organs? Spread of the tumor to other organs, such as the brain, liver, and bone marrow, always rules out a surgical cure. Spread within the chest cavity usually rules out a surgical cure. The techniques of performing staging change frequently, and not all physicians agree on the utility of various tests. Furthermore, there is no universal consensus on how best to treat tumors that can't be surgically removed.

However, there is general agreement that by obtaining a biopsy and doing a thorough staging evaluation, non-small cell tumors can be properly staged for both therapeutic and prognostic purposes. Staging is now based on the "TNM" classification. "T" relates to the size of the tumor, "N" to any spread to lymph nodes within the thorax, and "M" to any distant metastases (tumors that have spread beyond the lungs). Because oat cell cancer has invariably spread by the time of diagnosis, it is not staged this way. Examples of staging for non-oat cell lung cancers:

Stage 1 A lung cancer smaller than three cm on X-ray, with no apparent spread to lymph nodes. The best prognosis.
Stage 2 A tumor larger than three cm that has spread only to lymph nodes on the same side of the chest as the tumor. Intermediate prognosis.
Stage 3 A lung cancer of any size that has spread to the brain or liver. The worst prognosis.

The above are only examples and not meant to define each stage; this is often a complex process that must take into account all available tests and their proper interpretation. Prognosis is directly related to stage. For example, non-oat cell cancers that are stage 1 and less than two cm in diameter have an approximately 80 percent five-year survival rate after surgical removal! All stage 3 lung cancers carry less than a 10 percent survival rate after five years, regardless of treatment. The reason the overall statistics for lung cancer are so dismal is that only a small minority of patients fall into the earliest of stage 1 lung cancers.

WHAT IS THE ROLE OF RADIATION AND CHEMOTHERAPY IN LUNG CANCER?

The answer to this question is different for small (oat) cell and non-small cell cancers. Non-small cell will be discussed first.

This includes the sub-types squamous cell, large cell, and adenocarcinoma. Included in this group also is alveolar cell carcinoma. Complete surgical removal of these cancers is the only definitive cure available today, but most patients are not amenable to surgical care at the time of diagnosis. At present other modalities of treatment, such as radiation therapy and chemotherapy, are considered palliative.

Radiation therapy consists of aiming high voltage X-ray beams at the tumor. Treatment is usually given over a course of weeks, until a maximal amount of radiation has been delivered to the tumor. This form of therapy is not considered curative, though an occasional patient does seem to be cured. Radiation therapy is used mainly to slow down tumor growth or to relieve tumor-caused symptoms such as pain and shortness of breath. There is some controversy about when patients should receive radiation therapy, since it can damage the healthy lung tissue around the tumor. In practice, most unresectable patients are offered radiation therapy in the belief it may help somewhat.

Chemotherapy or treatment with anti-cancer drugs differs from radiation therapy in several aspects. It is a relatively recent modality, being widely used only in the past decade for lung cancers. Experience with non-small cell cancer is still very dismal; to better evaluate existing drugs, treatment for this type of lung cancer should only be given as part of an experimental protocol. This way groups of patients can be followed closely to detect any slight advantage of treatment among various regimens.

The situation with small (oat) cell lung cancer is different, as discussed in the next section.

HOW DOES THE TREATMENT OF OAT CELL DIFFER FROM OTHER FORMS OF LUNG CANCER?

Until a few years ago, small (oat) cell lung cancer carried the worst possible prognosis. It is a rapidly growing tumor, faster than any other lung cancer, and tends to spread far and wide very early in its growth. For this reason, at the time of diagnosis, small cell lung cancer has invariably spread elsewhere and cannot be removed surgically. Until recently this form of lung cancer was universally fatal within two years from the time of diagnosis.

In fact, growth of oat cell cancer is so rapid that researchers began regarding it almost like a lymphoma, a tumor of the lymph glands that also grows quickly and spreads widely. Because some lymphomas are amenable to chemotherapy and radiation therapy, these treatments were also given to oat cell cancer patients. Radiation therapy alone does in fact shrink oat cell cancer considerably, but it always recurs and death ensues within two years.

However, systematic trials using up to four cancer-killing drugs showed remarkable results. One group of patients receiving the drugs was compared to a group not receiving drugs; the former lived a few weeks longer, a difference that, in this deadly tumor, was highly significant! Using more potent drug combinations, a small minority of patients with the disease is now living more than two years beyond diagnosis—and can guardedly be considered "cured." In less than a decade chemotherapy has changed this cancer from one always fatal to, in a few instances, possibly curable. This is a dramatic breakthrough, one ironically not available for other inoperable lung cancers that used to have a better outcome than oat cell. For non-oat cell tumors that can't be surgically removed, the dismal outlook has not changed.

WHAT IS THE DIFFERENCE BETWEEN BEING OPERABLE AND RESECTABLE?

Clinicians and surgeons make this distinction on every patient they see with lung cancer. Essentially the distinction is as follows:

Operable A patent is operable if he or she can successfully undergo the surgery necessary to remove the tumor. Operable refers mainly to the condition of the patient. Examples of patients *not* operable, despite the presence of a lung cancer, are those who have recently suffered a heart attack, anyone in a coma or in another unstable situation such as uncontrolled diabetes, and patients with compromised lung function in whom the surgeon would have to remove functioning lung along with the tumor to the point where there would not be enough good lung left to sustain life.

Resectable This applies to the technical aspects of whether or not the tumor could be removed totally from the patient's chest. It does no good if the patient is operable but the tumor has spread so far that it cannot be entirely resected. Examples of unresectable tumors include small (oat) cell cancers, tumors with distant metastases, tumors that have spread to the pleura (lining) of the chest cavity, and tumors that have spread to the area between the two lungs (the mediastinum). If the tumor has spread from one part of the lung to another part of the *same* lung it *may* be resectable, depending on its extent, size, and what other structures are involved.

Richard T.—A Case of Lung Cancer

Mr. T., 48 and president of his own company, was always in good health until the morning he awoke and coughed up blood. As he told it, shortly after awakening he felt this "welling up" of liquid in his mouth and the need to cough; he expectorated about a tablespoonful of bright red blood into the sink. At first he tried to ignore it, thinking he might have bronchitis. Moreover, he did not feel ill and had no other coughing spells. By mid-morning however, he could no longer rationalize the symptom and called his doctor. He was told to come for a chest X-ray immediately. The X-ray revealed a large mass in his right lung, about five cm (two inches) in diameter, appearing to arise from one of the large bronchi (see Figure 21-2). He was admitted to the hospital the same evening. Mr. T. had smoked about a pack of cigarettes a day for 28 years. He made it clear to the examining physician that he never intended to smoke again, regardless of what was found. On examination, despite the large mass seen in his X-ray, he appeared healthy and no abnormalities were found. He coughed up no blood in the hospital and when asked to give a sputum sample could cough nothing up. Routine blood and urine tests were normal. The next morning he underwent fiberoptic bronchoscopy. A large tumor was seen occluding the lower lobe bronchus of his right lung. Multiple tiny biopsies were taken and sent to the pathology laboratory. The pathologic diagnosis was "lung carcinoma (cancer), small cell type." This is the most rapidly growing lung cancer and not amenable to surgical removal; at the time of diagnosis it had invariably spread to other parts of the body. An oncologist (cancer specialist) was consulted who recommend some other tests, including a bone marrow examination. This showed a few areas of cancer cells, confirming spread of the lung cancer. Thus, despite Mr. T.'s feeling of well-being, he had inoperable, metastatic lung cancer. He was begun on a regimen of radiotherapy and chemotherapy treatments and did well for about 18 months. At that time he had a seizure, and a computerized brain scan showed a cancer focus. Treatments were continued, but Mr. T. had a rapid downhill course and died six weeks later.

Comment: Mr. T.'s death was due to a preventable cause: cigarettes.

WHAT ARE THE SIDE EFFECTS OF LUNG CANCER TREATMENT?

Lung cancer is a deadly disease. Doing nothing offers no chance of cure. At the same time doing something may make the patient miserable and may not affect the outcome.

All effective treatments, either for palliation or cure, carry substantial morbidity (discomfort and/or pain). Surgery, the only cure for most lung cancer, requires opening the chest cavity (thoracotomy)—a major operation lasting one to several hours. In otherwise healthy people with normal lungs except for the cancer, the risk of dying from the surgery is probably less than 1 percent. The sicker the patient or the more diseased the lungs, the greater the risk. In addition, pain and

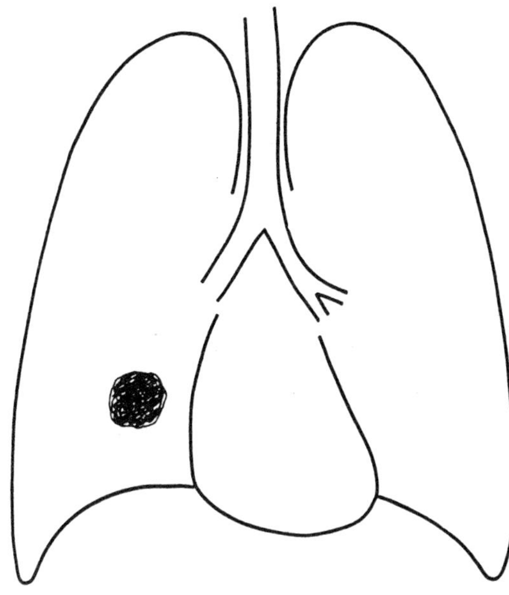

FIGURE 21-2 Chest x-ray on Mr. T. showing large tumor in lower third of right lung.

discomfort in the first few days after surgery are substantial. Worst of all, surgery is *not* curative for the majority of people who come under the knife.

Thus, taking into account the morbidity and mortality inherent in surgery, doctors would like to refer for operation only those patients likely to be cured. This determination is part of the staging process. Although staging becomes more sophisticated with each diagnostic advance (such as CAT scanners), it is still an imperfect process. Given the possibility of cure, therefore, most physicians recommend surgery if resection is thought possible and the patient is operable.

Radiation therapy is the best tolerated treatment, at least initially. It is painless and causes no side effects at the time of treatment. With time there is variable destruction of surrounding, previously healthy lung tissue, which may make the patient sick or produce shortness of breath. In patients with already compromised lung function this can be devasting. For this reason, it remains controversial about exactly when and to what extent radiotherapy should be given for lung cancer.

Chemotherapy involves giving cancer-killing drugs, all of which have serious potential side effects. Drugs currently in use can cause symptoms ranging from nausea, baldness, weakness, and skin rashes to lung scarring and heart damage. They should obviously be used in a cautious manner. For oat cell cancer the risk of these symptoms is considered a small price for the definite chance of improved longevity and possible cure. For non-oat cell cancer the results are not nearly as encouraging and drugs should only be given as part of a research protocol. This allows treatment programs to be compared so slight differences in improvement can be appreciated. (In some hospitals patients may be offered unusual treatments, such as surgery for oat cell carcinoma, investigational drugs, immunotherapy, and possibly other unconventional treatments. This is the only way to find out about such modalities, and informed consent should always be obtained.)

Sometimes physicians lose sight of the symptoms and side effects of their therapy and forget that treatment may be worse than the disease. Although lung cancer is incurable without treatment, many patients clearly do not benefit, and the subsequent morbidity only makes some patients feel worse than if they had no treatment. This seems to be particularly true for patients with inoperable non-small cell cancer.

Dr. B. J. McNeil and colleagues, in a 1978 article called "Fallacy of the Five-Year Survival in Lung Cancer," also argued that some patients should be given the alternative of choosing between treatments for lung cancer, recognizing that one type (radiation) offers relative comfort and less chance for cure while the other (surgery) offers relative discomfort and better chance for cure. Physicians cannot automatically assume all patients want to take the chance of living five years (that is, of being cured) if the chance of success is not guaranteed and the treatment is risky. Patients should be given an opportunity to decide this for themselves, after all the facts are presented. This does not solve the problem of inherent physician bias in presenting "facts." It does suggest an alternative and perhaps more humane approach.

WHAT IS THE FUTURE FOR LUNG CANCER?

Despite 50 years of international experience treating lung cancer, including all forms of surgery, drugs, and radiotherapy, the overall five-year survival rate has not changed!

We know how to prevent most cases of lung cancer (see Epilogue). We don't know how to cure most of it. It is possible that all cancers, including lung cancer, will become amenable to effective chemotherapy within a generation. Perhaps lung cancer will go the way of tuberculosis–from being a major killer to becoming a controllable problem. Unfortunately, this is not on the horizon.

On the horizon are better and newer drugs for some forms of lung cancer, particularly oat cell carcinoma, that will slow down the tumor in a larger number of patients; earlier diagnosis in selected individuals, that may allow cure in situations that otherwise would progress and prove fatal; and a future decrease in the incidence of lung cancer as a decreasing percentage of adults take up the smoking habit.

CHAPTER TWENTY-TWO

Diseases of the Pulmonary Circulation

WHAT IS THE PULMONARY CIRCULATION?

In Chapter 1 you learned that the left side of the heart pumps oxygenated blood to all the body's tissues (organs, muscles, bones, skin, and so forth). On its way this bright-red, oxygenated blood travels in the systemic arterial system. You can feel one of the arteries of this system—the radial artery—pulsating by placing your fingers over the wrist, behind your thumb.

Each of the body's many systemic arteries ends in a meshwork of tiny systemic capillaries. At the capillary level, oxygen is given off from the blood cells, to be used for metabolism, and carbon dioxide is taken up by the same blood cells. From this point, the blood, now *dark red* and *de-oxygenated*, is called *venous* because it returns to the right side of the heart via the systemic veins. This path, from left side of the heart to systemic capillaries and back to the heart's right side, describes the systemic circulation.

There is *another* circulatory system *between* the right and left sides of the heart, called the pulmonary circulatory system or "pulmonary circulation." In this system de-oxygenated blood leaves the right heart and travels in the pulmonary artery that branches into smaller and smaller arteries, finally ending in an extensive meshwork of pulmonary capillaries. Once in the pulmonary capillaries blood picks up oxygen (from the alveolar sacs) and gives off CO_2 (the process of gas exchange—see Chapter 1). The newly oxygenated blood then travels to the left side of the heart via the pulmonary veins. From the left heart blood is pumped out to once again begin its journey through the systemic circulation.

Before proceeding it will be helpful to review Figure 1-4 (Chapter 1) and Table 22-1.

Compared to the systemic circulation, the pulmonary circulation operates under a much lower pressure. Pulmonary artery pressure is normally about one-quarter to one-fifth as high as the systemic artery pressure (the pressure you feel when you take your pulse). Of course the systemic artery pressure is also what is measured when "blood pressure" is taken with the familiar blood pressure cuff.

Unfortunately, pulmonary artery pressure is not so easy to measure. Because the entire pulmonary circulation is within the thoracic cavity, pressure measurements can only be accomplished by catheterization of the heart and pulmonary vessels. This is obviously a sophisticated technique and not done routinely (see Chapter 8). In many lung and heart conditions the pulmonary artery pressure is elevated; when there is a need to know this pressure, catheterization will be performed.

There are many diseases and disorders that can afflict the pulmonary circulation; the two most important are *pulmonary hypertension* and *pulmonary thromboembolism.*

TABLE 22-1 Systemic and pulmonary circulations (See also Figure 1-4)

	Systemic Circulation	Pulmonary Circulation
Path of Blood	Left side of heart → s.* arteries → s. capillaries → s. veins → right side of heart.	Right side of heart → p.* arteries → p. capillaries → p. veins → left side of heart.
Function	1. Carries oxygenated blood from left side of heart, via systemic arteries, to all organs and tissues. 2. After giving up O_2 and receiving CO_2, de-oxygenated blood returns, via systemic veins, to right side of the heart from where the pulmonary circulations begins.	1. Carries de-oxygenated blood from right side of heart, via pulmonary arteries, to the lungs. 2. After O_2 is picked up and CO_2 given off in the lung capillaries, oxygenated blood is returned, via pulmonary veins, to left side of the heart from where the systemic circulation begins.
Pressure	Relatively high pressure system; can easily be measured with blood pressure cuff.	Relatively low pressure system; can only be measured with catheterization and sophisticated instruments.
Treatment of Elevated Pressure	High blood pressure pills, taken by millions of hypertensive people.	Depends on cause; for some forms there is no effective treatment. For other types heart pills or oxygen may be beneficial (see text).

*s. = systemic
p. = pulmonary

WHAT IS PULMONARY HYPERTENSION?

Pulmonary hypertension is an increase in the pressure within the pulmonary arteries, the blood vessels that carry de-oxygenated blood from the right heart to the lungs. Except for the relatively rare condition of "primary pulmonary hypertension," all cases of pulmonary hypertension are secondary to some other disease or condition. Thus, pulmonary hypertension is not a single disease entity, but rather the result of a variety of abnormal conditions. Nonetheless, pulmonary hypertension can be every bit as debilitating as the more common (and more easily measured) systemic hypertension. (Patients who are "hypertensive" or have high blood pressure suffer from systemic hypertension. Pulmonary hypertension is not ordinarily a component of systemic hypertension.)

The danger from pulmonary hypertension of any cause is the strain put on the right side of the heart; this makes it more difficult to pump blood to and through the lungs. Because the right heart has to pump harder against the high pressure system, the heart muscle enlarges and this can eventually lead to right heart failure. The end result in severe pulmonary hypertension is inability to pump enough blood through the lungs to pick up oxygen.

The causes of pulmonary hypertension can be conveniently divided into "heart" and "lung" disease.

Heart Disease

Any disease or disorder of the left side of the heart may cause pressure to build up within the pulmonary circulation, leading to pulmonary hypertension. Since heart disease is so common, it is a major cause of pulmonary hypertension. Treatment will be discussed below.

Lung Disease

Any type of severe or chronic lung disease may lead to pulmonary hypertension, especially chronic obstructive lung disease and chronic interstitial lung diseases.

WHAT IS PRIMARY PULMONARY HYPERTENSION?

This is a rare form of pulmonary hypertension that, for unknown reasons, mainly occurs in women between the ages of 20 and 40. Its cause is also unknown. As its name implies it is not due to any detectable lung or heart disease. The pulmonary hypertension appears to occur *de novo*, unrelated to diet, weight, dust exposure, or any other environmental or genetic factors.

WHAT IS THE TREATMENT FOR PULMONARY HYPERTENSION?

Because there are diverse causes of pulmonary hypertension, the treatment varies considerably. When *heart disease* is the cause drugs may be employed to strengthen the heart muscle and relieve the "back pressure" that results from the failing or damaged heart. In some cases pulmonary hypertension can be caused by an abnormality of the mitral heart valve, for which surgery may be recommended.

Lung diseases usually cause pulmonary hypertension via one of two mechanisms. In emphysema many of the blood capillaries are destroyed along with the rest of the lung tissue. The remaining blood vessels must then carry the full load of blood, but because there are fewer vessels the resulting pressure is increased. In this situation there is no effective treatment.

Another mechanism whereby lung disease can lead to pulmonary hypertension is hypoxemia—not enough oxygen in the blood. The blood vessels in the lungs tend to constrict and narrow when there is chronically low oxygen tension; over a period of time this can lead to pulmonary hypertension. Treatment in such conditions is chronic oxygen administration (see Chapter 13).

At present there is no effective treatment for the primary form of pulmonary hypertension. Several experimental drugs have been tried, with transient success. Unfortunately, the condition is usually severe and relentlessly downhill.

WHAT IS PULMONARY THROMBOEMBOLISM?

A thrombosis is a blood clot. An embolus is any foreign matter, such as a blood clot or air bubble or piece of fat, that is carried in the blood stream. Pulmonary thromboembolism is a condition where the blood clot forms somewhere in the body (usually in the deep veins of the legs) and then travels to the lungs. It is a common, and often fatal, condition in sick and debilitated patients, though it can occur in anyone.

Normally our blood, made up of both fluid and cells, is a freely flowing liquid and does not clot unless exposed to air outside the body. This happens when we bleed from a cut or bruise. In many patients, for reasons not fully understood, blood tends to form clots (thrombi) abnormally within the body. This occurs most commonly in the deep veins of the legs and in patients who are immobilized or confined to bed.

Moreover, these clots can form without patients feeling any pain or the legs showing any abnormality. If the clots stay in the leg they usually cause no major damage. They either do not completely obstruct the vein or the blood finds some other vein to flow through; the leg veins are numerous and venous collaterals—connections between veins—form easily.

The real danger comes when one or more of these clots break off from the walls of the vein and travel to the lungs. The clots travel with the normal flow of blood returning to the heart; thus, the clots go from the leg up to the right side of the heart, which they pass through, and lodge in the narrower pulmonary arteries within the lungs. When this happens the patient has sustained a pulmonary embolism. The symptoms are usually some combination of chest pain, shortness of breath, and cough.

The size of the blood clots seems to be critical. Tiny blood clots probably flow to the lungs in many people; normally they are captured in the pulmonary capillaries where they are easily dissolved and cause no problems. However, clots in some patients are of sufficient size to cause symptoms and even prove fatal. They may be up to several inches in length and as wide as the deepest veins of the leg—

half an inch or more! When these travel to the lungs they can cause pain, cough, shortness of breath, fast heartbeat—and sudden death.

WHO ARE AT RISK FOR PULMONARY EMBOLISM?

Serious pulmonary embolism, enough to cause symptoms and illness, is largely but not exclusively a condition of people who have some underlying disability or disease. It is distinctly unusual in active, healthy people unless they are taking medication or have some risk factor that predisposes them to form blood clots in their legs.

Pulmonary embolism occurs predominantly in the following groups of people:

1. Those who are sedentary for long periods of time, including patients at prolonged bed rest, people who drive long periods of time without standing, very obese people, and patients who are chronically ill from any cause.
2. Patients with underlying cardiac and pulmonary disease; this includes patients suffering from chronic obstructive lung disease and congestive heart failure.
3. Patients who have diseases of the deep veins of the legs, especially a history of deep vein phlebitis (inflammation of the veins). Varicose veins and phlebitis of the superficial veins of the legs (those you can see) do not, by themselves, predispose to pulmonary embolism.
4. Any patient who has undergone major surgery.
5. Women taking birth control pills, especially if they smoke cigarettes.

These groups have an increased risk of getting pulmonary embolism. Although most people within these groups will never experience pulmonary embolism, it is important to be aware of the increased risk so that, should symptoms occur, appropriate tests can be done to make the diagnosis.

HOW DO DOCTORS DIAGNOSE PULMONARY EMBOLISM?

Pulmonary embolism (PE) is difficult to diagnose without doing specialized tests called lung scans. In fact many medical studies over the years have shown that the diagnostic accuracy of PE without these tests is no better than flipping a coin. (That is, without lung scans physicians have about a 50 percent accuracy in making the correct diagnosis.) This is because the symptoms of pulmonary embolism—chest pain, shortness of breath, cough, fast heart rate—are entirely non-specific. They may be due to any heart or lung condition.

Even lung scans are not 100 percent accurate. Using both the ventilation and perfusion lung scans (see Chapter 8), physicians can arrive at a "probability" of the diagnosis of pulmonary embolism for many patients. If the probability is high, treatment may be instituted without further studies.

The currently accepted definitive test to make the diagnosis of pulmonary embolism is pulmonary angiography (see Chapter 8). This is a dye study that involves catheterizing the right side of the heart and injecting dye into the pulmonary circulation to outline the clots. Because it is an invasive test and requires special expertise to perform and interpret, pulmonary angiography is not available in all hospitals. Also, if the probability from lung scans is very high, pulmonary angiography may not be warranted. Whether or not angiography is done in a patient suspected of having PE will depend on the condition of the patient, the results of the lung scans, and the facilities in the hospital.

HOW IS PULMONARY EMBOLISM TREATED?

The current treatment of this condition is anti-coagulants, or blood thinners. Two are commonly used, heparin and coumadin. Heparin is begun immediately after the diagnosis is suspected or confirmed, and is usually given intravenously; an alternative and less preferred route is subcutaneously (injecting into the fat under the skin). Heparin cannot be given by mouth.

Coumadin is given only by mouth, in tablet form. It is begun within a few days of heparin and is used for long-term anticoagulation. The ability of both coumadin and heparin to thin the blood is usually monitored by a simple blood test.

How long to treat a patient who has suffered a pulmonary embolism depends on several factors. If the patient is only at risk for PE a short time, such as a post-operative patient who is experiencing rapid recovery, then treatment may be for only a few weeks. However, if the patient is at risk forever—as in some patients with chronic heart failure—treatment may be for life. Each patient's treatment must be individualized.

Unfortunately, there is always a risk of serious bleeding while on anti-coagulants. These risks must be made known to every patient and appropriate counseling given about how to minimize them.

CHAPTER TWENTY-THREE

Cystic Fibrosis

WHAT IS CYSTIC FIBROSIS?

Cystic fibrosis (CF) is an inherited disease that occurs in about one out of every 2,000 white births and much less commonly in black births. CF affects the gland secretions in a variety of organs, including the lungs, intestines, pancreas, and reproductive system. In CF the ductal secretions, normally thin and freely flowing, become thick and tenacious, leading to blockage of the ducts. In the lungs, for example, CF commonly leads to thick mucus and airway obstruction similar to that found in chronic bronchitis.

An old name for this condition was "cystic fibrosis of the pancreas," but CF always involves other organs as well. In fact the lungs are the most commonly affected organ in CF.

The basic cause of cystic fibrosis is unknown.

WHAT HAPPENS TO PATIENTS WITH CF?

First described in 1938, CF is now known to be the most common of the life-threatening genetic diseases. Before World War II no child with CF lived past puberty! Since then, with the advent of antibiotics and modern respiratory care, CF patients have been living longer and more productive lives. Now the median survival is to age 20 and over half of all CF patients alive today are over 15. Dismal as this sounds, it is a remarkable improvement over the pre-antibiotic era. An estimated 20,000 patients with CF live in the United States.

Cystic fibrosis usually manifests itself in the first years of life, presenting either as an acute gastrointestinal problem such as bowel obstruction or an acute lung infection such as bronchitis. These and other complications are directly related to obstruction of the mucus ducts in the organs. Most adult patients who die from CF do so from respiratory failure (see Chapter 25). Bowel obstruction and other severe gastrointestinal problems are another cause of death, mainly in children.

CF children who survive early complications may grow and develop normally, although their height and weight will be at the lower end of the normal range. Today, many CF patients are alive past age 30 and able to lead a reasonably normal life. However, since the disease is never cured, they remain at risk for chronic pulmonary infections as well as other CF complications. The increased longevity of CF patients has extended their care beyond the province of the pediatrician, into that of the internist and family practitioner. Any patient with CF should be under the care of a physician familiar with the possible complications.

HOW IS CF DIAGNOSED?

In the past the disease was often detected by the mother who, on kissing her baby, noted a salty taste to the sweat. This lead researchers in the 1950s to develop the "sweat chloride" test, now the diagnostic test for CF. In this test a small electric current is passed through the skin of the patient's arm. This current causes an increased production of sweat that is then collected and analyzed for its content of sodium and chloride. If the sodium and chloride are above a certain level the diagnosis is confirmed, as long as there is a compatible clinical history. In this way CF is usually diagnosed before puberty, although occasionally the diagnosis is not made until later in life.

WHO SHOULD HAVE THE SWEAT CHLORIDE TEST?

The test is routinely performed in children with chronic bowel or pulmonary problems, since the cause may be cystic fibrosis. It should also be considered in young adults with similar complaints, since CF is occasionally not diagnosed until after puberty. In addition, the test is recommended in siblings of CF patients since their chance of having the disease is much higher than for the general population.

HOW IS CF INHERITED?

Cystic fibrosis is autosomal recessive (*both* parents have to be carriers of the CF gene before a child can inherit CF). CF carriers have *no symptoms* and *do not develop CF*, so it would be helpful if they could be diagnosed before conceiving a child. Unfortunately, there is no easily performed method for detecting CF carriers today. The sweat chloride test in CF carriers is normal.

Based on the recessive mode of inheritance, the chance of any one child of

CF carrier parents inheriting the disease (that is, receiving the gene from each parent), is one in four, or 25 percent. This risk is the same for each birth, regardless of the number of previous children born with or without cystic fibrosis.

In the example shown in Figure 23-1, two parents are carriers of the cystic fibrosis gene; they are represented by Cc in the top row. "C" indicates the gene for cystic fibrosis, "c" the normal gene. In genetic terms the parents are *heterozygous* (possessing different genes for a given trait). If they have four children they could be expected to distribute the genes as shown, with one of the two genes going to each of their children.

For a child to inherit CF he or she must receive a CF gene from both parents. The result is one child with cystic fibrosis (CC), two children who are carriers like their parents (Cc), and one child who is not a carrier (cc). Both the carrier children (Cc) and the non-carrier child (cc) would be expected to have a normal life span. If a cystic fibrosis carrier (Cc) marries a non-carrier (cc), none of their children will have cystic fibrosis, since both parents must contribute a cystic fibrosis gene for the disease to be inherited.

IS THERE A CURE FOR CYSTIC FIBROSIS?

No. The disease is inherited and there is no cure at present. However, treatment with antibiotics and modern respiratory care have made a difference between children dying before puberty and many of them living a reasonably normal life into adulthood. "Cystics," as patients with this disease are often called, go to school, work, and play just like other people except that they have to take special precautions because of their difficulty with secretions.

Treatment is mainly antibiotics for any infection, plus careful attention to lung hygiene and mobilizing secretions. One useful technique is postural drainage, whereby the patient leans over his bed so the lung secretions can be mobilized by gravity. This can be aided by someone else percussing or tapping the patient's back. CF patients may also require intestinal enzyme replacement, which can be taken orally.

These and other aspects of treatment have lead to the development of several cystic fibrosis centers where skilled help is concentrated. A list of these centers is available from the Cystic Fibrosis Foundation (see Appendix A).

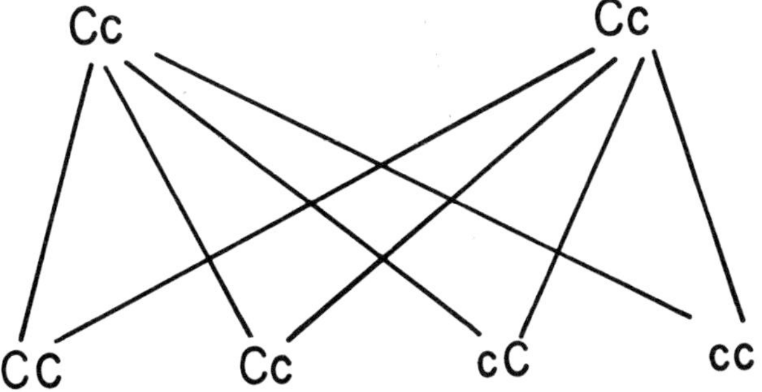

FIGURE 23-1
Inheritance of cystic fibrosis. See text for discussion.

CAN CYSTIC FIBROSIS PATIENTS HAVE CHILDREN?

Most cystic fibrosis patients are sterile. Up to 97 percent of all the males are sterile and most women cannot bear children. However, there are reports of CF women giving birth to healthy children. Because of the inherited nature of CF, as well as the difficulties cystic fibrosis women often have during childbirth, any female CF patient should be counseled thoroughly before deciding to bear children.

If a CF woman gives birth and the father is not a carrier, the children will not inherit CF. The same is true if a CF man fathers a child and the mother is not a carrier.

CAN GENETIC ENGINEERING PREVENT CF?

Genetic engineering is currently in its embryonic stage, with most of the research and development yet to come. By definition, it has the potential to prevent inherited diseases and CF is the most common, fatal inherited disease. Yet at present, CF is so poorly understood that speculation about *cure* would be an insult to its many victims. When a method is developed to detect CF carriers, and there is now much research in this area, we will be able to give reliable genetic counseling to potential parents; if followed, such counseling could lead to considerably fewer CF births.

CHAPTER TWENTY-FOUR

Trouble Breathing During Sleep

WHY STUDY BREATHING DURING SLEEP?

We spend roughly one-third of our lives asleep. What happens during sleep can affect our performance while awake, yet little was known about sleep disorders until recently. Now the study of sleep is a multidisciplined, growing area of research with articles published in many different specialties of medicine, such as psychiatry, neurology, and pulmonary disease. This research has found that many people do indeed have trouble breathing during sleep.

There is a wide range of sleep disorders. Insomnia, sleep-walking, recurring bad dreams, excessive snoring, and nocturnal leg cramps are some of the most familiar disorders. This chapter will concentrate on specific breathing disorders during sleep, most of which have been elucidated only in the last few years by using sensitive medical instruments. In some patients the pattern of nighttime breathing disorders has been diagnostically helpful in solving specific daytime medical problems.

Just the fact we spend so much time asleep seems to warrant a better understanding of this activity. Although sleep research is still in its infancy, a few examples of the potential benefits are already apparent:

1. The sudden infant death syndrome occurs eight to ten thousand times a year in the United States. Suddenly, without warning, an infant dies in his crib. Why this occurs is one of the major, agonizing questions of medicine.

Research is now pointing toward a central nervous system problem that either causes the infant to stop breathing or makes the infant unable to overcome obstruction of the upper airway. There are special instruments that may protect some children by making them wake up when their breathing starts to slow down. Other research is aimed toward identifying infants at particular risk for sudden crib death.

2. Adults with chronic obstructive pulmonary disease seem to have worse problems at night; their blood oxygen tension drops, sometimes so low as to cause heart beat irregularities and possibly sudden death. Once high-risk patients have been identified with special instruments, oxygen therapy can be instituted, preventing this nocturnal hypoxia.
3. Some patients, particularly the very obese, stop breathing at night because of upper airway obstruction. Presumably the muscles in the upper airway come together and occlude the opening so that no air can enter the lungs. When this happens the patient wakes up, snorts, and goes back to sleep again. Over a period of time this may lead to respiratory failure. Losing weight is one treatment, but for a small number of patients tracheostomy has proven most beneficial. Bypassing the obstructed upper airway by placing a breathing opening directly in the neck, a procedure known as tracheostomy, allows much better exchange of air. In many of these patients desirable weight loss will follow the tracheostomy.

HOW DO I KNOW IF I HAVE TROUBLE BREATHING DURING SLEEP?

Although special testing is needed to diagnose nocturnal sleep disorders there are certain clues. Any of the following suggests the possibility of trouble breathing during sleep:

1. Excessive daytime sleepiness.
2. Marked obesity, particularly when accompanied by excessive snoring at night.
3. Any irregular breathing pattern detected by a bed partner (such as irregular snoring or gasping respirations).

In addition, patients who have chronic respiratory failure (as may occur from chronic bronchitis or emphysema) often have breathing irregularities during sleep.

Almost all information we know about breathing disorders during sleep comes from special testing. The patient or volunteer is brought to the sleep lab before bedtime and connected, via wires, to a variety of sensitive instruments. These record brain waves and also measure the movement of air through the mouth and nostrils, the movement of the chest wall, and the amount of oxygen in the blood (this last is done with a special skin sensor; no needles are used). All of these are continuous measurements, recorded on graph paper. By the end of the sleep period the investigator has an excellent idea of just what breathing problems occurred and how long they lasted.

Obviously, this is not a routine test and is currently performed in relatively few hospitals.

WHAT IS SLEEP APNEA?

There are a variety of abnormal breathing patterns that may occur during sleep but the most important is called "apnea"–literally cessation of all breathing activity. It appears we all normally have brief apneic periods throughout sleep, each episode lasting only a few seconds or less. Any apneic period 10 seconds or longer is abnormal; these abnormal apneic periods are easy to diagnose since there is no airflow at the mouth or nose. Apnea is the most studied breathing disorder during sleep and is classified into two broad types:

Central Sleep Apnea

The defect here is somewhere in the central nervous system. No effort is made to breathe during central apneic periods, so there is no movement of the chest cage. These patients usually have associated neurologic diseases such as polio or spinal cord injuries. They may be of any age, weight, and of either sex.

Obstructive Sleep Apnea

Here apneic episodes are caused by abnormal relaxation of the pharyngeal muscles that make up the throat and hence part of the upper airway. This relaxation leads to airway blockage. The result is a breathing effort (the chest cage is moved in and out) but no movement of air in and out of the lungs.

Obstructive sleep apnea is a common finding in patients with chronic bronchitis and emphysema. In addition, researchers at the University of Florida have uncovered this pattern in some middle-aged men who are stocky (but not grossly overweight) and who have short, thick necks.

Most patients with obstructive sleep apnea are overweight; this presumably affects the upper airway muscles. However, this cause of sleep apnea is highly variable and its severity cannot be predicted by body weight, routine breathing tests, or clinical history. Special sleep studies are needed to characterize accurately its severity and prescribe proper treatment. For many patients simply losing weight may be the most beneficial therapy. A few extreme cases have been treated successfully with tracheostomy.

Combined Central and Obstructive Apnea

The results of sleep studies show that some patients have both causes present, further reinforcing the need for accurate studies in anyone suspected of a sleep disorder.

WHAT ARE PICKWICKIAN SYNDROME AND ONDINE'S CURSE?

The Pickwickian syndrome is a term applied to patients who are very obese, have a decreased drive to breathe, and have a tendency to fall asleep during the day. When a patient with these characteristics was first described there was noticed a striking resemblance to the fat boy Joe, a character in Charles Dickens' *The Posthumous*

Papers of the Pickwick Club (1837). Since the original clinical description in 1956, much has been learned about the Pickwickian syndrome. We now know that the decreased drive to breathe, and not the obesity, is the major underlying problem. The decreased breathing drive seems to be aggravated by the obesity and the symptoms can often be reversed by losing weight. As might be expected Pickwickian patients suffer from sleep apnea episodes.

Ondine's curse refers to a condition where the lungs and chest bellows are normal, but patients stop breathing, usually during sleep. It gets its name from a legend about an ondine, or water nymph. This ondine was jilted by a mortal man who married her, but then left for another woman (not an ondine). His punishment, according to legend, was to lose automatic control of body functions, including breathing. Unless he thought about it, he would forget to breathe. When the jilter finally did fall asleep he died of apnea.

Pickwickian syndrome and Ondine's curse do not refer to specific diseases or causes of disease but are merely descriptive terms used by physicians to describe certain groups of patients.

CHAPTER TWENTY-FIVE

Respiratory Failure: The Ultimate Catastrophe

WHAT IS RESPIRATORY FAILURE?

The role of the respiratory system is simple and vital: to bring in oxygen and excrete carbon dioxide. As discussed in Chapter 1, this process of gas exchange is *the* function of the respiratory system. When the system no longer exchanges these gases efficiently, it has failed and the patient has respiratory failure (RF). RF is not a specific disease but rather a "failed state of respiratory function," that in turn may be due to a variety of diseases.

Obviously, if there were *no* exchange of O_2 and CO_2 between the atmosphere and the blood, there could be no life. Thus RF represents a condition, in terms of the system's gas exchange function, between normalcy and death. Although most respiratory illnesses interfere somewhat with exchange of O_2 and CO_2, respiratory failure is said to be present when gas exchange is *severely* impaired. The severity of impairment, and thus the diagnosis of RF, are determined with the aid of arterial blood gas analysis (see Chapter 8).

WHAT DISEASES CAN LEAD TO RESPIRATORY FAILURE?

The respiratory system is made up of three components (see below, and Chapter 1). Disease or abnormality of any of the three parts of the respiratory system can, if severe, lead to respiratory failure. The three components are:

1. The area of the brain that regulates our breathing. RF may result from depression of this area. Clinical examples include: overdose from any narcotic, sedative, or tranquilizer; strokes that affect the brain's breathing center; Ondine's curse; and Pickwickian syndrome (see Chapter 24).
2. The nerves, muscles, bones, and connective tissue that make up the chest bellows portion of the respiratory system. Conditions that may affect this part of the respiratory system are listed in Chapter 14.
3. The lungs, including the airways. Diseases of the lungs and airways, such as asthma, bronchitis, emphysema, pneumonia, and pulmonary edema, make up the bulk of this book and account for the majority of all serious respiratory conditions. They also account for most causes of respiratory failure.

In summary, disease or malfunction of any component of the respiratory system can lead to respiratory failure, including any of the diseases discussed in this book. The relationship of RF to *all* respiratory illness is shown in Figure 25-1. Note that most respiratory conditions do not manifest or cause respiratory failure in most patients. However, all RF occurs because of some respiratory problem—even though the primary cause may originate in another organ such as the heart.

DOES SEVERE LUNG DISEASE ALWAYS MEAN RESPIRATORY FAILURE?

No. Patients can have severe, even life-threatening lung disease without having RF at the time of diagnosis. Such patients may be at increased risk for developing RF, but unless gas exchange is seriously impaired they are not considered to have respiratory failure. The distinction is important therapeutically. Failure of gas

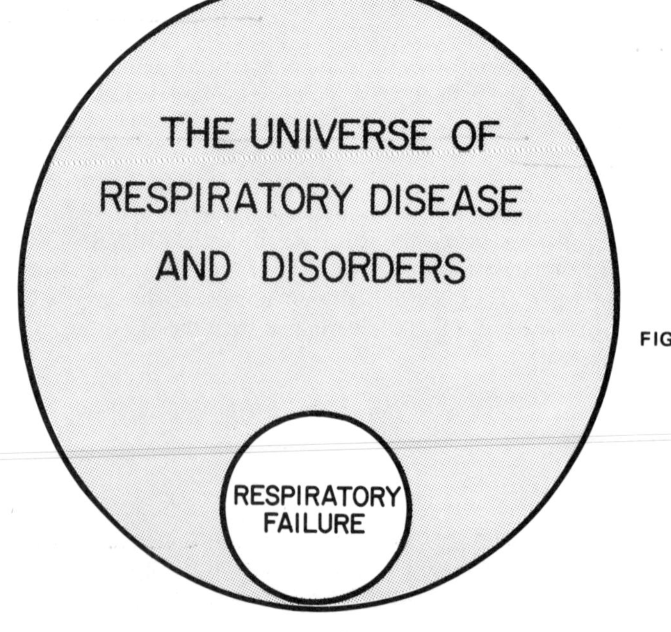

FIGURE 25-1 Diagrammatic relationship of respiratory failure to all respiratory illness. Only a small fraction respiratory illness ever lea[ds] to respiratory failure.

exchange (RF) requires special treatment. When RF occurs acutely, patients often must receive artificial ventilation to sustain life. If RF occurs chronically, patients may have to receive long term oxygen therapy, even at home. At the least, chronic RF implies a very limited state of activity.

Respiratory failure is the "worst clinical state" a patient can have for any particular respiratory condition. Once RF sets in, the prognosis for any patient is poor, unless it is acute and easily reversible. Examples of patients who may recover completely from RF include those suffering from drug overdose, severe asthma, severe pneumonia, and trauma affecting the respiratory system.

HOW IS RESPIRATORY FAILURE DIAGNOSED?

Unless a patient has stopped breathing altogether, there is no reliable way to diagnose respiratory failure by history and physical examination. The only reliable way to diagnose *and* treat RF is with the aid of arterial blood gas analysis as discussed in Chapter 8. This test measures the pressures or tensions of O_2 and CO_2 in the blood (which together define the state of RF), plus the amount of blood acidity. Clinically, patients in respiratory failure may present with an extremely varied clinical picture, depending on three important circumstances:

1. Underlying clinical condition. The clinical diseases that lead to RF are varied and wide ranging, as indicated above. Each may have its own charactertistic findings without necessarily indicating RF. For example, the majority of very obese people have no problem with gas exchange, yet complain of shortness of breath on stair climbing. The same may be true of the obese patient with RF.
2. Rapidity of onset. "Acute" RF occurs over a period of hours to a few days, and is usually characterized by shortness of breath and obvious breathing difficulty if the patient is awake (see below). "Chronic" RF occurs over months to years; the patient may have no visible signs and offer no complaints, in part because of chronic adaptation to the condition.
3. Patient's mental status. Mental status will be altered when RF is due to brain depression, as by an overdose of sleeping pills. At the same time the patient's drive to breathe is reduced, so the usual picture of difficult breathing is absent. This is why it is so important to think of RF in patients who are obtunded or confused—they won't complain of trouble breathing and may not appear short of breath.

In summary, shortness of breath, confusion, or coma should be a tip-off to possible respiratory failure; these signs may indicate not enough O_2, or too much CO_2, in the blood. However patients with RF may *not* show these signs, particularly those with chronic respiratory failure.

HOW IS RESPIRATORY FAILURE TREATED?

There are two basic aspects of treating respiratory failure. Because RF is a state of not enough O_2 and/or too much CO_2 in the blood, the first aspect is aimed at correcting this imbalance. This is called non-specific or "supportive" treatment because it doesn't treat the underlying cause and only supports the patient until recovery from the underlying illness.

Depending on the type and severity of RF, supportive treatment may range from using only supplemental oxygen all the way to intubation and artificial ventilation (see Chapter 8). Artifical ventilators are available in every hospital that cares for acutely ill patients. Not all patients with RF receive artificial ventilation, but all patients who receive artificial ventilation have RF. (Patients undergoing surgery or other procedures requiring general anesthesia are artificially ventilated to prevent the transient RF that occurs from anesthesia).

If the cause of RF is unknown, as in some cases of paralysis, the patient may receive only supportive treatment—correction of O_2 and/or CO_2 imbalance. More commonly a treatable cause is diagnosed and along with supportive measures, the second aspect of management is added—specific therapy of the underlying disease. For example, if pneumonia is the cause of RF, antibiotics are given; if asthma, bronchodilators and corticosteroids; if drug overdose, the appropriate antidotes, and so forth. Specific treatment of many common conditions that may lead to RF is discussed elsewhere in this book (see Index).

Treatment of RF, regardless of whether or not the cause is known, is best handled by physicians who deal with the problem regularly. Patients with acute RF, especially those intubated and receiving artificial ventilation, need continuous monitoring and close availability of a physician 24 hours a day. Special duty nurses are required, often at a ratio of one nurse to one patient. This type of care is usually given in specially equipped and staffed areas of the hospital called intensive care units (ICU's). ICU's for acute RF have been standard in all large hospitals for over a decade and have themselves become sub-specialized. In addition to general medical and surgical ICU's, many hospitals have intensive care units devoted to cardiovascular, neonatal, and neurosurgical patients. The idea behind all such units is *intensive* care, providing close nurse and physician monitoring for patients whose condition is unstable and potentially reversible. This characterizes many patients with respiratory failure.

Tom R.—A Patient with Chronic Obstructive Pulmonary Disease and Respiratory Failure

Mr. R. had chronic obstructive pulmonary disease first diagnosed at age 59. He continued to smoke until age 67 when he developed pneumonia that required hospitalization for two weeks. After recovery his level of pulmonary function was only 30 percent of predicted, but he maintained adequate O_2 and CO_2 tension in his blood—he was not in respiratory failure. He supported himself from Social Security and a small pension and had a very limited lifestyle. Mr. R. spent most of his time reading and gardening, but became increasingly short of breath with exertion. At age 69, a little less than two years following his last hospitalization, he developed acute bronchitis and wheezing. Two days of treatment at home with antibiotics and bronchodilators provided no relief and his condition rapidly deteriorated. He became extremely short of breath and confused and was rushed to the hospital.

On admission he was found to be in severe respiratory failure, with a very low PO_2 and high PCO_2 in the arterial blood, plus increased acidity from the excess

CO_2. Because of these life-threatening blood changes and his confused state he was intubated and given artificial ventilation. In addition to this supportive treatment Mr. R. also received several medications to combat the obstructive lung disease: corticosteroids, bronchodilators, and antibiotics.

Despite maximal ventilatory support and treatment for his underlying lung disease, improvement was slow. After one week Mr. R. still could not tolerate breathing on his own. When disconnected from the ventilator he failed to maintain adequate O_2 and CO_2 levels in his blood. Because of the need for prolonged ventilatory support he was advised to have a tracheostomy. (A tracheostomy allows removal of the endotracheal (throat) tube from the mouth and placement of another tube through a hole in the trachea. With this procedure a patient can eat and still receive artificial ventilation.) He agreed and the procedure was done on his eighth hosptial day.

It took another two weeks to wean him from the ventilator and one additional week before the tracheostomy tube could be pulled out of his neck. Altogether he was in the hospital 31 days. Prior to discharge his PO_2 and PCO_2 tensions were considerably better than on admission, although only boderline.

Mr. R. remains in a state of chronic respiratory failure at home and uses oxygen when he sleeps. Another episode of acute RF may be fatal.

WHAT IS NON-CARDIAC PULMONARY EDEMA?

Non-cardiac pulmonary edema is a condition of abnormal accumulation of fluid within the alveolar spaces, not due to heart disease (hence, "non-cardiac"). It must be distinguished from the more common cardiac pulmonary edema (see Chapter 17), since the causes and treatment are different. Another term for non-cardiac pulmonary edema in adults is "adult respiratory distress syndrome," or ARDS.

ARDS is a very common and severe form of respiratory failure. This syndrome may be due to a variety of separate and specific causes such as:

- severe viral pneumonia
- aspiration pneumonia (aspiration of stomach contents into the lungs)
- trauma to any region of the body (head, thorax, abdomen, or legs)
- severe hemorrhage (blood loss from any cause)
- sepsis (blood poisoning)
- pancreatitis (severe inflammation of the pancreas)
- drug overdose (virtually any drug, but particularly morphine, heroin, and other narcotics)
- shock (severe or sudden drop in blood pressure from any cause)
- fat embolism (travel of bone marrow fat from the long bones of the body to the lungs, as may occur following trauma)

Despite the widespread prevalence and severity of ARDS the syndrome was not fully characterized and named until the late 1960s.

The features that characterize the adult respiratory distress syndrome are:

1. sudden shortness of breath in a previously healthy and functioning person; this always follows the onset of an acute illness or injury such as those listed above;
2. very low PO_2 in the arterial blood; and
3. a chest X-ray showing pulmonary edema (see Figure 25-2).

In contrast to cardiac pulmonary edema, fluid in the lungs of ARDS patients is not due to backup from a failing heart; rather, it is due to damage of the pulmonary capillaries and leakage of fluid through these injured blood vessels. Although much research is underway to determine how this occurs, the mechanism leading to capillary damage and pulmonary edema from any of the above conditions remains unknown.

ARDS is a common syndrome. In the early 1970s the National Heart and Lung Institute estimated 150,000 cases per year in the United States, and there are probably more cases annually in the 1980s. The mortality rate depends on the underlying cause but overall is approximately 50 percent. Thus, about 75,000 people die each year from ARDS. Since ARDS is not a specific disease entity, the reason for death is more likely to be listed by the underlying cause, such as trauma, pneumonia, drug overdose, and so forth.

Since the national speed limit was lowered to 55 mph in the early 1970s, an esimated several thousand deaths have been prevented yearly, simply by preventing accidents that no doubt would have resulted in acute respiratory failure. Any other measures to prevent the causes of ARDS will likewise decrease the number of respiratory failure deaths.

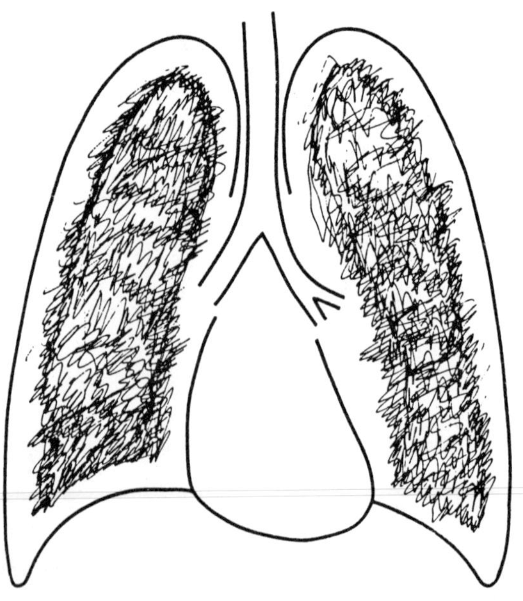

FIGURE 25-2 Chest x-ray of non-cardiac pulmonary edema, or adult respiratory distress syndrome (ARDS). Note similarity to x-ray of cardiac pulmonary edema (Figure 17-1d). Heart size (normal here) is only distinguishing feature. In some ARDS cases, the heart may appear enlarged even though heart failure is not present.

ARDS is one of the most severe forms of respiratory failure and almost always requires intubation and artificial ventilation for proper management. Fortunately, patients who recover do so almost completely—there is little if any residual lung damage in most surviors of ARDS.

Delores G.—A Case of Adult Respiratory Distress Syndrome

Delores G., a 28-year-old woman, was in good health prior to an automobile accident in which the car she was driving flipped over and rolled into a ditch. When the rescue squad arrived she was alert, but she could not move her right leg. X-rays in the emergency room revealed a fractured thigh bone; her chest X-ray was normal. Vital signs showed normal blood pressure, breathing rate, and temperature.

She was given intravenous fluids and operated on to set the fractured bone. During surgery she required two units of blood. In the immediate post-operative period she did well.

Approximately 30 hours after her accident and 24 hours after surgery she developed a temperature of 101°. The nurse also noted an increase in her breathing rate, from a normal of 14 to 24 breaths per minute. She was given an aspirin suppository. Two hours later she was breathing 30 times a minute and complained of shortness of breath for the first time. A physician examined her, heard some abnormal breath sounds, and ordered an immediate chest X-ray. This confirmed the clinical suspicion of non-cardiac pulmonary edema or the adult respiratory distress syndrome (see Figure 25-2). An arterial blood gas showed a very low O_2 tension. At this point Mrs. G. was in severe, acute respiratory failure.

She was moved to the intensive care unit and begun on high flow oxygen and corticosteroids. However, she deteriorated rapidly and two hours later required intubation and artificial ventilation. This was maintained for two days before her X-ray began to clear and blood oxygen tension improve. By the end of the fourth intensive care day Mrs. G. was able to come off the ventilator and breathe on her own. She made an uneventful recovery and was discharged from the hospital a week later.

Although ARDS in Mrs. G. was obviously related to the accident, the immediate precipitating event was unclear. It could have been one of several events in her case: the trauma, per se; the blood she received during the operation; embolization of fat from the fractured bone to her lungs (so-called fat embolism syndrome); or excessive intravenous fluids given to her before or after the operation. Because she had suffered a fractured thigh bone, fat embolism was considered the most likely cause.

WHAT IS THE FUTURE FOR RESPIRATORY FAILURE?

The first reported case of human lung transplantation was in 1963. The 38th reported case was published in October, 1980. Neither the first nor the 38th case lived longer than 18 days after surgery. The median survival for all 38 patients was 8.5 days after surgery, although two patients lived for 6 and 10 months respectively. Interestingly, the 38 transplants were performed by 26 different surgical teams working on five continents. Contrast this with heart transplants. The first was performed by Dr. Christian Barnard in 1969. Through 1980 several hundred had been done worldwide, with 70 percent had surviving the first year (in the Standford experience).*

Why the difficulty with lung transplants? There appear to be three reasons for their failure. First, the lung transplant patients were so sick to begin with that about a third did not survive the immediate surgical and post-surgical period. Second, a number of the patients rejected the transplanted lung, which was a cadaver lung. This tissue rejection is similar to what plagues heart and kidney transplants, but in the lung it is apparently more devastating. Third, in some patients the main air tube of the transplanted lung (main bronchus) suffered from inadequate blood supply.

Clearly the problems are enormous, leading one to conclude that lung transplants will not become feasible in the near future.

Much more feasible in the long run is the artificial lung, models of which already exist. An artificial lung is not to be confused with the older, now outmoded iron lung, a huge metal cylinder surrounding the patient that served to expand the chest cage. Patients in an iron lung still needed their own lungs for gas exchange.

Nor should an artificial lung be confused with the widely used artificial ventilator that pumps air into and out of the patient's own lungs. Although artificial ventilators are life-saving in patients with severe lung disease, they still require the patient to have *some* intrinsic lung function.

True artificial lungs are gas exchangers that effectively bypass the need to pump air into and out of the patient's lungs. They work by exchanging O_2 and CO_2 directly with the blood. In this sense they are analogous to kidney dialysis machines, which can support patients without kidneys indefinitely.

The problem with current artificial lungs is a matter of technology. They are too bulky and difficult to use; they require a large team of highly trained personnel to implement; and worse, they have not been shown to be effective in preventing mortality in critically ill patients. However, it is only a matter of time before technological improvements allow for an easy to use, portable, and effective artificial lung. While it may not allow for indefinite existence, it should provide for short-term maintenance until the patient's own lungs can heal from whatever insult caused respiratory failure. For patients with irreversible lung damage, totally effective artificial lungs are not on the horizon.

*A number of combined heart and lung transplants have also been done. It appears that patients with combined heart-lung transplants may have better survival than those with lung transplant alone.

Epilog

WHAT IS THE OUTLOOK FOR PREVENTION OF RESPIRATORY DISEASE?

The future for lung disease is underscored by one dramatic fact: THE MAJOR LUNG DISEASES ARE PREVENTABLE! Diseases responsible for most pulmonary disability and death could become uncommon in a generation by eliminating the single predominant cause: *cigarette smoking.* Alone, or acting in concert with industrial and auto pollution, cigarette smoking accounts for over 90 percent of lung cancers and chronic obstructive lung disease, the major respiratory killers. In addition, smoking accounts for an unknown amount of *increased morbidity* from all types of respiratory infections.

Eliminating cigarette smoking is not about to happen. Reasons are numerous and complex, but not the least is the matter of individual freedom. Banning cigarettes would be as counter-productive and unsuccessful as was Prohibition in the 1920s. The best that can (and perhaps should) be hoped for is sufficient smoking education so everyone can make his or her own decision, ideally as adults and not as teenagers under peer pressure. This method alone has been successful in decreasing the percentage of adults who smoke from almost one-half to about one-third over the past 2 decades.

It is unlikely technology will come to the rescue of smokers. There is not now, nor likely to be, any safe, widely accepted cigarette that will satisfy the addiction. Some reasons for this are discussed in Chapter 2.

The many lung diseases that are caused by industrial exposure are largely preventable using modern techniques of pollution control. However, because of enormous costs, and because new industrial processes are constantly being introduced, it is difficult to say what the future holds for industrial air pollution. The Three-Mile Island nuclear accident in 1979, while not directly responsible for any loss of life, exemplifies the challenges faced by new technologies in controlling safety and the work environment. Again however, it must be emphasized that the majority of patients adversely affected by industrial exposure of any kind, from mining to chemicals to fire fighting, are cigarette smokers! All too often, it is the combination of industrial exposure *plus* cigarette smoking that is harmful; for most people, eliminating cigarettes would minimize, if not eliminate, the harmful effects of industrial pollution.

It is likely the next 20 years will see only a gradual abatement in all forms of pollution. No breakthroughs are on the horizon. This assessment is based on extrapolating from the last few years, taking into account the smaller-sized autos now being produced. It obviously does not account for any cataclysmic event such as nuclear accidents.

Controlling air pollution may prevent some lung conditions; this is certainly more feasible than eliminating cigarettes. Although smog from automobiles continues to plague American cities, gradual improvement is occurring. Nonsmokers who suffer from chronic or recurrent lung conditions such as asthma should certainly benefit by an overall decrease in air pollution. However, so pervasive are the effects of cigarettes as a contributor to inhalation diseases that controlling air pollution will be most beneficial for smokers!

APPENDIX A

Sources of Additional Information

Following is a list of addresses and phone numbers of agencies that provide information to the public about various aspects of lung disease. The American Lung Association, in particular, has a wealth of free pamphlets, booklets, and books on virtually every aspect of respiratory disease. You may write them directly or call your local chapter listed in the phone book. There is an ALA chapter in every state and large metropolitan region.

Action on Smoking and Health
2013 H Street, N.W., Suite #301
Washington, DC 20006
(202) 659-4310
A national non-profit group that serves as the "legal action arm of the anti-smoking community." ASH provides information on harmful effects of cigarettes and sells non-smoking decals, bumper stickers and buttons.

American Cancer Society
777 Third Avenue
New York, NY 10017
(212) 371-2900
Publishes many booklets on all types of cancer; issues guidelines for cancer check-ups; offers assistance with employment problems.

American Heart Association
National Center
7320 Greenville Avenue
Dallas, TX 75231
The major national heart organization; sponsors no-smoking program; distributes material on all aspects of heart and blood pressure-related diseases; AHA chapter in most areas.

American Lung Association
1740 Broadway
New York, NY 10019
(212) 245-8000
The major national lung organization; sponsors stop-smoking program

and publishers scores of pamphlets and booklets on every aspect of lung disease; ALA chapter in most areas.

American Medical Association
535 North Dearborn St.
Chicago, IL 60610
(312) 751-6000

Keeps records on location and credentials of every physician in U.S.; also publishes *Journal of American Medical Association (JAMA),* most widely circulated medical journal.

Asthma and Allergy Foundation of America
801 Second Avenue
New York, NY 10017
(212) 867-8875

Provides information to the public, including names of physicians who specialize in allergy-related problems.

Center for Disease Control
Public Inquiries, Building 4, Room B-9
1600 Clifton Road, N.E.
Atlanta, GA 30333
(404) 633-3311

Information on communicable diseases; publishes *Morbidity and Mortality Weekly.*

Consumer Information Center
Pueblo, CO 81009

Government agency that issues dozens of free pamphlets on wide variety of health and consumer topics; publishes consumer information catalogue several times a year.

Cystic Fibrosis Foundation
3379 Peachtree Rd., N.E.
Atlanta, GA 30326
(404) 262-1100

Information on CF and location of CF clubs around the country.

Emphysema Anonymous, Inc.
P.O.Box 66
1364 Palmetto Avenue
Ft. Myers, FL 33902

Non-profit organization that sponsors self-help groups for emphysema and chronic bronchitis patients who have trouble breathing. Publishes a quarterly newsletter, *Batting the Breeze*; EAI will send a sample copy and descriptive brochure on request.

National Heart, Lung, and Blood Institute
Public Inquiries and Reports Section
9000 Rocksville Pike
Bethesda, MD 20014
(301) 496-4236

Major government-sponsored research institute, with special interest in interstitial lung diseases.

National Institute of Allergy and Infectious Diseases
Information Office
Room 7A-32, Building 31
9000 Rockville Pike
Bethesda, MD 20014
(301) 496-4000

Major government-sponsored research institute for study of allergy and infectious diseases.

National Institute for Occupational Safety and Health
Center for Disease Control
1600 Clifton Road, N.E.
Atlanta, GA 30333
(404) 633-3311

Government agency charged with enforcing occupational safety and health.

National Interagency Council on Smoking and Health
419 Park Avenue South
New York, NY 10016
(212) 532-6035

Represents 33 organizations (including the American Medical Association) concerned with diseases associated with tobacco use. Under contract from federal government to promote smoking education programs in schools.

National Jewish Hospital and Research Center/National Asthma Center
3800 East Colfax Avenue
Denver, CO 80206
Attn: Public Relations Dept.
(303) 388-4461

Large referral hospital for difficult cases of asthma.

Office on Smoking and Health
5600 Fishers Lane, Room 1-58
Rockville, MD 20857
(301) 443-1575

The federal agency directed to prepare the Surgeon General Reports on *Smoking and Health.*

Superintendent of Documents
Government Printing Office
Washington, DC 20402

This address (or the Consumer Information Center–see above) is where to send for most government publications.

Tel-Med Corporation
P.O. Box 22700
Cooley Drive
Colton, CA 92324
(714) 825-6034

Maintains tape library that can be accessed over local phone numbers across the country. Carries short tapes on subjects ranging from lung cancer to hay fever and shortness of breath.

APPENDIX B

Glossary

Adenocarcinoma—A type of *cancer*; one of the four types of primary lung cancer.

Adrenergic—Pertaining to the adrenal gland. Beta-adrenergic drugs are commonly used in asthma to help open up the airways. Such drugs are *bronchodilators*, one of the most powerful being epinephrine, a hormone also secreted by the adrenal gland.

Airways—A general term for the conducting tubes of the lungs. The largest airway is the trachea, followed in order by the *bronchi*, *bronchioles*, and *alveoli*.

Albuterol—A beta-adrenergic drug useful in treating asthma.

Allergy—A hypersensitive state manifested by altered reaction to a substance to which a person has been previously exposed.

Alveolar-capillary—Refers to the unit of *gas exchange*. Air is brought into the *alveolus*; then oxygen diffuses into the capillary and *carbon dioxide* diffuses out of the *capillary*.

Alveolar ventilation—That part of the air breathed in each minute that reaches the alveoli and takes part in *gas exchange*. Contrast with *dead space ventilation*.

Alveolus—The air sac of the lung, where gas exchange occurs. Plural is alveoli. There are normally over 300,000,000 alveoli in both lungs, each situated next to one or more pulmonary *capillaries*. The alveolus delivers *oxygen* to the capillary and takes up *carbon dioxide* from it.

Aminophylline—The generic term for diethyl-theophylline. Theophylline is one of the three major drug classes

*Words italicized in the definition may be found in the glossary, in either singular or plural form.

for treating *asthma* and aminophylline is one important type of theophylline preparation. It is the only theophylline preparation available for intravenous use, but also comes in tablet form.

Anemia–A red blood cell count below normal. Red blood cells contain *hemoglobin,* responsible for carrying most of the *oxygen* in the blood. Anemia, if severe, may lead to lack of oxygen for the body's tissues.

Antibiotic–A drug that is used to fight bacteria infections.

Apnea–Absence of breathing.

ARDS–*A*dult *R*espiratory *D*istress *S*yndrome, a syndrome of severe, non-cardiac pulmonary edema.

Arterial–Refers to the artery on arteries, blood vessels that carry bright-red (oxygen-rich) blood from the heart to the organs and tissues. See *venous.*

Arterial blood gas test–A measurement of oxygen and carbon dioxide gas *tensions* in a sample of *arterial* blood.

Asbestos–Material commonly used for insulation and fireproofing. When inhaled over years may lead to *asbestosis* or lung *cancer.* The risk of lung cancer is greatly increased in cigarette smokers exposed to asbestos.

Asbestosis–A form of lung scarring due to long-term inhalation of asbestos fibers. Asbestosis scarring shows up on the chest X-ray usually at the bottom portion of the lungs.

Aspiration–Breathing or drawing in. Air, fluid, or cells may be aspirated from the body by thin needles or tubes. Aspiration also refers to breathing in food, dusts, or chemicals into the lung, where they may cause *pneumonia.*

Asthma–A medical condition characterized by hyper-reactive *airways*; sometimes defined as "twitchy airways." During an asthma attack airways narrow and there may be increased mucus production. The result is usually shortness of breath, chest congestion, and *wheezing.*

Asymptomatic–Without symptoms.

Atelectasis–Collapse of part of the lung. Atelectasis is usually an X-ray finding; it can be due to many different causes. The amount of atelectasis may range from small and of no consequence to the patient, all the way to massive and enough to cause trouble breathing.

Bacillus–Another term for bacterium (the terms bacilli and bacteria are also interchangeable).

Bacteria–Micro-organisms responsible for many infections; they can only be seen with aid of a microscope (hence are microscopic). Bacteria are larger than *viruses. Antibiotics* are effective against many bacterial infections.

Benign–A term for a non-malignant (that is, not cancerous) disease or condition. A tumor, mass, or growth may be benign or *malignant* (cancer). Also, sometimes used as a descriptive term for a mild or harmless disease or condition.

Biopsy–Removal of piece of tissue for purpose of diagnosis. Several types of biopsies are used in pulmonary medicine.

Black Lung–See Coal Workers' Pneumoconiosis.

Bronchi–The larger (greater than 2 mm diameter) air tubes or *airways* of the lungs, that bring air from the *trachea* down to the alveoli. Singular is bronchus. The bronchi are affected in many lung diseases such as *asthma.* See *bronchioles.*

Bronchiectasis–A lung condition where the air tubes *(bronchi)* are permanently weakened and dilated. It is characterized by chronic cough with copious amounts of sputum. Accurate diagnosis usually requires a *bronchogram.*

Bronchioles–After bronchi, the next smallest airways; they are less than

2 mm in diameter. Bronchioles lead into *alveoli,* the smallest airspaces.

Bronchiolitis–Inflammation of the bronchioles. Bronchiolitis is more common in children than in adults, who are more apt to suffer from *bronchitis.*

Bronchitis–Inflammation of the lining of the bronchial tubes. May be acute on chronic. The latter, usually due to cigarette smoking, is one type of *chronic obstructive lung disease.*

Bronchoconstrictor–Something that constricts, or narrows, the *bronchi.* This may be a drug, dust, pollen, noxious gas, and so forth.

Bronchodilator–Something (usually a drug) that dilates, or opens up, the bronchial tubes. Bronchodilators are a mainstay of treatment in *asthma* and reversible airways diseases.

Bronchogenic–Arising from the bronchus. Bronchogenic *carcinoma* is cancer arising from the cells that line the *bronchi.*

Bronchogram–An X-ray study that outlines the bronchi with a dye that is inhaled or injected into the airways. Bronchograms are rarely ordered today.

Bronchoscopy–A diagnostic and/or therapeutic procedure whereby a long, thin tube (the bronchoscope) is inserted into the bronchi, via either the nose or mouth. Modern bronchoscopes are narrow and flexible and hence better tolerated than the older "rigid" models.

Bronchospasm–Contraction of the muscles in the airway leading to narrowing and airway obstruction. Bronchospasm plays a major role in asthma attacks and commonly causes the patient to wheeze.

Brown Lung–See byssinosis.

Byssinosis–Lung disease from inhaling cotton dust; also known as "brown lung." In early stages byssinosis can present like *asthma* or acute *bronchitis.* In chronic stages it can lead to irreversible respiratory impairment.

Cancer–A malignant growth of any type. As a group of diseases cancer is the second largest cause of death in the United States, after heart disease. More Americans die from lung cancer than any other type.

Cannula–A small bore tubing; nasal cannula are small plastic tubes that fit in the nostrils through which oxygen is commonly delivered.

Capillary–Smallest blood vessel. There are two major capillary systems in the body, the *pulmonary* and the *systemic.* The former carries blood that takes up O_2 and gives off CO_2. The opposite occurs in the systemic capillary.

Carbon Dioxide–Chemical abbreviation: CO_2. An odorless gas produced as part of normal metabolism. One of the two main functions of the lung is to excrete CO_2 (the other is to bring in O_2).

Carbon Monoxide–Chemical abbreviation: CO. A colorless, odorless, poisonous gas. CO binds avidly with *hemoglobin,* displacing *oxygen* from the blood. A small amount of CO is normally present in the blood. Much greater amounts are present in the blood of all *cigarette* and cigar smokers.

Carcinogen–Any chemical, organism, or substance capable of causing *cancer.*

Carcinoma–The most common form of *cancer*, carcinoma may arise from many any of the body's organs. Most usual sites are the lungs, intestines, breast, uterus, and skin. Other types of cancer are sarcoma (arising from muscle), leukemia (from blood cells), lymphoma (from lymph nodes), and glioma (from brain tissue). A cancer arising from the lining of the lung is called a *mesothelioma.*

Carina–The point at which the airways divide. The main carina is the point at which the trachea divides into the right and left main *bronchi.*

CAT Scan–"Computerized Axial Tomography" Scan, a relatively new computerized *X-ray* device that scans the body with X-rays and reconstructs the pictures so that all organs and structures can be viewed in cross section.

Chemotherapy–Any treatment with drugs. Also used as a general term for "cancer chemotherapy" (treating cancer with drugs in contrast to surgery or radiation). This is an active area of research for many types of *cancer.*

Cigarettes–A form of rolled tobacco responsible for most lung cancer and chronic obstructive pulmonary disease, as well as a major portion of *coronary* heart disease. The smoke from cigarettes contains many *carcinogens* plus other chemicals that may deprive the heart of oxygen.

Cilia–Tiny hair-like projections that line the airways (also found in other organs). Covered by a blanket of mucus cilia help sweep out inhaled dusts. This ciliary sweeping mechanism is damaged or impaired by chronic inhalation of cigarette smoke.

CO–Chemical abbreviation for *carbon monoxide.*

CO_2–Chemical abbreviation for *carbon dioxide.*

Coal Workers' Pneumoconiosis–Lung disease in coal workers caused by chronic inhalation of coal dust. A more common name for this condition is "Black Lung" disease.

COPD–Chronic Obstructive Pulmonary Disease. Includes *chronic bronchitis* and *emphysema,* some cases of chronic *asthma,* and other less common conditions such as *cystic fibrosis.*

Coronary–The coronary arteries supply blood to the heart; coronary heart disease (CHD) refers to narrowing or blockage of these vessels and is the cause of heart attacks, the number one killer in the U.S. A major risk factor for CHD is *cigarette* smoking.

Corticosteroids–A major group of drugs used in treating severe *asthma* and *COPD.* Often referred to as "steroids," these drugs can be taken by mouth or given intravenously. See Appendix C.

Croup–Common childhood infection of the upper airway that leads to swelling and edema of the area above the vocal cords. This often gives *stridor*, a high pitched, inspiratory *wheeze.*

Cyanosis–A term for the blue skin color that occurs with severe lack of *oxygen.* Not all patients who lack oxygen will show cyanosis, so it is an unreliable guide to *hypoxia.*

Cystic Fibrosis–An inherited disorder that affects the lungs, intestines, and reproductive organs. Before antibiotics CF patients invariably died before puberty; now many survive well into adulthood.

Cytology–Laboratory method of looking at cells taken from the body. Under the microscope these cells can often be diagnosed as *benign* or *malignant,* and if the latter, diagnoses as to what type of *cancer.*

Dead Space Ventilation–That part of the air breathed in each minute that does not reach the alveoli and take part in *gas exchange.* The bulk of this dead space air stays in the mouth, throat, *trachea,* and *bronchi.*

Diaphragm–The main muscles of breathing. They also separate the chest cavity from the abdominal cavity. In normal breathing the diaphragms move down as we inspire, up as we expire. Paralysis of the diaphragms is one cause of dyspnea.

Dyphylline–A *bronchodilator* chemically similar to *theophylline.*

Dyspnea–Difficult breathing. Commonly used synonyms are "shortness of breath," "short-winded," and "can't catch my breath." A patient who has these symptoms is said to be dyspneic.

Edema–Excess fluid within the tissues. Leg edema (with resultant swelling) often results from failure of the right side of the heart. Pulmonary edema often results from failure of the left side of the heart, and is a common cause of *dyspnea.* Pulmonary edema can also occur from non-cardiac causes (see *ARDS*).

Embolus–A clot that travels through the bloodstream. The most common form is pulmonary embolus, a blood clot that usually travels from the legs to the lungs where it may cause chest pain or shortness of breath. See *thromboembolism.*

Emphysema–Dilation of the airspaces due to destruction of alveolar and capillary walls. This is one type of chronic obstructive pulmonary disease *(COPD)* and is almost always due to cigarette smoking.

Empyema–Pus in the pleural space; a more general definition is any infected pleural fluid, especially when a chest tube is required for treatment.

Endemic–A disease or condition constantly present in a defined population or community. *Histoplasmosis* is considered endemic in some parts of the U.S.

Epidemic–A disease or condition only occasionally present but that has high morbidity and attacks many people at the same time. The influenza syndrome *(flu)* may occur as an epidemic.

Epinephrine–An adrenal hormone that increases during periods of stress. Also a drug used in treating acute *asthma* attacks.

Etiology–The cause of a disease or condition. When the etiology is not known it is said to be *idiopathic.*

Expectorant–Any medication or solution that helps mobilize and clear secretions from the airway.

Fibrosis–Formation of fibrous material (scar tissue) in an organ. Pulmonary fibrosis is one common form of lung disease. Although *cystic fibrosis* usually involves the lungs, the scar tissue is in the pancreas, not the lungs.

Flu–The influenza syndrome, an infection characterized by fever and malaise, along with other symptoms. Caused by a virus.

Gallium Scan–A nuclear medicine scan that picks up tumor tissue and inflammatory tissue, but does not distinguish between the two. It is useful in diagnosing *sarcoidosis* and in staging some lung *carcinomas.*

Gas Exchange–The main function of the lungs. *Oxygen* is brought from the air into the blood and *carbon dioxide* is excreted from the blood into the air.

Generic–In biology a genus is a large group sharing common characteristics; generic means "of this class or group." Generic drugs have a common chemical name and composition, but carry no brand name (theophylline is available as a generic drug or under the brand name of several drug companies).

Goodpasture's Syndrome–An uncommon medical condition characterized by kidney and lung disease occurring together. Patients with this disease may present with *hemoptysis.*

Granuloma–A microscopic collection of cells found in the body's organs in certain diseases, such as *sarcoidosis* and *tuberculosis.* Granulomas occur when the body tries to wall off or defend against a foreign substance, such as the organism causing tuberculosis. The cause of the granulomas in sarcoidosis, and hence of the disease itself, is unknown.

Guaifenesin–An *expectorant* drug frequently combined with *bronchodilators* and prescribed for asthma and conditions associated with cough.

Hemoglobin–The red blood cell molecules that carry oxygen to the tissues. People with reduced amounts of hemoglobin have *anemia.*

Hemoptysis–Coughing up blood. Hemoptysis should be distinguished from vomiting up blood, "hematemesis." Hemoptysis can range from minimum ("blood streaking") to massive, requiring emergency transfusions and possibly lung surgery. As a new symptom it always warrants medical evaluation.

Histoplasmosis–A fungal infection that commonly affects the lungs. Only found in certain areas of the country, mainly the Mississippi and Ohio Valley regions. May cause many symptoms similar to *tuberculosis.*

Hormone–A substance secreted from one organ that travels via the blood stream to exert its action on another organ. *Corticosteroids* are hormones secreted by the adrenal gland; synthetic steroids are commonly used in treating severe *asthma.* As well as being affected by some hormones, the lungs also play a role in their synthesis and metabolism.

Hyperbaric–Greater than normal atmospheric pressure. In medicine a hyperbaric chamber is one that can surround the patient with air at greater than normal atmospheric pressure. This can effectively increase the pressure of inspired oxygen as well. Hyperbaric chambers are rarely used in respiratory disease, more commonly employed for some types of gangrene.

Hyperventilation–Refers to blowing off carbon dioxide at a rate so that the level in the blood remains lower than normal. This is done by increasing effective or *alveolar ventilation.* Healthy people can do this voluntarily by breathing deeper and faster than normal. Contrast with *hypoventilation.*

Hypoventilation–Refers to retaining CO_2 in the blood by decreasing effective or *alveolar ventilation.* Although normal people can voluntarily *hyperventilate,* they cannot voluntarily hypoventilate. Finding an elevated CO_2 tension in the blood is diagnostic of hypoventilation and always indicates a respiratory problem.

Hypoxemia–A term for lack of oxygen in the blood, usually due to lung disease or anemia. It is one of the causes of *hypoxia,* a more general term for lack of oxygen.

Hypoxia–A general term for lack of *oxygen.* May be due to heart or lung disease or anemia, as well as other causes such as shock. Encompasses the term *hypoxemia.*

Idiopathic–Of unknown cause.

Immunology–The science that deals with the body's defenses against foreign material. Immunologic responses play a role in many lung diseases, including *tuberculosis, sarcoidosis,* and some cases of *asthma.*

Incidence–The rate at which a certain event occurs. For example, the incidence of lung cancer in a study population is two cases per 1,000 people per year. See *prevalence.*

Infection–Invasion of the body with organisms that cause an abnormal tissue or blood reaction. Not all patients with infection have symptoms. Infection by the tuberculosis organism means only the presence of it in the body; when the organism causes symptoms, the term tuberculosis *disease* is used.

Influenza–A viral infection caused by the influenza virus. Generally associated with respiratory symptoms; may also lead to pneumonia.

Interstitial–Refers to the interstitium of the lung, that part that contains pulmonary capillaries, connective tissue, and lymphatic drainage. The interstitium lies between the *alveolar* air spaces. Interstitial lung disease is a major cause of respiratory morbidity and mortality.

Isoetharine–A beta-*adrenergic* drug used for treating bronchospasm; given only as an inhaled medication.

Isoproterenol–A beta-*adrenergic* drug used for treating bronchospasm. Usually given as an inhaled medication.

Lower Respiratory Tract—That portion of the airways that begins at the main carina and ends at the alveoli. By definition all cases of asthma and most lung infections and lung disease involve the LRT. Contrast with *Upper Respiratory Tract.*

Lung Cancer—See *cancer.*

Lungs—The two organs inside the chest cavity whose main function is *gas exchange.* The lungs are part of the body's *respiratory system.*

Malignant—When applied to a tumor or growth, "malignant" is synonymous with *cancer.* Also sometimes used as a descriptive term for a serious or potentially fatal disease or condition, such as malignant hypertension.

Marijuana—A drug obtained from the flowering tops, stems, and leaves of the plant *Cannabis sativa.* It is usually smoked for its euphoric effect. The major active ingredient is tetrahydrocannabinol.

Mediastinoscopy—A surgical operation, performed under general anesthesia, that is used to remove lymph nodes from the *mediastinum.* These nodes can then be examined under the microscope and allow for diagnosis of some lung diseases, mainly cancer.

Mediastinum—The space between the two lungs in the thoracic cavity. The mediastinum contains the heart and the great blood vessels, the trachea, esophagus, many lymph nodes, and other structures. Lung tumors have a tendency to invade the mediastinum, making surgical removal difficult or impossible.

Mesothelioma—A tumor from the mesothelial cells that are found in the *pleura* covering the lungs. These tumors can be *benign* or *malignant.* Malignant mesotheliomas cannot be removed surgically and do not respond to *radio-* or *chemotherapy;* they are often related to asbestos exposure.

Metaproterenol—A beta-*adrenergic* agent used to treat *asthma.*

Metastasis—The spread of disease from one organ or tissue to another area of the body. When a cancer has metastasized it has spread from the originating organ to another, distant organ or tissue and is therefore unresectable.

Morbidity—Negative characteristics of any illness or disease while a patient is alive. Pain, discomfort, lost work days, and so forth represent the morbidity of any illness. See *mortality.*

Mortality—In any disease or illness, mortality refers either to the rate or number of deaths. In discussing the impact of any illness, both its *morbidity* and mortality are usually examined.

Mucus—Normal secretions of ductal glands. In many lung diseases mucus becomes thickened, infected, or difficult to mobilize.

Mycobacteria—Name for a group of *bacteria* that cause tuberculosis and other infectious diseases.

Mycoplasma—A type of *bacterium* that has some characteristics of viruses, but responds to antibiotics. Mycoplasma is a common cause of respiratory *infections,* including *pneumonia.*

Nebulizer—A device that converts a liquid into a spray. Nebulizers are commonly used in respiratory diseases to deliver medication in the form of sprays.

Nicotine—Compound in cigarette smoke known to constrict blood vessels. Nicotine is also responsible for the addicting aspect of cigarettes. The major harm from nicotine and cigarettes is cardiovascular damage.

Nitrogen—21 percent of air is *oxygen.* Nitrogen is an inert gas and the largest single component of air—78 percent. The last 1 percent is made up of other inert gases, such as argon.

Oat Cell Carcinoma–A highly malignant form of lung *cancer;* it has almost always *metastasized* by the time of diagnosis. Some cases respond to *chemotherapy* and *radiotherapy.*

Obstructive–Refers to a pulmonary condition manifested by difficulty getting the air out (difficulty on expiration). *Asthma,* chronic *bronchitis,* and *emphysema* are the most common conditions causing obstructive lung disease.

Operable–Able to withstand surgery. See *resectable.*

Oxygen–Chemical abbreviation: O_2. A component of the air we breathe and necessary for life. 21 percent of the air is oxygen; most of the rest is *nitrogen.* After delivery to the blood by the lungs, O_2 is transported to the tissues by *hemoglobin.*

Oxygen Extractor–A device which operates by electricity and concentrates O_2 in room air for delivery to the patient. Also called oxygen concentrator, oxygen enricher.

Oxygen Tank–A green tank or cylinder that holds either compressed, dry oxygen or liquid oxygen.

Palliative–Refers to any treatment that lessens symptoms or slows down progression of a condition, but does not cure.

Perfusion–Passage of fluid through vessels; pulmonary perfusion refers to circulation of blood through the lungs.

Perfusion lung scan–A diagnostic test for the uniformity of pulmonary perfusion.

Pleura–Thin membranes that cover the lungs and the insides of the *thoracic cage;* there is a potential space between these membranes (the pleural space) into which abnormal collections of fluid may occur in many conditions. See *pleural effusion.*

Pleural Effusion–An abnormal collection of fluid in the *pleural* space; may be due to a variety of conditions, the most common of which are *congestive heart failure, pneumonia,* and *cancer.*

Pleurisy–A general term for inflammation of the *pleural* membranes that line the *lungs* and inside part of *thoracic cage.* Pleurisy can occur from many causes, the most common being viral infection; *pleural effusion* may accompany pleurisy.

Pneumococcus–The organism responsible for the most common type of *bacterial* pneumonia.

Pneumoconiosis–Lung disease due to inhalation of inorganic dusts such as silica and carbon. When it occurs in coal workers, it is also known as black lung disease.

Pneumonectomy–A surgical operation that removes one lung; done most commonly for lung *cancer.*

Pneumonia–*Infection* of the airspaces (alveoli) of the lungs. May be due to *bacteria, viruses,* or other organisms. Most common bacterial cause is *pneumococcus.* See *pneumonitis.*

Pneumonitis–Inflammation of the airspaces; a more general term than *pneumonia,* which is inflammation due to infection.

Pneumothorax–Collapse of all or part of a lung that occurs when air enters the *pleural* space; common in trauma, but may also occur spontaneously.

PPD–Purified protein derivative; contains *tuberculin* material derived from tuberculous *bacilli* that is purified and used as skin test for tuberculosis.

Prednisone–A form of oral *corticosteroid* useful in treating asthma and other diseases.

Prevalence–The number of cases of a disease in existence at a certain time in a designated area. For example, if in surveying 10,000 subjects, 20 are found to have lung cancer, the prevalence is 20/10,000 or .2 percent. See *incidence.*

Prospective–A prospective study is one that looks at data or events as they occur; hence investigators can decide, in advance, exactly what to measure or look for; contrast with *retrospective.*

Prostaglandins–A group of chemical compounds that serve many different bodily functions. Some prostaglandins (PG) are bronchoconstrictors (PGF), others bronchodilators (PGE). Aspirin may inhibit PG formation in some asthmatics, leading to bronchoconstriction and wheezing.

Pulmonary–Refers to the lungs or to components within the lungs, such as pulmonary blood flow, pulmonary *fibrosis,* pulmonary vessels, pulmonary *edema.*

Radiotherapy–Treatment with X-rays; a common method of treating many cancers, including lung *cancer,* for which it is considered only *palliative.* For some cancers, such as Hodgkin's Disease, radiotherapy may be curative.

Resectable–Able to be removed completely. A resectable lung tumor is one that can be removed by surgery, thus offering the chance of cure. Contrast with *operable.*

Respiratory Failure–Failure of the respiratory system in its gas exchange function. The result is a build-up of carbon dioxide and/or lowering of oxygen tension in the arterial blood.

Respiratory System–One of the body's major organ systems, responsible for gas exchange. Lungs are one of three components of this system; others are the chest *bellows* and parts of the central nervous system that control breathing. All components must function for normal breathing to occur.

Restrictive–One of two major patterns of breathing abnormality. Patients with restrictive disease are unable to expand their lungs to normal full capacity. See *Obstructive.*

Retrospective–A retrospective study looks at data or events after they have occurred; hence investigators cannot control what has happened or how the data was collected. Contrast with *prospective.*

Sarcoidosis–A disease of unknown cause that involves the lungs in over 90 percent of all cases. The clinical course is variable and any part of the body may be affected. Characteristic of the disease are microscopic *granulomas* in involved organs.

Scan–In medicine, a test whereby some device travels over part or all of the body taking pictures or readings. Many X-ray tests are scans, such as *CAT scan, gallium scan,* and *ventilation and perfusion lung scan.*

Sign–In medicine, something that is observed about a patient, such as *cyanosis* or *tachypnea.* Contrast with *symptom.*

Silicosis–A lung disease due to inhaling silica dust. It is a type of *pneumoconiosis* and usually work-related.

Skin test–Skin tests are commonly performed to check the body's immunologic response to something injected under the skin. The most useful of all skin tests is the tuberculin skin test or PPD, which looks for *tuberculosis infection.*

Sputum–Also known as phlegm, sputum is the material coughed up in many lung conditions. Sputum may be white, yellow, brown, bloody, and so forth. Examination of the sputum is often a valuable diagnostic test.

Squamous cell–A common type of cell that makes up the outer layer of our skin and lines many hollow organs. Squamous cell lung *cancer* arises from the lining of the *bronchi* and hence is a form of *bronchogenic carcinoma.*

Steroids–See corticosteroids.

Stridor–A high pitched, inspiratory sound that indicates obstruction of the upper airway. Stridor is a common finding in children suffering from croup.

Symptom–Something the patient notices or complains about, such as chest pain or shortness of breath; contrast with *sign.* A patient without symptoms is *asymptomatic.*

Syndrome–A group of *symptoms* and *signs* that occur together in certain disease conditions, such as *adult respiratory distress syndrome.*

Synergistic–When the effect of two things is greater than would be expected from just adding them together, they are said to be synergistic. For example, the risk of lung cancer from smoking and asbestos exposure combined is greater than you would get from just adding their individual risks.

Systemic–Refers to the entire body. A systemic illness is one involving multiple organs, an example being sarcoidosis. Systemic capillaries and blood vessels are those outside the lungs. See also *pulmonary.*

Tar–Usually written "tar," it is a term used to represent all of the particulate matter found in cigarette smoke, after moisture and *nicotine* have been removed. "Tar" contains the *carcinogens* responsible for lung cancer.

Tension–In referring to oxygen (O_2) and carbon dioxide (CO_2) in the blood, tension is the pressure exerted by these gases. Their tension reflects (but doesn't exactly equal) the amount of O_2 and CO_2 in the blood. Thus, the higher the tension, the more gas is present, and vice versa. O_2 and CO_2 tensions are routinely measured in the arterial blood gas test.

Terbutaline–A beta-adrenergic bronchodilator useful in treating asthma.

Theophylline–One of the three major types of drugs used to treat asthma and chronic obstructive lung disease. Theophylline is closely related chemically to caffeine, and is a powerful *bronchodilator.*

Thoracic Cage–The bony chest cage in which the lungs are situated; it is a major part of the chest bellows. The lungs, chest bellows, and those parts of the central nervous system that control breathing make up the *respiratory system.* Disease in any part of this system may affect breathing.

Thoracotomy–Surgical opening of the chest cavity.

Thromboembolism–Condition present when a blood clot travels from one part of the body to another. Most commonly the clot, or *embolus,* arises in the deep veins of the leg and breaks off to travel and lodge in the lungs.

Trachea–The main windpipe that connects the mouth and nose to the lungs. The trachea begins just below the Adam's apple in the neck and ends at the main carina, where it divides into the right and left main *bronchi.*

Tracheostomy–A surgical operation whereby an opening is placed in the neck, through the trachea. Patients requiring prolonged artificial ventilation often have this operation so the breathing tube can be removed from the mouth and placed in the neck.

Tuberculin–A sterile liquid containing substances extracted from the tuberculosis bacillus; purified protein derivative (PPD) is the most commonly used tuberculin test today. If positive, the patient is said to be infected with the TB organism. See *infection.*

Tuberculosis–Disease caused by the *bacillus mycobacterium tuberculosis.*

Although tuberculosis most commonly involves the lungs, virtually any organ may become infected.

Upper Respiratory Tract–That portion of the airways that starts at the mouth and nose and extends to the main *carina.* The URT is the site of all colds and many other common viral infections. Contrast with *lower respiratory tract.*

Vaccine–A substance derived from living organisms which, when injected into people, protects against developing disease from that organism. Vaccines may be live organisms that have been considerabl attenuated or weakened (such as Sabin polio vaccine) or non-living material derived from the organisms (such as Salk polio vaccine). Flu and pneumococcal vaccines are used to prevent respiratory disease among susceptible popluations.

Venous–Refers to the veins, which carry de-oxygenated (oxygen-poor) blood from the tissues and organs back to the heart.

Ventilation–Movement of air in and out of the lungs. A ventilation or ventilatory breathing test measures how much air moves in or out in a given time period.

Ventilation lung scan–A diagnostic test for the uniformity of air distribution in the lungs.

Ventilator–A device that can take over the breathing function of the respiratory system. Also called "artificial ventilator," these devices are commonly used to treat *respiratory failure.*

Virus–The smallest organism that can cause *infections.* Viruses are responsible for most *upper respiratory* infections and many *pneumonias.* Except for some *influenza* infections, viruses are not responsive to drug treatment.

Wheeze–A high pitched breathing sound that may be heard on inspiration or expiration. It is usually heard in asthma and in patients with chronic obstructive pulmonary disease who have an asthmatic component.

Xenon–An element commonly used in its radioactive form for diagnosis. Radioactive xenon, when inhaled as a gas, travels to the airspaces and can be viewed with a special camera to develop a *ventilation scan.* The pattern of distribution is helpful in diagnosing some cases of pulmonary embolism.

X-ray–A form of radiation discovered in 1895 by Konrad Wilhelm Roentgen; it revolutionized medical diagnosis and treatment and continues to prove invaluable. A chest X-ray is the most widely used diagnostic X-ray test. See also *radiotherapy, CAT scan.*

APPENDIX C

Drugs Used in Asthma and Reversible Airways Disease

TABLE 1–Oral adrenergic drugs–tablets and inhalation agents

TABLE 2–Oral theophylline preparations and derivatives, including combination drugs

TABLE 3–Oral and inhalation corticosteroids

TABLE 4–Inhalation cromolyn sodium

*Principal sources for these listings are the *Physician's Desk Reference* and *Facts and Comparisons* (see Appendix D, under Chapter 11).

TABLE C-1 Oral adrenergic drugs: Tablets, capsules and inhalation sprays[1]

Brand Name	Bronchodilator[2] Medication	Comment	Rx[2] or O.T.C.
Adrenalin Chloride	Epinephrine 1:100 Solution	Solution for nebulization	Rx
Aerolone	Isoproterenol 0.25%	Solution for nebulization	Rx
Alupent Inhalent Solution	Metaproterenol 5%	Liquid that may be used diluted or undiluted	Rx
Alupent Metered Dose Inhaler	Metaproterenol .65 mg/inhalation	Hand-held nebulizer for inhalation use	Rx
Alupent Tablets	Metaproterenol 10 & 20 mg	–	Rx
Alupent Syrup	Metaproterenol 10 mg/5 ml	–	Rx
AsthmaHaler	Epinephrine 0.3 mg/inhalation	Hand-held nebulizer for inhalation use	O.T.C.
AsthmaNefrin	Racemic epinephrine	For use with nebulizer, undiluted	Rx
Brethine Tablets	Terbutaline 2.5 & 5 mg	–	Rx
Bricanyl Tablets	Terbutaline 2.5 & 5 mg	–	Rx
Bronitin Mist	Epinephrine 0.3 mg/inhalation	Hand-held nebulizer for inhalation use	O.T.C.
Bronkaid Mist	Epinephrine .27 mg/dose	Hand-held nebulizer for inhalation use	O.T.C.
Bronkometer	Isoetharine .34 mg/dose	Hand-held nebulizer for inhalation use, comes in 10 and 20 ml size	Rx

[1]This list includes prescription and over-the-counter beta-adrenergic drugs indicated for asthma and reversible airways disease. Except under physician supervision, no patient should use more than one beta-adrenergic agent for treatment of asthma.

NOTE: Combination asthma drugs that include beta-adrenergic components are listed under the Oral Theophylline Preparations, Table 2.

[2]Mg = milligrams. For tablets the mg shown is the amount of drug in the tablet. For mists and sprays the mg shown is the amount delivered with each depression of the nebulizer (each inhalation). For liquids the mg amount is per 4 or 5 ml, as indicated.

NOTE: THERAPEUTIC DOSE OF EACH DRUG IS NOT SHOWN IN THIS TABLE. The therapeutic dose must be individualized. See Chapter 11 on Asthma Treatment for further discussion of therapeutic dose.

RX = Available only by prescription.

OTC = Available over-the-counter, that is, without a doctor's prescription.

[3]Generic Name. Although this drug is marked under several brand names, it is also available generically.

[4]Ephedrine is combined with various antihistamines or barbiturate sedatives and marketed by several manufacturers for relief of "allergic conditions such as mild to moderate attacks of asthma, hay fever, and vasomotor rhinitis." However, ***Facts and Comparisons*** lists these combinations under the heading "Upper Respiratory Combinations—Decongestants" and recommends their use only in colds and other upper respiratory problems, not in asthma.

TABLE C-1 (continued)

Brand Name	Bronchodilator[2] Medication	Comment	Rx[2] or O.T.C.
Bronkosol Solution	Isoetharine 1.0%	Liquid that is diluted with water prior to use in a nebulizer	Rx
Bronkosol Unit Dose	Isoetharine 0.25%	Liquid that comes in 2 ml syringes and is pre-diluted by manufacturer for use in a nebulizer	Rx
Duo-Medihaler	Isoproterenol .16 mg/inhalation	Hand-held nebulizer for inhalation use; contains phenylephrine for constricting blood vessels in mucous membranes	Rx
[3]Ephedrine capsules	Ephedrine 25 & 50 mg	Available as generic	Rx & O.T.C.
[3]Ephedrine syrup	Ephedrine 11 & 20 mg/5 ml	Available as generic	Rx & O.T.C.
[4]Ephedrine & antihistamine	Ephedrine, various doses	See footnote #4	Rx
[4]Ephedrine & sedative	Ephedrine, various doses	See footnote #4	Rx
Isoetharine HCl	Isoetharine 0.125%	Solution for nebulization	Rx
[3]Isoproterenol	Isoproterenol 0.5%	Solution for nebulization, available as generic	Rx
Isoproterenol HCl	Isoproterenol 0.25%	Aerosol for inhalation use	Rx
Isuprel Mistometer .125 mg/inhalation	Isoproterenol	–	Rx
Isuprel Hydrochloride	Isoproterenol 0.5 & 1.0%	Solution for nebulization	Rx
Isuprel Hydrochloride	Isoproterenol 0.25%	Hand-held nebulizer for inhalation use	Rx
KIE Syrup	Ephedrine 8 mg/5 ml	Also contains potassium iodide 150 mg/5 ml	Rx
KIE Tablets	Ephedrine 24 mg	Also contains potassium iodide 400 mg/5 ml	RX
Medihaler-Epi	Epinephrine .3 mg/inhalation	Hand-held nebulizer for inhalation use	O.T.C.
Medihaler-Iso	Isoproterenol .075 mg/inhalation	Hand-held nebulizer for inhalation use	Rx
Metaprel Metered Dose Inhaler	Metaproterenol .65 mg/inhalation	Hand-held nebulizer for inhalation use	Rx
Metaprel Syrup	Metaproterenol 10 mg/5 ml	–	Rx

TABLE C-1 (continued)

Brand Name	Bronchodilator[2] Medication	Comment	Rx[2] or O.T.C.
Metaprel Tablets	Metaproterenol 10 & 20 mg	–	Rx
microNEFRIN	Racemic Epinephrine 2.25%	Comes as liquid that is diluted with saline or water prior to inhalation	Rx
Mucomyst with Isoproterenol	Isoproterenol 0.05%	Comes as liquid for nebulization and inhalation; contains 10% acetylcystein (mucomyst), a mucolytic agent	Rx
Norisodrine Aerotrol	Isoproterenol 0.25%	Hand-held nebulizer for inhalation use	Rx
Norisodrine Sulfate Aerohaler	Isoproterenol .045 & .110 mg/ inhalation	Comes as 10 & 25 mg cartridges to be used with an Aerohaler provided by manufacturer	Rx
Primatene Mist Solution	Epinephrine .2 mg/inhalation	Hand-held nebulizer for inhalation use	O.T.C.
Primatene Mist Suspension	Epinephrine .3 mg/inhalation	Hand-held nebulizer for inhalation use	O.T.C.
Proventil	Albuterol	Hand-held nebulizer for inhalation use	Rx
Proventil Tablets	Albuterol 2 & 4 mg	–	Rx
Vapo-Iso	Isoproterenol 0.5%	Solution for nebulization	Rx
Vaponefrin Solution	Racemic Epinephrine	For use with nebulizer, undiluted	O.T.C.
Ventolin	Albuterol	Hand-held nebulizer for inhalation use	Rx
Ventolin Tablets	Albuterol 2 & 4 mg	–	Rx

TABLE C-2 Oral theophylline preparations and derivatives, including combination drugs

Brand Name	Bronchodilator[1] Medication	Equivalent Amt. Theophylline	Other Active Medication	Rx or[2] O.T.C.
Accurbron Liquid	Theophylline 150 mg	same	7.5% Alcohol	Rx
Aerolate Liquid	Theophylline 160 mg	same	–	Rx
[3]Aerolate Capsules	Theophylline 65, 130, & 260 mg	same	–	Rx
Aminodur Dura-tabs	Aminophylline 300 mg	236 mg	–	Rx
Aminophylline Tablets	Aminophylline 100 & 200 mg	79 & 158 mg	–	Rx
Aminophylline Generic	Aminophylline 100 & 200 mg	79 & 158 mg	–	Rx
Amodrine Tablets	Aminophylline 100 mg Racephedrine 25 mg	70 mg	Phenobarbital 25 mg	O.T.C.
Aquaphyllin Syrup	Theophylline 80 mg	same	–	Rx
Asbron G Inlay Tabs	Theophylline Sodium Glycinate 300 mg	150 mg	Guaifenesin 100 mg	Rx
Asbron G Elixir	Theophylline Sodium Glycinate 300 mg	150 mg	Guaifenesin 100 mg 15% Alcohol	Rx
Asma Syrup	Theophylline Sodium Alxanate 300 mg	150 mg	Guaifenesin 100 mg 10% alcohol	Rx
Asmalix elixir	Theophylline 80 mg	same	20% alcohol	O.T.C.

[1]Mg = milligrams. The mg of each drug shown is per single tablet or capsule. When more than one mg amount is shown, the drug is available in both dosages, such as Aminophylline 100 & 200 mg. When a derivative of theophylline is listed under Bronchodilator Medication, the equivalent amount of active drug (pur theophylline) is shown, such as Theophylline 85 & 170 mg. Except for dyphylline, all other "phylline" bronchodilators are active only by virtue of their theophylline content. Dyphylline is similar to theophylline, and is about 70 percent as effective on a milligram for milligram basis.

For liquids, elixirs, and syrups the amount of milligrams shown is per 15 ml (= 1 tablespoon).

NOTE: THE THERAPEUTIC DOSE OF EACH DRUG IS NOT SHOWN IN THIS TABLE. The therapeutic dose must be individualized for each patient. See Chapter 11 on Asthma Treatment for further discussion of dosage.

[2]RX = Prescription drug only. OTC = Sold "Over The Counter" (without a prescription). Some OTC drugs may not be sold this way in every state (the decision is up to individual state pharmacy boards). For any given drug listed OTC, check with your local pharmacy.

[3]Several theophylline preparations are formulated to be long-acting. This is done by arranging the drug in the tablet or capsule so the active compound is released slowly in the stomach or intestines after it is swallowed. Synonyms used by various drug companies for long acting are "SA" (sustained action) and "SR" (sustained release).

[4]Combination drug (contains more than one active bronchodilator). All combination drugs for asthma contain theophylllie or a theophylline derivative.

TABLE C-2 (continued)

Brand Name	Bronchodilator[1] Medication	Equivalent Amt. Theophylline	Other Active Medication	Rx or[2] O.T.C.
[4]Asminyl Tablets	Theophylline 130 mg Ephedrine 32 mg	same	–	Rx
[4]Bronchobid Duracap (Capusles)	Theophylline 260 mg Ephedrine 35 mg	same	–	Rx
Brondecon Tablets	Oxtriphylline 200 mg	128 mg	Guaifenesin 100 mg	Rx
Brondecon Elixir	Oxtriphylline 300 mg	192 mg	Guaifenesin 150 mg 20% alcohol	Rx
Brondelate Elixir	Oxtriphylline 300 mg	192 mg	Guaifenesin 150 mg	Rx
[4]Bronitin Tablets	Theophylline 120 mg Ephedrine 24 mg	same	Guaifenesin 100 mg Pyrilamine maleate 16.6 mg	O.T.C.
[4]Bronkaid Tablets	Theophylline 100 mg Ephedrine 24 mg	same	Guaifenesin 100 mg	O.T.C.
Bronkodyl Capsules	Theophylline 100 & 200 mg	same	–	Rx
Bronkodyl Elixir	Theophylline 80 mg	same	2% alcohol	Rx
[3]Bronkodyl S-R	Theophylline 300 mg	same	–	Rx
Bronkolixir Liquid	Theophylline 36 mg Ephedrine 36 mg	same	Guaifenesin 150 mg Phenobarbital 8 mg 19% alcohol	O.T.C.
[4]Bronkotabs Tablets	Theophylline 100 mg Ephedrine 24 mg	same	Guaifenesin 100 mg Phenobarbital 8 mg	O.T.C.
Cerylin Capsules	Theophylline 150 mg	same	Guaifenesin 90 mg	Rx
Cerylin Liquid	Theophylline 150 mg	same	Guaifenesin 90 mg	Rx
Choledyl Tablets	Oxtriphylline 100 & 200 mg	64 & 128 mg	–	Rx
Choledyl	Oxtriphylline Elixir 300 mg	192 mg	20% alcohol	Rx
Choledyl Syrup	Oxtriphylline 150 mg	96 mg	–	Rx
[3]Choledyl-SA	Oxtriphylline 400 & 600 mg	256 & 384 mg	–	Rx
[3]Constant-T	Theophylline 200 & 300 mg	same	–	Rx

TABLE C-2 (continued)

Brand Name	Bronchodilator[1] Medication	Equivalent Amt. Theophylline	Other Active Medication	Rx or[2] O.T.C.
Dialixir	Theophylline Glycinate 300 mg	150 mg	Guaifenesin 10% alcohol	Rx
Dilor Tablets	Dyphylline 200 & 400 mg	140 & 280 mg	–	Rx
Dilor Elixir	Dyphylline 160 mg	112 mg	–	Rx
Dilor-G Tablets	Dyphylline 200 mg	140 mg	Guaifenesin 200 mg	Rx
Dilor-G Liquid	Dyphylline 300 mg	220 mg	Guaifenesin 300 mg	Rx
Duovent Tablets	Theophylline 130 mg Ephedrine 24 mg	same	Guaifensin 100 mg Phenobarbital 8 mg	Rx
Dyflex Tablets	Dyphylline 200 & 400 mg	140 & 280 mg	–	Rx
Dyflex-G Tablets	Dyphylline 200 mg	140 mg	Guaifenesin 200 mg	Rx
Dyline-GG Tablets	Dyphylline 200 mg	140 mg	Guaifenesin 200 mg	Rx
Elixicon (Liquid)	Theophylline 300 mg	same	–	Rx
Elixophylline Capsules	Theophylline 100 & 200 mg	same	–	Rx
[3]Elixo-phylline SR Capsules	Theophylline 125 & 250 mg	same	–	Rx
Elixo-phylline Elixir	Theophylline 80 mg	same	20% alcohol	Rx
Elixo-phylline-KI Elixir	Theophylline 80 mg	same	Potassium 130 mg 10% alcohol	Tx
Glyceryl-T Capsules	Theophylline 150 mg	same	Guaifenesin 90 mg	Rx
Hylate Tablets	Theophylline Sodium Glycinate 400 mg	200 mg	Guaifenesin 100 mg	Rx
[3]La-Bid Tablets	Theophylline 250 mg	same	–	Rx
Lanophyllin Elixir	Theophylline 80 mg	same	20% alcohol	Rx
Liquo-phylline Elixir	Theophylline 80 mg	same	20% alcohol	Rx
Lixaminol Elixir	Aminophylline 250 mg	215 mg	20% alcohol	Rx
Lufyllin Elixir	Dyphylline 100 mg	70 mg	20% alochol	Rx

TABLE C-2 (continued)

Brand Name	Bronchodilator[1] Medication	Equivalent Amt. Theophylline	Other Active Medication	Rx or[2] O.T.C.
Lufyllin Tablets	Dyphylline 200 & 400 mg	140 & 280 mg	-	Rx
Lufyllin EPG Tablets	Dyphylline 100 mg Ephedrine 16 mg	70 mg	Guaifenesin 200 mg Phenobarbital 16 mg	Rx
Lufyllin-GG Tablets	Dyphylline 200 mg	140 mg	Guaifenesin 200 mg	Rx
Lufyllin-GG Elixir	Dyphylline 100 mg	70 mg	Guaifenesin 100 mg 17% alcohol	Rx
[4]Marax DF Syrup	Theophylline 97.5 mg Ephedrine 18.75 mg	same	Hydroxyzine 5% alcohol	Rx
[4]Marax Tablets	Theophylline 130 mg Ephedrine 25 mg	same	Hydroxyzine 10 mg	Rx
[4]Mudrane Tablets	Aminophylline Ephedrine 16 mg	110.5 mg	Potassium Phenobarbital 8 mg	Rx
Mudrane-2 Tablets	Aminophylline 130 mg	110.5 mg	Potassium Iodide 195 mg	Rx
[4]Mudrane GG Tablets	Aminophylline Ephedrine 16 mg	110.5 mg	Guaifenesin Phenobarbital 8 mg	Rx
Mudrane GG-2 Tablets	Aminophylline 130 mg	110.5 mg	Guaifenesin 100 mg	Rx
[4]Mudrane GG Elixir	Theophylline Ephedrine 12 mg	same	Guaifenesin Phenobarbital 7.5 mg 20% alcohol	Rx
Neothylline Tablets	Dyphylline 200 & 400 mg	140 & 280 mg	-	Rx
Neothylline Elixir	Dyphylline 160 mg	112 mg	-	Rx
Neothylline GG Tablets	Dyphylline 200 mg	140 mg	Guaifenesin 200 mg	Rx
Neothylline GG Elixir	Dyphylline 100 mg	70 mg	Guaifenesin 100 mg 10% alcohol	Rx
Norophylline Elixir	Theophylline 80 mg	same	20% alcohol	Rx
Oralphylline Elixir	Theophylline 80 mg	same	20% alcohol	Rx
[4]Phyllocontin Tablets	Aminophylline	182 mg	-	Rx
[3]Physpan Capsules	Theophylline 130 & 260 mg	same	-	Rx

TABLE C-2 (continued)

Brand Name	Bronchodilator[1] Medication	Equivalent Amt. Theophylline	Other Active Medication	Rx or[2] O.T.C.
[4]Primatene 'M' Tablets	Theophylline 130 mg Ephedrine 24 mg	same	Pyrilamine 16.6 mg	O.T.C.
[4]Primatene 'P' Tablets	Theophylline Ephedrine 24 mg	same	Phenobarbital 8 mg	O.T.C.
[4]Quadrinal Tablets	Theophylline salicylate 130 mg Ephedrine 24 mg	65 mg	Potassium Iodide 320 mg Phenobarbital 24 mg	Rx
[4]Quadrinal Suspension (Liquid)	Theophylline salicylate 195 mg Ephedrine 36 mg	97.5 mg	Potassium Iodine 480 mg Phenobarbital 36 mg	Rx
Quibron Capsules	Theophylline 150 & 300 mg	same	Guaifenesin 180 mg	Rx
Quibron Liquid	Theophylline 150 mg	same	Guaifenesin 90 mg	Rx
[3]Quibron SR Tablets	Theophylline 300 mg	same	-	Rx
Quibron Tablets	Theophylline 300 mg	same	-	Rx
[4]Quibron Plus Capsules	Theophylline Ephedrine 25 mg	same	Guaifenesin Butabarbital 20 mg	Rx
[4]Quibron Plus Elixir	Theophylline 150 mg Ephedrine 25 mg	same	Guaifenesin Butabarbital 20 mg 15% alcohol	Rx
[3]Respbid Tablets	Theophylline 250 & 500 mg	same	-	Rx
[3]Slo-bid Gyrocaps	Theophylline 100, 200, & 300 mg	same	-	Rx
[3]Slo-phyllin Gyrocaps	Theophylline 60, 125, & 250 mg	same	-	Rx
Slo-phyllin Tablets	Theophylline 100 & 200 mg	same	-	Rx
Slo-phyllin 80 Syrup	Theophylline 80 mg	same	-	Rx
Slo-Phyllin GG Capsules	Theophylline 150 mg	same	Guaifenesin 90 mg	Rx
Slo-Phyllin GG Syrup	Theophylline 150 mg	same	Guaifenesin 90 mg	Rx
Somophyllin DF Liquid	Aminophylline 315 mg	270 mg	-	Rx
Somophyllin	Theophylline	same	-	Rx

TABLE C-2 (continued)

Brand Name	Bronchodilator[1] Medication	Equivalent Amt. Theophylline	Other Active Medication	Rx or[2] O.T.C.
T Capsules	100, 200, & 250 mg			
[3]Somo-phyllin-CRT Capsules	Theophylline 50, 100, & 250 mg	same	–	Rx
[3]Sustaire Tablets	Theophylline 100 & 300 mg	same	–	Rx
Synophylate Tablets	Theophylline Sodium Glycinate 330 mg	165 mg	–	Rx
Synophylate Elixir	Theophylline Glycinate 330 mg	165 mg	20% alcohol	Rx
Synophylate-GG Tablets	Theophylline Glycinate 300 mg	150 mg	Guaifenesin 100 mg	Rx
Synophylate-GG Syrup	Theophylline Sodium Glycinate 300 mg	150 mg	Guaifenesin 100 mg 10% alcohol	Rx
[4]Tedral Elixir	Theophylline 97.5 mg Ephedrine 18 mg	same	Phenobarbital 15% alcohol	O.T.C.
[4]Tedral Suspension (Liquid)	Theophylline 195 mg Ephedrine 36 mg	same	Phenobarbital 12 mg	O.T.C.
[4]Tedral Tablets	Theophylline 130 mg Ephedrine 24 mg	same	Phenobarbital 8 mg	O.T.C.
[3,4]Tedral SA Tablets	Theophylline 180 mg Ephedrine 48 mg	same	Phenobarbital 25 mg	Rx
[4]Tedral 25 Tablets	Theophylline 130 mg Ephedrine 24 mg	same	Butabarbital 25 mg	Rx
[4]Tedral Expectorant Tablets	Theophylline 130 mg Ephedrine 24 mg	same	Phenobarbital 8 mg Guaifenesin 100 mg	Rx
[4]T.E.H. Tablets	Theophylline 130 mg Ephedrine 25 mg	same	Hydroxyzine 10 mg	Rx
[4]Thalfed Tablets	Theophylline 120 mg Ephedrine 25 mg	same	Phenobarbital 8 mg	O.T.C.
[3]Theobid Duracap Capsules	Theophylline 130 & 260 mg	same	–	Rx
Theocap Capsules	Theophylline 200 mg	same	–	Rx
[3]Theoclear L.A. Cenules	Theophylline 130 & 260 mg	same	–	Rx
Theoclear 80 Syrup	Theophylline 80 mg	same	–	Rx

TABLE C-2 (continued)

Brand Name	Bronchodilator[1] Medication	Equivalent Amt. Theophylline	Other Active Medication	Rx or[2] O.T.C.
Theoclear Tablets	Theophylline 100 & 200 mg	same	–	Rx
Theo-Col Elixir	Theophylline 150 mg	same	Guaifenesin 90 mg	Rx
[3]Theo-Dur Tablets	Theophylline 100, 200, & 300 mg	same	–	Rx
[3]Theo-Dur Sprinkle Capsules	Theophylline 50, 75, 125, & 200 mg	same	–	Rx
[3]Theo-24	Theophylline 100, 200, & 300 mg	same	–	Rx
[4]Theofedral Tablets	Theophylline 130 mg Ephedrine 24 mg	same	Phenobarbital 8 mg	O.T.C.
[4]Theofenal Tablets	Theophylline 130 mg Ephedrine 24 mg	same	Phenobarbital 8 mg	O.T.C.
Theokin Elixir	Theophylline calcium salicylate 450 mg	225 mg	9.5% alcohol	Rx
Theokin Tablets	Theophylline calcium salicylate 450 mg	225 mg	450 mg potassium iodide	Rx
Theolair Liquid	Theophylline 80 mg	same	–	Rx
[3]Theolair SR Tablets	Theophylline 250 & 500 mg	same	–	Rx
Theolair Tablets	Theophylline 125 & 250 mg	same	–	Rx
Theolair-Plus Liquid	Theophylline 125 mg	same	Guaifenesin 100 mg	Rx
Theolair-Plus Tablets	Theophylline 125 & 250 mg	same	Guaifenesin 100 & 200 mg	Rx
Theo-Lix Elixir	Theophylline 80 mg	same	20% alcohol	Rx
Theolixir	Theophylline 80 mg	same	20% alcohol	Rx
[3]Theo-nar	Theophylline 200 mg	same	Noscapine 30 mg	Rx
Theon Liquid	Theophylline 150 mg	same	10% alcohol	Rx
[3]Theon 300 Capsules	Theophylline 300 mg	same	–	Rx
Theo-Organidin Elixir	Theophylline 120 mg	same	Iodinated Glycerol 30 mg 15% alcohol	Rx

TABLE C-2 (continued)

Brand Name	Bronchodilator[1] Medication	Equivalent Amt. Theophylline	Other Active Medication	Rx or[2] O.T.C.
[4]Theophed Tablets	Theophylline 130 mg Ephedrine 24 mg	same	Phenobarbital 8 mg	Rx
Theophyl Chewable Tablets	Theophylline 100 mg	same	–	Rx
[3]Theophyl SR Capsules	Thophylline 125 & 250 mg	same	–	Rx
Theophyl 225 Tablets	Theophylline 225 mg	same	–	Rx
Theophyl 225 Elixir	Theophylline 112.5 mg	same	Calcium salicylate 112.5 mg 5% alcohol	Rx
Theophylline Tablets Generic	Theophylline 100, 200, & 300 mg	same	–	Rx
Theophylline Elixir, Generic	Theophylline 80 mg	same	–	Rx
Theophylline Timed Release Capsules, Generic	Theophylline 125 & 250 mg	same	–	Rx
[3]Theospan SR Capsules	Theophylline 65, 130, & 260 mg	same	–	Rx
Theostat 80 Syrup	Theophylline 80 mg	same	1% alcohol	Rx
Theostat Tablets	Theophylline 100 & 200 mg	same	–	Rx
[3]Theovent Capsules	Theophylline 125 & 250 mg	same	–	Rx
[3]Uniphyl Tablets	Theophyllin 200 & 400 mg	same	–	Rx
[4]Veraquad Tablets	Theophylline Calcium Salicylate 130 mg Ephedrine 24 mg	65 mg	Guaifenesin 100 mg Phenobarbital 8 mg	Rx
[4]Veraquad Suspension	Theophylline Calcium Salicylate 195 mg Ephedrine 36 mg	97.5 mg	Guaifenesin Phenobarbital 12 mg	O.T.C.

TABLE C-3 Oral and inhalation corticosteroids for asthma

Generic Corticosteroid[1]	Milligram Tablets Available[2]	Brand Name
Tablets		
Cortisone	5, 10, 20	Cortisone Acetate Tablets[3]
Betamethasone	0.6	Celestone Tablets
Dexamethasone	0.25, 0.5, 0.75, 1.5, 4	Decadron Tablets Dexamethasone Tablets[3] Dexone Tablets Hexadrol Tablets SK-Dexamethasone Tablets
Fluprednisolone	1.5	Alphadrol Tablets
Hydrocortisone	5, 10, 20	Cortef Tablets Hydrocortisone Tablets[3] Hydrocortone Tablets

[1]Corticosteroids are listed by generic name. This is different from tables 1 and 2, where beta-adrenergic and theophylline preparations are arranged by brand name. Reasons for generic arrangement are: a) the drugs are usually prescribed by generic name rather than brand name, and b) many manufacturers market only generic corticosteroids and advertise no unique brand name for the drug. In addition, corticosteroids are never included as part of combination asthma medication so there are fewer varieties of medication to choose from.

[2]Not all dosages are available from all manufacturers. Corticosteroid tablets are manufactured so that a tablet of one drug type is equal in anti-inflammatory potency to a tablet of any other drug type, in the following dosages:

	Equivalent Doses
Betamethasone	0.6 mg
Dexamethasone	0.75
Fluprednisone	1.5
Paramethasone	2
Meprednisone	4
Triamcinolone	4
Methylprednisolone	4
Prednisolone	5
Prednisone	5
Hydrocortisone	20
Cortisone	25

Thus, a patient taking 3 prednisone tablets of 5 mg each could substitute 3 methylprednisolone tablets of 4 mg each with no change in effective steroid dose. Similarly, 3 dexamethasone tablets of 0.75 mg each could substitute for 3 cortisone tablets of 25 mg each. Looked at another way, dexamethasone tablets are ***milligram for milligram*** over 33 times as potent as cortisone tablets. However, since tablet size for all the above drugs is about the same, there is no inherent advantage of choosing one preparation over another. (Note: Some of these compounds cause salt and water retention more than others. The equivalent dosages listed above apply to anti-inflammatory activity only.)

[3]The drug is distributed under its generic name by several pharmaceutical companies. The drug may be manufactured by one company that sells it both under its own brand name to the public and in bulk lots to other drug companies that may then distribute the drug as a generic product. In such cases the generic product will be the same as the brand name product. Because of frequent changes in the drug industry, generic drugs cannot be readily identified as to source.

TABLE C-3 (continued)

Generic Corticosteroid[1]	Milligram Tablets Available[2]	Brand Name
Meprednisone	4	Betapar Tablets
Methylprednisolone	2, 4, 8, 16, 24, 32	Medrol Tablets Methylprednisolone[3]
Paramethasone	1, 2	Haldrone Tablets
Prednisolone	1, 2.5, 5	Predoxine Panisolone Delta Cortef Tablets Prednisolone Tablets[3] Stearane Tablets Cortalone Fernisolone
Prednisone	1, 2.5, 5, 10, 20, 50	Deltasone Tablets Meticorten Tablets Orasone Tablets Prednisone Tablets[3] SK-Prednisone Tablets Sterapred Uni-Pak Cortan Tablets Fernisone Tablets Panasol Tablets Paracort Tablets Prednicen-M Tablets
Triamcinolone	1, 2, 4, 8, 16	Aristocort Tablets Kenacort Tablets SK-Triamcinolone Tablets Triamcinolone Tablets[3] Tricilone Tablets Spencart Tablets Cino Tablets
Liquids		
Betamethasone	0.6 mg/5 ml	Celestone Syrup
Dexamethasone	0.5 mg/5 ml	Decadron Elixir Hexadrol Elixir
Triamcinolone	4 mg/5 ml	Kenacort Diacetate Syrup
Inhalation Sprays		
Beclomethasone dipropionate	.042 mg/inhalation	Beclovent Inhaler Vanceril Inhaler
Dexamethasone sodium phosphate Respihaler	.084 mg/inhalation	Decadrin Phosphate

TABLE C-4 Inhalation cromolyn sodium

Cromolyn sodium is marketed only to prevent asthma attacks, not to treat them once begun. This drug is not classified as a bronchodilator. It is available only by prescription.

Brand Name	How Supplied	Comment
Intal Capsules	As a powder inside a capsule; each capsule contains 20 mg cromolyn sodium	For inhalation only; requires a hand-held device called a spinhaler
Intal Nebulizer Solution	In a double-ended glass capsule containing 20 mg cromolyn sodium in 2 ml purified water	For inhalation only; requires a power driven nebulizer

APPENDIX D

References and Bibliography

References cited in the text are listed under each chapter heading. Additional references are provided for the reader who wishes further information. Those marked by "*" were written specifically for a lay or non-medical audience. Others contain medical or scientific language. The American Lung Association (ALA) also publishes, for the general reader, information pamphlets on many respiratory conditions. They are available free by writing the ALA in New York or through your local ALA branch.

GENERAL

*ALA Bulletin. American Lung Association, 1740 Broadway, N.Y., NY 10019.

A bimonthly, lay-oriented publication. Each issue covers two or three topics related to respiratory diseases.

FRASER, R.G., and PARE, J.A.P. *Diagnosis of Diseases of the Chest.* 4 volumes (Philadelphia: W. B. Saunders Co., 1979).

FISHMAN, A.P., editor. *Pulmonary Diseases and Disorders.* (New York: McGraw-Hill, 1980).

BAUM, G.L., and WOLINSKY, E. *Textbook of Pulmonary Diseases.* (Boston: Little, Brown, 1983).

Three comprehensive textbooks in the field of respiratory disease.

NETTER, F.H. *The Ciba Collection of Medical Illustrations, Volume 7, Respiratory System.* (Summit, NJ, Ciba Pharmaceutical Company, 1979).

Pulmonary Disease Reviews. R.C. Bone, editor (New York: John Wiley & Sons).

Seminars in Respiratory Medicine. (New York: Brian C. Decker).

Clinics in Chest Medicine. (Philadelphia: W. B. Saunders Co.).

Reviews is an annual publication that contains summaries of recent medical articles on all aspects of respiratory disease, along with editorial comments by experts in each area. *Seminars* and *Clinics,* published several times each year, contain in-depth reviews of selected respiratory topics.

Report of Task Force on Epidemiology of Respiratory Diseases. State of Knowledge. Problems. Needs. NIH Publication No. 81-2019, October, 1980.

The Merck Manual of Diagnosis and Therapy. 14th Edition. Berkow, Robert, Editor-in-Chief. (Rahway, NJ, Merck and Co., 1982).

Although designed as a brief synopsis of medicine for physicians, the *Merck Manual* has proved popular with lay readers; it offers concise descriptions of most medical illnesses.

CHAPTER 1–HOW OUR LUNGS AND RESPIRATORY SYSTEM WORK

**Book of the Body. The Way Things Work.* (New York: Simon and Schuster, 1980).

*BEVAN, JAMES. *The Simon and Schuster Handbook of Anatomy and Physiology.* (New York: Simon and Schuster, 1978).

These two books, illustrated and written in nontechnical language, contain chapters on the respiratory system. They are available in many bookstores.

MURRAY, J.F. *The Normal Lung.* (Philadelphia: W. B. Saunders Co., 1976).

SAID, S.I. "The lung in relation to hormones: an update," *Basics of RD,* American Thoracic Society, Medical Section of ALA, 9:3 (Jan. 1981).

CHAPTER 2–SMOKING AND YOUR HEALTH

**The Smoking Digest. Progress Report on a Nation Kicking the Habit.* (U.S. Department of Health, Education and Welfare, Office of Cancer Communications, National Cancer Institute, 1977).

*WINTER, RUTH. *The Scientific Case Against Smoking. Based on the Latest Surgeon General's Report.* (New York: Crown Publishers, Inc., 1980).

*HARRIS, ROGER W. *How to Keep on Smoking and Live.* (New York: St. Martin's Press, 1978).

Written in an entertaining and breezy style, this book is also interesting for its reproductions of old cigarette ads.

*DOYLE, N.C. *Smoking Among Women–An Equal Opportunity Tragedy.* American Lung Association Bulletin (July-August, 1980).

*Freedom From Smoking in 20 Days. (New York: American Lung Association).

The ALA's stop-smoking program. Available from the ALA in New York or through your local branch.

Smoking and Health. Report of the Advisory Committee to the Surgeon General of the Public Health Service, 1964. U.S. Department of Health, Education and Welfare, Publication No. 1103. *Smoking and Health. A Report of the Surgeon General.* DHEW Publication No. 79-50066 (1979).

The original Surgeon General's Report was in 1964. Updates were periodically issued until the next full Report in 1979.

The Health Consequences of Smoking. The Changing Cigarette. A Report of the Surgeon General. Dept. Health and Human Services, Publication No. 81-50156 (1981). *The Health Consequences of Smoking Cancer.* A report of the Surgeon General. U.S. Dept. of Health and Human Services (1982).

The 1981 Surgeon General's Report deals with changes in cigarette "tar" and nicotine, and the health effects of cigarette additives. The 1982 Report deals with the relation of cigarettes to cancer and concludes: "Cigarette smoking . . . is the chief, single avoidable cause of death in our society . . ."

WHITE, J.R. and FROEB, H.F. "Small airways dysfunction in non-smokers chemically exposed to tobacco smoke," *New England Journal of Medicine* 302 (1980), 720-23.

FRIEDMAN, G.D., PETITTI, D.B., BAWOL, R.D. et al. "Mortality in cigarette smokers and quitters," *New England Journal of Medicine* 304 (1981), 1407.

Marijuana Smoking

*JANECZEK, CURTIS L. *Marijuana. Time For A Closer Look.* (Columbus, Ohio: Healthstar Publications, 1980).

*DUPONT, R.L. *Marijuana Smoking–A National Epidemic.* American Lung Association Bulletin. (September, 1980).

*DOYLE, NANCY C. *Marijuana and the Lungs.* American Lung Association Bulletin. (November, 1979).

**Marijuana–What are the Risks?* The Harvard Medical School Health Letter, 79 Garden St., Cambridge, Mass. 02138. (June, 1980).

*MANN, PEGGY and LEHMANN, WALTER X. "Marijuana Alert. I. Brain and Sex Damage. II. Enemy of Youth," *Readers Digest* (December, 1979).

Marijuana and Health. Report from the National Academy of Sciences, 1982. (Washington, DC: National Academy Press.

A comprehensive report on health affects of marijuana.

TASHKIN, D.P., SHAPIRO, B.J., and LEE, E.L. "Subacute effects of heavy marijuana smoking on pulmonary function in healthy young males," *New England Journal of Medicine* 294 (January 15, 1976), 125-129.

TASHKIN, D.P., CALVARESE, B.M., SIMMONS, M.S. et al. "Respiratory status of seventy-four habitual marijuana smokers," *Chest* 78 (November, 1980), 699-706.

CHAPTER 3–AIR POLLUTION

**Your Health and Air Pollution.* Pamphlet published by the American Lung Association, 1980.

MITCHELL, ROGER S. et al: "Health effects of urban air pollution," *Journal American Medical Association* 242 (September 14, 1979), 1163-68.

Air Pollution Primer. Booklet published by the American Lung Association, 1978.

ZWILLICH, C.W. and CHERNIAK, R.R. "The 23rd Aspen Lung Conference: The Environment and the Lung," *Chest* 80: No. 1, Supplement (July, 1981).

A collection of brief scientific articles dealing with both general and workplace air pollution.

CHAPTER 4–OCCUPATIONAL LUNG DISEASE

Asbestos-Related Diseases

*"The Asbestos Problem," *The Harvard Medical School Health Letter.* Vol. V: 10 (August, 1980).

BECKLAKE, M.R. "Asbestos-related diseases of the lung and other organs. Their epidemiology and implications for clinical practice. State of the Art review," *American Review Respiratory Disease* 114 (1976), 187.

SELIKOFF, I.J. and HAMMOND, E.C. "Health Hazards of Asbestos Exposure," *Annals New York Academy of Sciences* 330 (1979), 1-814.

A compendium of scientific papers presented at an international conference on asbestos, June, 1978.

CRAIGHEAD, J.E. and MOSSMAN, B.T. "The pathogenesis of asbestos-associated disease," *New England Journal of Medicine* 306 (June 17, 1982), 1446-55.

SELIKOFF, I.J., CHURG, J., and HAMMOND, E.C. "Relation between exposure to asbestos and mesothelioma," *New England Journal of Medicine* 272 (1965), 560-65.

SELIKOFF, I.J., HAMMOND, E.C., and CHURG, J. "Asbestos exposure, smoking and neoplasia," *Journal American Medical Association* 204 (1968), 106-12.

CHURG, A.W. and WARNOCK, M.L. "Numbers of asbestos bodies in urban patients with lung cancer and gastrointestinal cancer and in matched controls," *Chest* 76 (1979), 143-49. (See also accompanying editorial by Becklake, M.R., pages 245-247, same issue).

SELIKOFF, I.J. and HAMMOND, E.C. "Asbestos and smoking," *Journal American Medical Association* 242 (1979), 458-59.

Coal Mining and Silicosis

*SHAMAN, DIANA. "Silicosis: The occupational disease that shouldn't exist," *ALA Bulletin* (March-April, 1983), 6-12.

ZISKIND, M., JONES, R.N., and WEILL, H. "Silicosis. State of the Art review," *American Review Respiratory Disease* 113 (1976), 643.

MORGAN, W.K.C. and LAPP, N. "Respiratory Disease in Coal Miners. State of the Art review," *American Review Respiratory Disease* 113 (1976), 531.

MORGAN, W.K.C., LAPP, N.L., and SEATON, D. "Respiratory disability in coal miners," *Journal American Medical Association* 243 (June 20, 1980), 2401-4. (See also accompanying editorial by Barclay, W.R., page 2427, same issue).

General and Miscellaneous

*Anderson, J. Marion. *Occupational Lung Diseases–An Introduction.* (American Lung Association, 1979).

An 80-page booklet that provides a reasonable overview of this complex field of medicine.

*"A case of deadly neglect," *ALA Bulletin* (June-July, 1981).

An article about "brown lung" or byssinoisis. Contains extracts of Pulitzer Prize winning series published in the Charlotte, North Carolina *Observer* in February, 1980.

MORGAN, W.K.C. "International Conference on Occupational Lung Diseases," *Chest* 78: 2, Supplement (August, 1980).

WEILL, HANS, guest editor. "International Conference on Byssinosis," *Chest* Supplement 79: 4, (April, 1981).

BROOKS, S.M., LOCKEY, J.E., and HARBER, P., guest editors. "Occupational Lung Diseases," *Clinics in Chest Medicine* 2: 2&3 (May & September, 1981).

The two issues of *Clinics in Chest Medicine* contain articles by experts, and are also an excellent source of references.

"NIOSH Recommendations for Occupational Health Standards," *MMWR* Supplement 32: 15, (October 7, 1983).

National Institute for Occupational Safety and Health recommendations for limits of exposure to potentially hazardous substances or conditions in the workplace. Many of these hazards affect the respiratory system.

HEYDEN, S. and PRATT, P. "Commentary: Exposure to cotton dust and respiratory disease," *Journal American Medical Association* 244 (October 17, 1980), 1797-8.

CHAPTER 5–COMMON RESPIRATORY EMERGENCIES

**Handbook of First Aid and Emergency Care.* (American Medical Association, 1980).

*HEIMLICH, HENRY J., with GALTON, LAWRENCE. *Dr. Heimlich's Home Guide To Emergency Medical Situations.* (New York: Simon and Schuster, 1980).

*WEISS, JEFFREY. *The People's Emergency Guide.* (New York: St. Martin's Press, 1980).

"Standards and Guidelines for Cardiopulmonary Resuscitation (CRP) and Emergency Cardiac Care (ECC)," *Journal American Medical Association* 244: 5 (August 1, 1980).

An entire issue of JAMA devoted to the results of a national conference on CPR and ECC. Discusses and illustrates technique of CPR; also goes into historical and medicolegal aspects.

HEIMLICH, H.J. and UHLEY, M.H. "The Heimlich maneuver," *Ciba Clinical Symposia (Illustrated)* 31: 3 (1979). (Summit, NJ: Ciba Pharmaceutical Co., 1979).

Textbook of Advanced Cardiac Life Support. (American Heart Association, 1981).

An excellent, in-depth manual on the subject. Includes chapters on resuscitation of infants and newborns, and medicolegal aspects of cardiopulmonary resuscitation. Available from local AHA chapters.

KIRK, BRYAN W. "Respiratory Emergencies," *Seminars in Respiratory Medicine* 2: 1 (July, 1980).

HAUGEN, R. "The cafe coronary," *Journal American Medical Association* 186: (1963), 142-43.

GANN, D.A. "Emergency management of the obstructed airway," *Journal American Medical Association* 143 (March 21, 1980), 1141-2.

WINTER, P.M. and MILLER, J.N. "Carbon monoxide poisoning," *Journal American Medical Association* 236 (September 27, 1976), 1502-1504.

JACKSON, D.L. and MENGES, H. "Accidental carbon monoxide poisoning," *Journal American Medical Association* 243 (February 22/29, 1980), 772-4.

"Carbon monoxide intoxication–A preventable environmental health hazard." *Morbidity Mortality Weekly Report* 31: 39 (October 8, 1982), 529-32.

A concise summary of the problem, with guidelines for prevention.

CHAPTER 6–SYMPTOMS AND SIGNS OF LUNG DISEASE

*GALTON, LAWRENCE. *The Complete Book of Symptoms and What They Can Mean.* (New York: Simon and Schuster, 1978).

IRWIN, R.S., ROSEN, M.J., and BRAMAN, S.S. "Cough, A Comprehensive Review," *Archives Internal Medicine* 137 (September, 1977), 1186-91.

CORRAO, W.M., BRAMAN, S.S., and IRWIN R.S. "Chronic cough as the sole presenting manifestation of bronchial asthma," *New England Journal of Medicine* 300, (March 22, 1979), 633-37.

MISSRI, J.C. and ALEXANDER, S. "Hyperventilation syndrome. A brief review," *Journal American Medical Association* 240 (1978), 2093.

WAITES, T.F. "Hyperventilation–chronic and acute," *Archives Internal Medicine* 138 (1978), 1700.

CHAPTER 7–HOW TO FIND A DOCTOR AND CHOOSE A HOSPITAL

*PEKKANEN, JOHN. *The Best Doctors in the U.S.* (New York: Seaview Books, 1981).

Directory of Medical Specialists. 21st Edition, 1983-1984. (Chicago, Illinois: Marquis Who's Who, Inc.).

American Medical Directory–1982. 28th Edition. (Chicago, Illinois: American Medical Association).

CHAPTER 8– DIAGNOSTIC TESTS AND PROCEDURES

PETTY, T.L. *Pulmonary Diagnostic Techniques.* (Philadelphia: Lea & Febiger, 1975).

FELSON, BENJAMIN. *Chest Roentgenography.* (Philadelphia: W. B. Saunders Co., 1973).

PUTMAN, CHARLES E. *Pulmonary Diagnosis. Imaging and Other Techniques.* (New York: Appleton-Century-Crofts, 1981).

CHUSID, E.L. "Diagnostic procedures in bronchopulmonary diseases." *Hospital Practice* (July, 1981), 99.

CHAPTER 9–PATTERNS OF LUNG DISEASE

See references under General.

CHAPTER 10–ASTHMA–"HYPERSENSITIVE AIRWAYS"

*Many pamphlets and booklets on the subject of asthma are available from the American Lung Association.

GERSHWIN, M. ERIC, edtior. *Bronchial Asthma. Principles of Diagnosis and Treatment.* (New York: Grune and Stratton, 1981).

WEISS, E.G. and SEGAL, M.S., editors. *Bronchial Asthma. Mechanism and Therapeutics.* (Boston: Little Brown and Co., 1976).

Asthma and other Allergic Diseases. NIAID Task Force Report. NIH Publication #79-387 (May, 1979).

WILLIAMS, M.H., Jr., editor. "Asthma and airways reactivity." *Seminars in Respiratory Medicine* 1(April, 1980).

An entire issue devoted to asthma, edited by one of the leaders in the field.

MATHEWS, K.P. "Respiratory atopic disease, *Journal American Medical Association* 248 (1982), 2587-2610.

A concise review of the subject of allergic lung diseases that also discusses non-allergic forms of asthma.

MARTIN, L. "Asthma: Current Concepts in Outpatient Management," *Hospital Medicine* (February, 1981).

MCFADDEN, E.R., INGRAN, R.H. "Exercise-induced asthma. Observations on the initiating stimulus," *New England Journal Medicine* 301 (1979), 763-9.

REBUCK, A.S. and READ, J. "Assessment and management of severe asthma." *American Journal Medicine* 51 (1971), 788-798.

MCFADDEN, E.R., JR., KISER, R., and DEGROOT, W.J. "Acute bronchial asthma. Relations between clinical and physiologic manifestations," *New England Journal Medicine* 288 (1973), 221.

SHERTER, C.B. and POLNITSKY, C.A. "The relationship of viral infections to subsequent asthma," *Clinics in Chest Medicine* 2 (1981), 67-78.

MCCOMBS, R.P., LOWELL, F.C., and OHMAN, J.L. "Myths, morbidity and mortality in asthma," *Journal American Medical Association* 242 (1979), 1521.

CHAPTER 11–TREATMENT OF ASTHMA AND OTHER REVERSIBLE AIRWAY PROBLEMS

**Physicians' Desk Reference for Nonprescription Drugs.* Published yearly by Medical Economics Company, Oradell, New Jersey.

**Physicians' Desk Reference for Prescription Drugs.* Published yearly by Medical Economics Company, Oradell, New Jersey.

Although both "PDR's" contain technical language, they are widely marketed in neighborhood bookstores; in addition to labeling information for many widely used drugs, they also contain pictures that can be useful for drug identification.

Facts and Comparisons Drug Information Updated Monthly. Facts and Comparisons Division, J.B. Lippincott Co., 111 West Port Plaza, St. Louis, Missouri 63141).

Facts and Comparisons has a much more extensive listing of medications than contained in the PDR. It also includes voluminous numbers of cough and cold medications.

ZIMENT, IRWIN. *Respiratory Pharmacology and Therapeutics.* (Philadelphia: W. B. Saunders Co., 1978).

AMA Drug Evaluation, Fifth Edition. (Chicago: American Medical Association, 1983).

GILMAN, A.G., GOODMAN, L.S., and GILMAN, A. *The Pharmacological Basis of Therapeutics.* (New York: MacMillan Publishing Company, 1980).

CHAPTER 12–CHRONIC BRONCHITIS AND EMPHYSEMA

*MOSER, K.M., ARCHIBALD, C., HANSEN, P. et al. *Better Living and Breathing. A Manual for Patients.* (St. Louis: C.V. Mosby Co., 1980).

**Help Yourself To Better Breathing.* (American Lung Association, 1980).

*PETTY, T.L. *Enjoying Life With Emphysema.* (Philadelphia: Lea & Febiger, 1983).

*SILVER, H.M. and FELDMAN, M. *Travel For The Patient With Chronic Obstructive Pulmonary Disease.* Washington, DC: George Washington University Medical Center, 20037.

The first three booklets are written and illustrated for patients who have trouble breathing from emphysema or chronic bronchitis. The fourth booklet covers all aspects of travel, including air travel.

*COOPER, K.H. *Aerobics.* (New York: Bantam Book, 1968).

*COOPER, K.H. *Aerobics for Women.* (New York: Bantam Book, 1972).

*COOPER, K.H. *The Aerobics Way.* (New York: Bantam Book, 1977).

Rationale and specific steps for aerobic exercise training.

HODGKIN, J.E. editor. *Chronic Obstructive Pulmonary Disease. Current Concepts in Diagnosis and Comprehensive Care.* (Park Ridge, Illinois: American College of Chest Physicians, 1979).

CHAPTER 13–OXYGEN: FOR SOME, A VITAL DRUG

"Continuous or nocturnal oxygen therapy in hypoxemic chronic obstrucive lung disease. A clinical trial." *Annals Internal Medicine* 93 (1980), 391-98. (See accompanying editiorial by Roberts, S.D., page 499, same issue).

A multicenter trial in which 203 COPD patients were treated with either 12 or 24 hours of continuous oxygen at home. The 24-hour group did much better.

PETTY, T.L. *Prescribing Home Oxygen for COPD.* (New York: Thieme-Stratton Inc., 1982).

An excellent, concise review of the subject. Contains pictures of patients using oxygen equipment.

PETTY, T.L. "Selection criteria for long-term oxygen," *American Review Respiratory Disease* 127 (April, 1983), 397-398.

CHAPTER 14–PROBLEMS OF THE CHEST BELLOWS

BERGOFSKY, E.H. "Respiratory failure in disorders of the thoracic cage," *American Review Respiratory Disease* 119 (1979), 643-69. State of the Art Review.

LUCE, J.M. "Respiratory complications of obesity," *Chest* 78 (October, 1980), 626-31.

LIGHT, R.M. Pleural effusions," *Medical Clinics North America* 61 (1977), 1339-52.

CHAPTER 15–INTERSTITIAL LUNG DISEASE

CRYSTAL, R.G., CADEK, J.E., FENANS, V.J. et al: "Interstitial lung disease: current concepts of pathogenesis, staging and therapy," *American Journal Medicine* 70 (March 1981), 542-68.

Report of Task Force on Epidemiology of Respiratory Diseases. State of Knowledge. Problems. Needs. NIH Publication No. 81-2019. (October, 1980).

TEIRSTEIN, A.S. and KLEINERMAN, J. "Diffuse interstitial lung disease," *Hospital Practice,* (June, 1981), 126-136.

ROSENOW, E.C., editor. "Drug-induced lung disease," *Seminars in Respiratory Medicine* 2: 2 (October, 1980).

Many cases of interstitial lung disease are drug-induced. This monograph covers the spectrum of all pulmonary drug reactions.

GROSS, N.J. "Pulmonary effects of radiation therapy," *Annals Internal Medicine* 86 (1977), 81-92.

CHAPTER 16–SARCOIDOSIS

SHARMA, O.P. *Sarcoidosis. A Clinical Approach.* (Springfield, Illinois: Charles C. Thomas, Publisher, 1975).

A concise book covering most manifestations of sarcoidosis. Many photographs, 471 references.

MITCHELL, D.N. and SCADDING, J.G. "Sarcoidosis. State of the Art." *American Review Respiratory Disease* 110 (1974), 774.

CRYSTAL, R.G., ROBERTS, W.C., HUNNINGHAKE, G.W. et al. "Pulmonary sarcoidosis: A disease characterized and perpetuated by activated T-lymphocytes," *Annals Internal Medicine* 94 (January, 1981), 73-94.

A review by investigators in the forefront of research on this enigmatic disease.

DEREMEE, R.A. "The present status of treatment of pulmonary sarcoidosis. A house divided," *Chest* 71 (1977), 388-93.

Discusses controversy over how best to give steroids in sarcoidosis and reviews literature on the subject.

CHAPTER 17–HEART DISEASE

*Many pamphlets and booklets on the subject of heart disease are available from the American Heart Association.

RAFFIN, T.A. and THEODORE, J.T. "Separating cardiac from pulmonary dyspnea," *Journal American Medical Association* 238 (1977), 2066.

CHAPTER 18—FROM COLDS TO INFLUENZA

*BENNETT, HAL Z. *Cold Comfort. Colds and Flu. Everybody's Guide to Self Treatment.* (New York: Clarkson N. Potter, Inc., 1979).

*PAULING, LINUS. *Vitamin C, the Common Cold and Flu.* (New York: Berkley Books, 1981). (Revision of the original 1970 edition).

Influenza Vaccines. Recommendation of the Public Health Service Immunization Practices Advisory Committee. Morbidity and Mortality Weekly Report (published yearly).

The PHS issues annual revisions of its influenza vaccine guidelines, which are first published in MMWR (issued by CDC, Atlanta).

Pneumococcal Polysaccharide Vaccine. Recommendation of the Immunization Practices Advisory Committee. Morbidity Mortality Weekly Report (August 28, 1981), 410.

KARK, J.D., LEBIUSH, M., and RANNON, L. "Cigarette smoking as a risk factor for epidemic A(HlNl) influenza in young men," *New England Journal of Medicine* 307 (October 21, 1982), 1042-46.

ARONSON, M., WEISS, S.T., BEN, R.L., and KOMAROFF, A.L. "Association between cigarette smoking and acute respiratory tract illness in young adults," *Journal American Medical Association* 248 (July 9, 1982), 181-83.

HURWITZ, E.S., SCHONBERGER, L.B., NELSON, D.B. et al. "Guillain Barre syndrome and the 1978-1979 influenza vaccine," *New England Journal Medicine* 304 (June 25, 1981), 1557-61.

"Amantadine: does it have a role in the prevention and treatment of influenza? A National Institutes of Health consensus development conference," *Annals Internal Medicine* 92 (Part 1) (1980), 256-8.

BARKER, W.H. and MULLOOLY, J.P. "Influenza vaccination of elderly persons. Reduction in pneumonia and influenza hospitalizations and deaths," *Journal American Medical Association* 244 (1980), 2547-9.

CHAPTER 19—PNEUMONIA AND PLEURISY

Reynolds, H.W., editor. "Respiratory Infections," *Clinics in Chest Medicine* 2 (January, 1981).

MEYER, R.D. and FINEGOLD, S.M. "Legionnaire's Disease," *Annual Review Medicine* 31 (1980), 219.

FRASER, D.W. "Legionnaire's disease. Four summers harvest," *American Journal Medicine* 68 (1980), 1.

WEINSTEIN, L. "The "new" pneumonias: The doctor's dilemma," (Editorial) *Annals Internal Medicine* 92 (1980), 559.

CHAPTER 20—TUBERCULOSIS AND OTHER LESS COMMON PULMONARY INFECTIONS

*STEAD, WILLIAM W. *Understanding Tuberculosis Today. A Handbook for Patients,* (Milwaukee, Wisconsin: Central Press, 1980).

A well-written, illustrated pamphlet by a recognized expert.

*American Lung Assoc. *Bulletin,* Special Anniversary Issue (March, 1982).

"Centennial: Koch's discovery of the tubercle bacillus," *Morbidity and Mortality Weekly Report* 31: 10 (March 19, 1982).

In 1882 Robert Koch discovered the organism responsible for tuberculosis. These issues of the *ALA Bulletin* and *MMWR* provide interesting historical accounts of tuberculosis control since then.

YOUMANS, GUY P. *Tuberculosis.* (Philadelphia: W. B. Saunders Co., 1979).

STEAD, W.W. and DUTT, A.K., editors. "Tuberculosis." *Clinics in Chest Medicine* I: 2 (Mary, 1980).

"Diagnostic Standards and Classification of Tuberculosis and other, Mycobacterial Disease," *American Review Respiratory Disease* 123 (1981), 343-51. "Treatment of Tuberculosis and other Mycobacterial Diseases", *American Review Respiratory Disease* 127 (1983), 790-96.

These are the official statements of the American Thoracic Society, medical section of the American Lung Association. They are also available directly from the ALA.

EINSTEIN, H.E., editor. *Handbook on Fungus Diseases.* (Park Ridge, Illinois: American College of Chest Physicians, 1981).

A succinct, well-written book on all the major fungal diseases.

CHAPTER 21–LUNG CANCER: A NATIONAL EPIDEMIC

MATTHAY, R., editor. "Recent Advances in Lung Cancer," *Clinics in Chest Medicine* 3: 2 (May, 1982).

Contains 16 review articles on the subject.

MITTMAN, C. and BRUDERMAN, I. "Lung Cancer: To operate or not? State of the Art review," *American Review Respiratory Disease* 116 (1977), 477.

The Health Consequences of Smoking. Cancer. A Report of the Surgeon General, 1982. (See listing under Chapter 2 references).

Guidelines For The Cancer-Related Check-Up. Recommendations and Rationale. Ca–A Cancer Journal for Clinicians. (American Cancer Society, July/August, 1980).

CARR, D.T. "Malignant lung disease." *Hospital Practice* (January, 1981), 97.

MCNEIL, B.J., WEICHSELBAUM, R., and PAUKER, S.G. "Fallacy of the five-year survival in lung cancer," *New England Journal Medicine* 299 (1978), 1397-1401.

CHAPTER 22–DISEASES OF THE PULMONARY CIRCULATION

MOSER, K.M. "Pulmonary Embolism. State of the Art review," *American Review Respiratory Disease* 115: (1977), 829.

ROSENOW, E.C., OSMUNDSON, P.J., and BROWN, M.L. "Pulmonary Embolism. Subject Review," *Mayo Clinic Proceddings* 76 (1981), 161.

FISHMAN, A.P. "Primary Pulmonary Hypertension: more light or more tunnel?" (Editorial) *Annals Internal Medicine* 94 (1981), 815-17.

REEVES, S.T. "Hope in primary pulmonary hypertension," (Editorial), *New England Journal Medicine* 302 (1981), 112-13.

ALPERT, J.S., IRWIN, R.S., and DALEN, J.E. "Pulmonary Hypertension," *Current Problems in Cardiology* V: 10 (January 1981).

CHAPTER 23—CYSTIC FIBROSIS

WOOD, R.E., BOAT, T.P., and DOERSHUK, C.F. "Cystic Fibrosis. State of the Art review," *American Review Respiratory Disease* 113 (1976), 833.

DI SANT'AGNESE, P.A. and DAVIS, P.B. "Cystic fibrosis in adults. 75 cases and a review of 232 cases in the literature." *American Journal Medicine* 66 (1979), 121-32.

SHWACHMAN, H., KOWALSKI, M., and KHAW, K.T. "Cystic fibrosis: A new outlook." *Medicine* 56 (1977), 129-149.

CHAPTER 24—TROUBLE BREATHING DURING SLEEP

CHERNIACK, N.S. "Respiratory dysrhythmias during sleep," *New England Journal Medicine* 305 (August 6, 1981) 325-30.

WYNNE, J.W., BLOCK, A.J., and BOYSEN, P.G. "Oxygen desaturation in sleep: sleep apnea and COPD," *Hospital Practice* (October, 1980), 77.

BLOCK, A.J., BOYSEN, P.G., WYNNE, J.W. et al. "Sleep apnea, hypopnea and oxygen desaturation in normal subjects. A strong male predominance," *New England Journal Medicine* 300 (1979), 513-17.

STROHL, K.P., HENSLEY, M.J., SAUNDERS, N.A. et al. "Progesterone administration and progressive sleep apneas," *Journal American Medical Association* 245 (1981), 1230-32. (See also editorial by Martin, R.J. "The problems of sleep-related respiratory disorders," pages 1250-1, same issue).

GUILLEMINAULT, C., SIMMONS, B., MOTTA, J. et al. "Obstructive sleep apnea syndrome and tracheostomy. Long-term follow-up experience," *Archives Internal Medicine* 141 (July, 1981), 985-88. (See also accompanying editorial by Drs. J.E. Remmers and A.M. Anch, page 989, same issue).

For 50 patients with severe symptoms from obstructive sleep apnea, tracheostomy was definitely beneficial.

COMROE, J.H., JR. "Frankenstein, Pickwick and Ondine." Chapter in *Retrospectroscope. Insights Into Medical Discovery.* (Menlo Park, California: Von Gehr Press, 1977).

WILLIAMS, A.J. "Dormouse Disease?" *Chest* 83 (1983), 591-2.

Drs. Comroe and Williams provide interesting editorial comments on the origin of terms used to characterize patients with sleep apnea syndrome.

CHAPTER 25—RESPIRATORY FAILURE: THE ULTIMATE CATASTROPHE

*FISCHE, L., and DAVIS, A.L. "Lung failure. How and why it happens," *American Lung Association Bulletin* (January-February 1980).

HUDSON, L.D., editor. "Adult respiratory distress syndrome." *Seminars in Respiratory Medicine* 2 (January, 1981).

This issue of seminars devoted to review articles on all aspects of ARDS.

MARTIN, L. "Respiratory Failure," *Medical Clinics N. America* 61 (November, 1977), 1369-96.

NELEMS, J.M.B., REBUCK, A.S., COOPER, J.D. et al. "Human lung transplanation," *Chest* 78 (October, 1980), 569.

"Heart-lung transplant may herald new era. AMA medical news," *Journal American Medical Association* 245 (April 10, 1981), 1397.

APPENDIX A—SOURCES OF ADDITIONAL INFORMATION

*ULENE, A. and FELDMAN, S. *Help Yourself to Health.* (New York: G.P. Putnam's Sons, 1980).

*KRUZAS, A.T., editor. *Medical and Health Information Directory.* 3rd Edition. Detroit, Michigan: Gale Research Co., 1983.

The first book contains addresses and phone numbers of the major national organizations, plus a listing of many services and publications available to the lay public. It is available in paperback at many bookstores. The *Directory* provides names, addresses, and phone numbers for local chapters of major national organizations (such as the American Cancer Society, Cystic Fibrosis Foundation, and American Lung Association).

BLUMBERG, B.D. and FLAHERTY, M. "Services available to persons with cancer—National and Regional Organizations," *Journal American Medical Association* 244 (October, 1980), 1715-17.

APPENDIX B—GLOSSARY OF MEDICAL TERMS

Four comprehensive medical dictionaries in print are listed below; at least one of these should be found in every school, college, or hospital library. Each is updated every few years.

Dorland's Illustrated Medical Dictionary. 26th edition. (Philadelphia: W. B. Saunders Co.).

Urdang Dictionary of Current Medical Terms. For Health and Science Professionals. (New York: John Wiley & Sons).

Steadman's Medical Dictionary. Illustrated. 24th edition. Baltimore: Williams and Wilkins Co.

Taber's Cyclopedic Medical Dictionary. 14th Edition. Philadelphia: F.A. Davis Co.

APPENDIX C—DRUGS USED IN ASTHMA AND REVERSIBLE AIRWAYS DISEASE

See references under Chapter 11, above.

ndex